Marine Bioactive Peptides—Structure, Function, and Application 2.0

Marine Bioactive Peptides—Structure, Function, and Application 2.0

Guest Editors

Bin Wang
Chang-Feng Chi

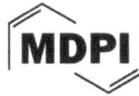

Basel • Beijing • Wuhan • Barcelona • Belgrade • Novi Sad • Cluj • Manchester

Guest Editors

Bin Wang
Zhejiang Provincial
Engineering Technology
Research Center of Marine
Biomedical Products
School of Food and Pharmacy
Zhejiang Ocean University
Zhoushan
China

Chang-Feng Chi
National and Provincial Joint
Laboratory of Exploration and
Utilization of Marine Aquatic
Genetic Resources
National Engineering
Research Center of Marine
Facilities Aquaculture
School of Marine Science and
Technology
Zhejiang Ocean University
Zhoushan
China

Editorial Office
MDPI AG
Grosspeteranlage 5
4052 Basel, Switzerland

This is a reprint of the Special Issue, published open access by the journal *Marine Drugs* (ISSN 1660-3397), freely accessible at: https://www.mdpi.com/journal/marinedrugs/special_issues/5XPG3GP5G0.

For citation purposes, cite each article independently as indicated on the article page online and as indicated below:

Lastname, A.A.; Lastname, B.B. Article Title. *Journal Name* **Year**, *Volume Number*, Page Range.

ISBN 978-3-7258-4115-8 (Hbk)
ISBN 978-3-7258-4116-5 (PDF)
https://doi.org/10.3390/books978-3-7258-4116-5

© 2025 by the authors. Articles in this book are Open Access and distributed under the Creative Commons Attribution (CC BY) license. The book as a whole is distributed by MDPI under the terms and conditions of the Creative Commons Attribution-NonCommercial-NoDerivs (CC BY-NC-ND) license (https://creativecommons.org/licenses/by-nc-nd/4.0/).

Contents

About the Editors vii

Bin Wang and Chang-Feng Chi
Marine Bioactive Peptides—Structure, Function, and Application 2.0
Reprinted from: *Mar. Drugs* **2025**, 23, 192, https://doi.org/10.3390/md23050192 1

Qiuting Wang, Gongming Wang, Chuyi Liu, Zuli Sun, Ruimin Li, Jiarun Gao, et al.
The Structural Characteristics and Bioactivity Stability of *Cucumaria frondosa* Intestines and Ovum Hydrolysates Obtained by Different Proteases
Reprinted from: *Mar. Drugs* **2023**, 21, 395, https://doi.org/10.3390/md21070395 7

Qianxia Lin, Yueping Guo, Jie Li, Shuqi He, Yan Chen and Huoxi Jin
Antidiabetic Effect of Collagen Peptides from *Harpadon nehereus* Bones in Streptozotocin-Induced Diabetes Mice by Regulating Oxidative Stress and Glucose Metabolism
Reprinted from: *Mar. Drugs* **2023**, 21, 518, https://doi.org/10.3390/md21100518 22

Ming-Xue Ge, Ru-Ping Chen, Lun Zhang, Yu-Mei Wang, Chang-Feng Chi and Bin Wang
Novel Ca-Chelating Peptides from Protein Hydrolysate of Antarctic Krill (*Euphausia superba*): Preparation, Characterization, and Calcium Absorption Efficiency in Caco-2 Cell Monolayer Model
Reprinted from: *Mar. Drugs* **2023**, 21, 579, https://doi.org/10.3390/md21110579 38

Christian Bjerknes, Sileshi Gizachew Wubshet, Sissel Beate Rønning, Nils Kristian Afseth, Crawford Currie, Bomi Framroze and Erland Hermansen
Glucoregulatory Properties of a Protein Hydrolysate from Atlantic Salmon (*Salmo salar*): Preliminary Characterization and Evaluation of DPP-IV Inhibition and Direct Glucose Uptake In Vitro
Reprinted from: *Mar. Drugs* **2024**, 22, 151, https://doi.org/10.3390/md22040151 57

Markus Tost and Uli Kazmaier
Synthesis and Late-Stage Modification of (−)-Doliculide Derivatives Using Matteson's Homologation Approach
Reprinted from: *Mar. Drugs* **2024**, 22, 165, https://doi.org/10.3390/md22040165 75

Claudio A. Álvarez, Teresa Toro-Araneda, Juan Pablo Cumillaf, Belinda Vega, María José Tapia, Tanya Roman, et al.
Evaluation of the Biological Activities of Peptides from Epidermal Mucus of Marine Fish Species from Chilean Aquaculture
Reprinted from: *Mar. Drugs* **2024**, 22, 248, https://doi.org/10.3390/md22060248 100

Sha-Yi Mao, Shi-Kun Suo, Yu-Mei Wang, Chang-Feng Chi and Bin Wang
Systematical Investigation on Anti-Fatigue Function and Underlying Mechanism of High Fischer Ratio Oligopeptides from Antarctic Krill on Exercise-Induced Fatigue in Mice
Reprinted from: *Mar. Drugs* **2024**, 22, 322, https://doi.org/10.3390/md22070322 117

Fei Li, Haisheng Lin, Xiaoming Qin, Jialong Gao, Zhongqin Chen, Wenhong Cao, et al.
In Silico Identification and Molecular Mechanism of Novel Tyrosinase Inhibitory Peptides Derived from Nacre of *Pinctada martensii*
Reprinted from: *Mar. Drugs* **2024**, 22, 359, https://doi.org/10.3390/md22080359 136

Zhiyong Li, Hongyan He, Jiasi Liu, Huiyue Gu, Caiwei Fu, Aurang Zeb, et al.
Preparation and Vasodilation Mechanism of Angiotensin-I-Converting Enzyme Inhibitory Peptide from *Ulva prolifera* Protein
Reprinted from: *Mar. Drugs* **2024**, *22*, 398, https://doi.org/10.3390/md22090398 . . . . **153**

Siyi Song, Wei Zhao, Qianxia Lin, Jinfeng Pei and Huoxi Jin
Peptides from *Harpadon nehereus* Bone Ameliorate Sodium Palmitate-Induced HepG2 Lipotoxicity by Regulating Oxidative Stress and Lipid Metabolism
Reprinted from: *Mar. Drugs* **2025**, *23*, 118, https://doi.org/10.3390/md23030118 . . . . **166**

About the Editors

Bin Wang

Bin Wang, PhD, studied Forestry at the College of Forestry, Shandong Agricultural University (Taian, China) from 1997 to 2001 and earned his Bachelors of Agronomy. From 2001 to 2004, he studied Biochemistry and Molecular Biology at the College of Life Science, Fujian Agriculture and Forestry University (Fuzhou, China). From 2004 to 2007, he continued his studies and research on pharmaceutical chemistry and earned his PhD degree from the Ocean University of China (Qingdao, China) under the guidance of Prof. Hua-Shi Guan. He joined the School of Food and Pharmacy, Zhejiang Ocean University (Zhoushan, China), as a lecturer in June 2007 and has been a professor since January 2015. His current research focuses on the preparation, identification, activity evaluation, and action mechanism of marine active peptides.

Chang-Feng Chi

Chang-Feng Chi, PhD, studied Forestry Science at the College of Forestry, Shandong Agricultural University (Taian, China), from 1997 to 2001 and obtained her bachelor's degree in Agronomy. From 2001 to 2004, she studied Plant Pathology at the College of Plant Protection, Shandong Agricultural University (Taian, China), and earned her master's degree in Agronomy. From 2004 to 2007, she continued her studies and research in Marine Biology and earned her PhD degree from the Ocean University of China (Qingdao, China) under the guidance of Prof. Qing-Yin Wang. From 2007 to 2009, she worked as a Biology Postdoctoral Fellow at Zhejiang University. She joined the Marine Science and Technology College, Zhejiang Ocean University (Zhoushan, China), as a lecturer in July 2009 and has been a professor since July 2015. Her current research focuses on the isolation, cloning, identification, function evaluation, and action mechanism of marine neuropeptides.

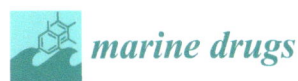

Editorial

Marine Bioactive Peptides—Structure, Function, and Application 2.0

Bin Wang [1,*] and Chang-Feng Chi [2,*]

1. Zhejiang Provincial Engineering Technology Research Center of Marine Biomedical Products, School of Food and Pharmacy, Zhejiang Ocean University, Zhoushan 316022, China
2. National and Provincial Joint Engineering Research Centre for Marine Germplasm Resources Exploration and Utilization, School of Marine Science and Technology, Zhejiang Ocean University, Zhoushan 316022, China
* Correspondence: wangbin@zjou.edu.cn (B.W.); chichangfeng@hotmail.com (C.-F.C.)

In recent years, people's lifestyles have undergone relatively significant changes. For instance, physical labor has decreased, and the number of people on a high-fat diet (HFD) has increased annually. This has also led to a year-on-year increase in the incidence and number of many diseases, such as non-alcoholic fatty liver disease (NAFLD), obesity, diabetes, hyperuricemia, etc. [1–4]. Therefore, people's demands for food are gradually changing, shifting from merely solving the problem of basic sustenance to a rapid shift towards nutrition and functionality [5,6]. Therefore, the discovery and preparation of functional components from natural foods have become a research hotspot.

The ocean is rich in biological resources, and its unique ecological environment makes the active components in marine organisms significantly different from those in terrestrial organisms [7,8]. Therefore, scientists in the fields of life sciences, pharmacy, chemistry, and others around the world have focused their attention on marine bioactive substances, hoping to discover more functional molecules beneficial to human health from them. Among the numerous active components, marine bioactive peptides have also become the focus of research due to their high nutritional value and significant biological activity, such as anticancer, antioxidant, antimicrobial, anti-inflammatory, anti-photoaging, antidiabetic, antifreeze, and immune-modulating characteristics [9–11]. Therefore, we are launching the Special Issue "Marine Bioactive Peptides—Structure, Function, and Application 2.0" (https://www.mdpi.com/journal/marinedrugs/special_issues/5XPG3GP5G0) in May 2023, to highlight the latest research in the field of marine active peptides. Herein, we introduce a brief overview of the ten research papers and their findings contributed by the authors.

The development of high-value active peptide products by utilizing bulk marine biological resources and their processing by-products has always been the focus of research [12]. This can not only solve the environmental pollution caused by the by-products but also increase the profits of enterprises. Therefore, this Special Issue begins with the article by Wang et al. dedicated to the structural characteristics and bioactivity stability of protein hydrolysates (CFHs) from *Cucumaria frondosa* intestines and ovum [13]. In this study, the effects of alcalase, papain, flavourzyme, and neutrase on the structural characteristics and antioxidant stability of CFHs are systematically investigated, and the selected enzyme is vital to the physicochemical properties and biological activities of the bioactive hydrolysates produced. According to the degree of hydrolysis (DH), primary structures, surface hydrophobicity, antioxidant activity, pancreatic lipase inhibitory activity, and the stability of CFHs, the authors found that flavourzyme is the optimal choice for the production of CFHs applied in functional foods because the flavourzyme-prepared CFHs had the highest DH and exhibited the highest DPPH radical scavenging activity, reduction capacity, and pancreatic lipase inhibitory activity. Moreover, flavourzyme-prepared CFHs showed excellent antioxidant stability and pancreatic lipase inhibitory activity during simulated gastrointestinal digestion in vitro. These findings, especially the significant antioxidant and lipid-lowering activities of CFHs, strongly support their application in functional foods, dietary supplements, and nutritional health products. This research has developed a new application for the intestines and ovum of *C. frondosa*, which can improve the comprehensive utilization of marine biological resources.

The number of diabetes patients worldwide with diabetes is as high as 589 million (accounting for 11.1%), which is equivalent to approximately one in every nine people. It is estimated that by 2050, the total number of adult patients with diabetes worldwide will increase to 853 million (accounting for 13.0%) [14]. Therefore, the treatment of diabetes, especially the development of new diabetes drugs, has attracted much attention. The second article by Lin et al. concerns the antidiabetic effect of collagen peptides (HNCP, Mw < 1 kDa) from *Harpadon nehereus* bones [15]. The authors found that HNCP can significantly reduce blood glucose levels by increasing insulin secretion and glucose tolerance in streptozotocin-induced type 1 diabetic mice. Research on the mechanism of action has proved HNCP's capability to improve antioxidant abilities by regulating the Keap1/Nrf2 pathway to increase the activity of antioxidant enzymes. Furthermore, HNCP can markedly ameliorate the glucose metabolism of type 1 diabetic mice by controlling the levels of glycosynthesis- and gluconeogenesis-related enzymes. This study explores the mechanism of HNCP in the treatment of diabetes from two aspects: oxidative stress and abnormal glucose metabolism, which are closely related to the occurrence and development of diabetes. This is an instructive study for the development of diabetes drugs.

Antarctic krill (*Euphausia superba*) has huge biomass and is regarded as the largest animal protein resource in the world [16]. Calcium (Ca) deficiency in the human body significantly influences cellular proliferation, neurotransmission, blood coagulation, muscle contraction, etc., and currently affects the health of about 900 million people in China [17]. The third article by Ge et al. concerns the preparation, characterization, and Ca absorption efficiency of Ca-chelating peptides from Antarctic krill protein hydrolysate [18]. In this study, the authors purify and identify 14 Ca-chelating peptides with the tetrapeptide (VERG), showing the highest chelating capability with Ca^{2+} in the groups of N-H, C=O, and -COOH. In addition, the VERG-Ca chelate remained stable in the simulated gastrointestinal digestion in vitro, and the monolayer experiment of Caco-2 cells proved that the VERG-Ca chelate could significantly improve calcium transport. The research results show that Ca-chelating peptides of Antarctic krill can be used as functional components to improve the bioavailability of Ca in healthy foods.

Metabolic syndrome (MetS) encompasses a series of metabolic abnormalities, such as hypertension, elevated triglycerides, hyperglycemia, low high-density lipoprotein cholesterol, and central obesity, and is associated with diabetes, cancer, neurodegenerative diseases, cardiovascular and cerebrovascular diseases, and NAFLD [19]. Focusing on improving diet to prevent MetS is a crucial aspect of enhancing human health. Therefore, the fifth article by Bjerknes et al. studies the glycemic regulatory characteristics of the protein hydrolysate (SPH) of Atlantic salmon (*Salmo salar*) through dipeptidyl peptidase-IV (DPP-IV) inhibition activity and the efficiency of direct glucose uptake in vitro [20]. The results indicate that SPH, especially the low-molecular-weight component prepared by membrane filtration (MW < 3 kDa), has a significant inhibitory effect on DPP-IV and can significantly increase the glucose uptake of L6 rat skeletal muscle cells, indicating that short-chained bioactive peptides in SPH mediate glucoregulatory activity. This study proves that the biotransformation of salmon processing by-products can provide high-quality nutrition and effective glycemic regulatory peptides, thereby significantly reducing the growing health burden of MetS. Moreover, bioactive peptides are promising functional tools that could be applied to future personalized medicine.

(-)-Doliculide is a marine cyclodepsipeptide isolated from *Dolabella auricularia* [21]. Due to its strong cytotoxicity, (−)-Doliculide has aroused the interest of researchers in the field of synthetic chemistry. Based on the structural characteristics of (−)-Doliculide, which is composed of peptide segments and polyketone segments, the fifth article by Tost and Kazmaier utilizes Matson's homology method and focuses on post-modification at the end positions of (−)-Doliculide polyketone fragments, successfully synthesizing various polyketone derivatives of (−)-Doliculide. In addition, the author also studies the activity of the synthesized (−)-Doliculide polyketone derivatives. The results prove that all modifications of the i-Pr fragment led to the inactivity of (−)-Doliculide polyketone derivatives against HepG2 [22]. This study lays a methodological foundation for the subsequent research of (-)-Doliculide, including the structure–activity relationship of its derivatives.

Antimicrobial peptides (AMPs), regarded as host defense peptides (HDPs), are small in size with a MW less than 10 kDa and can be encoded in the genome or produced by hydrolyzing proteins or larger polypeptides. Moreover, AMPs exhibit a variety of biological activities, such as antimicrobial, antifungal, antioxidant, antihypertensive, immunomodulatory, and anticoagulant properties [23]. Therefore, the sixth article by Álvarez et al. concerns the identification, characterization, and bioactivity evaluation of AMPs from the mucus of *Seriola lalandi* and *Seriolella violacea* [24]. Nine peptides with a disordered or random coil secondary structure were prepared and identified using chromatography and mass spectrometry techniques. The analysis of the structure–activity relationship indicated that the antimicrobial activity of prepared peptides is closely associated with basic and aromatic amino acid residues, while cysteine residue could remarkably enhance the peptides' antioxidant activity. In addition, the peptides with the highest antimicrobial activity also presented stimulated respiratory bursts in leukocytes. This study confirms the existence of bioactive peptides in the epidermal mucus of Chilean marine fish, providing a new source for the development of marine peptides.

Fatigue is a temporary decline in the functions of the body or brain due to continuous energy consumption, stress, or disease. It is divided into physiological fatigue and pathological fatigue [25]. Short-term fatigue can be relieved by rest, while long-term fatigue may be related to diseases and requires comprehensive intervention. High Fischer ratio oligopeptides (HFOs) are defined as peptide mixtures (2–9 peptides) with an F-ratio (branched-chain amino acids/aromatic amino acids) greater than 20. Due to their significant physiological activities, HFOs have aroused widespread interest and have been produced from grains, beans, meat, eggs, milk, and marine organisms [26]. Therefore, the seventh paper by Mao et al. systematically investigates the anti-fatigue function and mechanism of HFOs from Antarctic Krill (HFOs-AK) on exercise-induced fatigue [27]. HFOs-AK can significantly prolong the endurance of swimming time, improve physiological indicators, decrease metabolite levels, and protect the muscle tissues of exhausted mice. The research on the mechanism of action indicated that HFOs-AK could regulate AMPK and Keap1/Nrf2/ARE signaling pathways and ameliorate the energy metabolism and oxidative stress caused by intense exercise. In addition, HFOs-AK could improve the activity of Na^+-K^+-ATPase and Ca^{2+}-Mg^{2+}-ATPase to reduce tissue damage and increase ATP levels. Therefore, HFOs-AK can act as dietary ingredients applied in functional foods to resist the fatigue caused by intense exercise.

Melanin is a phenolic polymer that is widely present in animals and plants. Excessive melanin deposition can lead to a series of skin diseases, such as black and brown spots, and even cause melanoma and other skin cancers. Tyrosinase is the key enzyme for oxidizing tyrosine to generate melanin [28]. Therefore, screening safe and efficient tyrosinase inhibitors can effectively control melanin production. Therefore, the eighth article by Logesh et al. concerns the identification and mechanism of the tyrosinase inhibitory peptide AHYYD from *Pinctada martensii* nacre [29]. In this study, AHYYD, with an IC$_{50}$ value of 2.012 ± 0.088 mM, showed significant tyrosinase inhibitory activity through a reversible competitive model. In addition, AHYYD had a strong binding affinity to tyrosinase with a binding energy of −8.0 kcal/mol. Moreover, AHYYD could significantly decrease the melanin content by inhibiting tyrosinase activity and positively increasing the activity of antioxidant enzymes in mouse B16F10 melanoma cells. These findings suggest that AHYYD has the potential to be applied to cosmetic products due to its positive therapeutic efficacy in decreasing intracellular melanin production.

The physical health of more than 1.13 billion people worldwide is affected by hypertension. The angiotensin-I converting enzyme (ACE) is a key enzyme in the renin–angiotensin–aldosterone regulatory system (RAAS), which catalyzes the conversion of inactive angiotensin I (Ang I) into potent Ang II, thereby inactivating the vasodilator bradykinin [30]. Therefore, screening for small molecule compounds to inhibit ACE activity has become an effective method for the treatment of hypertension. The ninth article by Li et al. concerns ACE inhibitory peptides from the protein hydrolysate of *Ulva prolifera* [31]. Then, an anti-ACE peptide KAF with an IC$_{50}$ value of 0.63 ± 0.26 µM was separated and identified from the *U. prolifera* protein. KAF competes to bind ACE through two hydrogen bonds and inhibits its activity. Moreover, KAF could act on LTCC and RyR to increase Ca^{2+} levels in the endoplasmic reticulum of HUVECs and activate eNOS to promote the production of NO by regulating the Akt signaling pathway.

Saturated fatty acids play a significant role in maintaining human physiological functions. However, high concentrations of free fatty acids cause fat accumulation in the liver, promote the release of inflammatory factors and cellular dysfunction, induce liver cell damage and apoptosis, and thereby lead to the progression of NAFLD [32]. Therefore, the tenth paper by Song et al. investigates the effects of LALFVPR, KLHDEEVA, and PSRILYG from the bone collagen of *H. nehereus* on sodium palmitate (PANa)-induced hyperlipidemia in HepG2 cells [33]. The results demonstrate that LALFVPR, KLHDEEVA, and PSRILYG, particularly LALFVPR, can protect HepG2 cells against PANa-induced damage by up-regulating the level of Nrf2 to enhance the antioxidant enzyme activity. Compared with LALFVPR and PSRILYG, LALFVPR showed better effects in reducing oxidative stress and lipid accumulation by regulating the expression levels of proteins closely related to lipid metabolism, such as FASN, ACC1, ATGL, and CPT1. In addition, the inhibitory ability of LALFVPR on pancreatic lipase activity is stronger than that of orlistat. This research provides support for the functional food of fish bone collagen peptides used in the treatment of hyperlipidemia.

The papers in this Special Issue contain studies on bioactive peptides from *C. frondosa*, *H. nehereus*, Antarctic krill (*E. superba*), Atlantic Salmon (*S. salar*), the mucus of *S. lalandi* and *S. violacea* to *P. martensii* and *U. prolifera*. In addition, the derivatives of (−)-Doliculide were synthesized. Moreover, it is worth noting that more than half of the included papers focus on metabolism-related diseases such as hypertension, hyperlipidemia, and diabetes. This indicates that metabolism-related diseases require more highly effective drugs, and the significant activity of marine peptides in this regard shows their potential application value.

In conclusion, the Guest Editors thank all the authors who contributed to this Special Issue, all the reviewers for evaluating the submitted manuscripts, and the Editorial Board of *Marine Drugs*, especially Jane Qiao, Assistant Editor of this journal, for their continuous help in making this Special Issue a reality.

Funding: This research was funded the National Natural Science Foundation of China (No. 82073764).

Conflicts of Interest: The authors declare no conflicts of interest.

References

1. Zou, S.; Feng, G.; Li, D.; Ge, P.; Wang, S.; Liu, T.; Li, H.; Lai, Y.; Tan, Z.; Huang, Y.; et al. Lifestyles and health-related quality of life in Chinese people: A national family study. *BMC Public Health* **2022**, *22*, 2208. [CrossRef] [PubMed]
2. Anderson, E.; Durstine, J.L. Physical activity, exercise, and chronic diseases: A brief review. *Sports Med. Health Sci.* **2019**, *1*, 3–10. [CrossRef] [PubMed]
3. Huang, L.; Wang, Z.; Wang, H.; Zhao, L.; Jiang, H.; Zhang, B.; Ding, G. Nutrition transition and related health challenges over decades in China. *Eur. J. Clin. Nutr.* **2021**, *75*, 247–252. [CrossRef] [PubMed]
4. Wang, Y.-M.; Ge, M.-X.; Ran, S.-Z.; Pan, X.; Chi, C.-F.; Wang, B. Antioxidant Peptides from Miiuy Croaker Swim Bladders: Ameliorating Effect and Mechanism in NAFLD Cell Model through Regulation of Hypolipidemic and Antioxidant Capacity. *Mar. Drugs* **2025**, *23*, 63. [CrossRef]
5. Vermeulen, S.J.; Park, T.; Khoury, C.K.; Béné, C. Changing diets and the transformation of the global food system. *Ann. N. Y. Acad. Sci.* **2020**, *1478*, 3–17. [CrossRef]
6. Bodirsky, B.L.; Dietrich, J.P.; Martinelli, E.; Stenstad, A.; Pradhan, P.; Gabrysch, S.; Mishra, A.; Weindl, I.; Le Mouël, C.; Rolinski, S.; et al. The ongoing nutrition transition thwarts long-term targets for food security, public health and environmental protection. *Sci. Rep.* **2020**, *10*, 19778. [CrossRef]
7. Li, R.; Li, P. High-Value Utilization of Marine Biological Resources. *Foods* **2023**, *12*, 4054. [CrossRef] [PubMed]
8. Wang, S.; Fan, L.; Pan, H.; Li, Y.; Qiu, Y.; Lu, Y. Antimicrobial peptides from marine animals: Sources, structures, mechanisms and the potential for drug development. *Front. Mar. Sci.* **2023**, *9*, 1112595. [CrossRef]
9. Zheng, S.L.; Wang, Y.Z.; Zhao, Y.Q.; Chi, C.F.; Zhu, W.Y.; Wang, B. High Fischer ratio oligopeptides from hard-shelled mussel: Preparation and hepatoprotective effect against acetaminophen-induced liver injury in mice. *Food Biosci.* **2023**, *53*, 102638. [CrossRef]
10. Yang, H.; Zhang, Q.; Zhang, B.; Zhao, Y.; Wang, N. Potential Active Marine Peptides as Anti-Aging Drugs or Drug Candidates. *Mar. Drugs* **2023**, *21*, 144. [CrossRef]
11. Wang, P.; Zhang, Y.; Hu, J.; Tan, B.K. Bioactive Peptides from Marine Organisms. *Protein Pept. Lett.* **2024**, *31*, 569–585. [CrossRef] [PubMed]
12. Xu, S.; Zhao, Y.; Song, W.; Zhang, C.; Wang, Q.; Li, R.; Shen, Y.; Gong, S.; Li, M.; Sun, L. Improving the Sustainability of Processing By-Products: Extraction and Recent Biological Activities of Collagen Peptides. *Foods* **2023**, *12*, 1965. [CrossRef] [PubMed]
13. Wang, Q.; Wang, G.; Liu, C.; Sun, Z.; Li, R.; Gao, J.; Li, M.; Sun, L. The Structural Characteristics and Bioactivity Stability of *Cucumaria frondosa* Intestines and Ovum Hydrolysates Obtained by Different Proteases. *Mar. Drugs* **2023**, *21*, 395. [CrossRef]
14. IDF Diabetes Atlas 11th Edition. Available online: https://diabetesatlas.org/resources/idf-diabetes-atlas-2025/ (accessed on 7 April 2025).
15. Lin, Q.; Guo, Y.; Li, J.; He, S.; Chen, Y.; Jin, H. Antidiabetic Effect of Collagen Peptides from *Harpadon nehereus* Bones in Streptozotocin-Induced Diabetes Mice by Regulating Oxidative Stress and Glucose Metabolism. *Mar. Drugs* **2023**, *21*, 518. [CrossRef]
16. Dong, X.M.; Suo, S.K.; Wang, Y.M.; Zeng, Y.H.; Chi, C.F.; Wang, B. High Fischer ratio oligopeptides from Antarctic krill: Ameliorating function and mechanism to alcoholic liver injury through regulating AMPK/Nrf2/IκBα pathways. *J. Funct. Foods* **2024**, *122*, 106537. [CrossRef]
17. Yan, W.-Z.; Wang, J.; Wang, Y.-M.; Zeng, Y.-H.; Chi, C.-F.; Wang, B. Optimization of the preparation process and ameliorative efficacy in osteoporotic rats of peptide–calcium chelates from Skipjack tuna (*Katsuwonus pelamis*) meat. *Foods* **2024**, *13*, 2778. [CrossRef]
18. Ge, M.-X.; Chen, R.-P.; Zhang, L.; Wang, Y.-M.; Chi, C.-F.; Wang, B. Novel Ca-chelating peptides from protein hydrolysate of Antarctic krill (*Euphausia superba*): Preparation, characterization, and calcium absorption efficiency in Caco-2 cell monolayer model. *Mar. Drugs* **2023**, *21*, 579. [CrossRef] [PubMed]
19. Li, S.; Wen, C.P.; Tu, H.; Wang, S.; Li, X.; Xu, A.; Li, W.; Wu, X. Metabolic syndrome including both elevated blood pressure and elevated fasting plasma glucose is associated with higher mortality risk: A prospective study. *Diabetol Metab Syndr.* **2025**, *17*, 72. [CrossRef]
20. Bjerknes, C.; Wubshet, S.G.; Rønning, S.B.; Afseth, N.K.; Currie, C.; Framroze, B.; Hermansen, E. Glucoregulatory Properties of a Protein Hydrolysate from Atlantic Salmon (*Salmo salar*): Preliminary Characterization and Evaluation of DPP-IV Inhibition and Direct Glucose Uptake In Vitro. *Mar. Drugs* **2024**, *22*, 151. [CrossRef]
21. Harrigan, G.G.; Luesch, H.; Yoshida, W.Y.; Moore, R.E.; Nagle, D.G.; Paul, V.J. Symplostatin 1: A Dolastatin 10 Analogue from the Marine Cyanobacterium *Symploca hydnoides*. *J. Nat. Prod.* **1998**, *61*, 1075–1077. [CrossRef]

22. Tost, M.; Kazmaier, U. Synthesis and Late-Stage Modification of (−)-Doliculide Derivatives Using Matteson's Homologation Approach. *Mar. Drugs* **2024**, *22*, 165. [CrossRef] [PubMed]
23. Huan, Y.; Kong, Q.; Mou, H.; Yi, H. Antimicrobial Peptides: Classification, Design, Application and Research Progress in Multiple Fields. *Front. Microbiol.* **2020**, *11*, 582779. [CrossRef]
24. Álvarez, C.A.; Toro-Araneda, T.; Cumillaf, J.P.; Vega, B.; Tapia, M.J.; Roman, T.; Cárdenas, C.; Córdova-Alarcón, V.; Jara-Gutiérrez, C.; Santana, P.A.; et al. Evaluation of the Biological Activities of Peptides from Epidermal Mucus of Marine Fish Species from Chilean Aquaculture. *Mar. Drugs* **2024**, *22*, 248. [CrossRef]
25. Si, X.; Si, Y.; Lu, Z.; Zhong, T.; Xiao, Y.; Wang, Z.; Yu, X. Mechanisms of fatigue and molecular diagnostics: The application of bioactive compounds in fatigue relief research. *Food Biosci.* **2025**, *68*, 106523. [CrossRef]
26. Wang, Z.; Zhang, X.; Wang, L.; Ou, X.; Huang, J. High Fischer ratio oligopeptides in food: Sources, functions and application prospects. *J. Future Foods* **2024**, *4*, 128–134. [CrossRef]
27. Mao, S.-Y.; Suo, S.-K.; Wang, Y.-M.; Chi, C.-F.; Wang, B. Systematical Investigation on Anti-Fatigue Function and Underlying Mechanism of High Fischer Ratio Oligopeptides from Antarctic Krill on Exercise-Induced Fatigue in Mice. *Mar. Drugs* **2024**, *22*, 322. [CrossRef]
28. Logesh, R.; Prasad, S.R.; Chipurupalli, S.; Robinson, N.; Mohankumar, S.K. Natural tyrosinase enzyme inhibitors: A path from melanin to melanoma and its reported pharmacological activities. *Biochim. Biophys. Acta BBA-Rev. Cancer* **2023**, *1878*, 188968. [CrossRef] [PubMed]
29. Li, F.; Lin, H.; Qin, X.; Gao, J.; Chen, Z.; Cao, W.; Zheng, H.; Xie, S. In Silico Identification and Molecular Mechanism of Novel Tyrosinase Inhibitory Peptides Derived from Nacre of *Pinctada martensii*. *Mar. Drugs* **2024**, *22*, 359. [CrossRef]
30. Wu, Q.; Luo, F.; Wang, X.L.; Lin, Q.; Liu, G.Q. Angiotensin I-converting enzyme inhibitory peptide: An emerging candidate for vascular dysfunction therapy. *Crit. Rev. Biotechnol.* **2022**, *42*, 736–755. [CrossRef]
31. Li, Z.; He, H.; Liu, J.; Gu, H.; Fu, C.; Zeb, A.; Che, T.; Shen, S. Preparation and Vasodilation Mechanism of Angiotensin-I-Converting Enzyme Inhibitory Peptide from *Ulva prolifera* Protein. *Mar. Drugs* **2024**, *22*, 398. [CrossRef]
32. Leamy, A.K.; Egnatchik, R.A.; Young, J.D. Molecular mechanisms and the role of saturated fatty acids in the progression of non-alcoholic fatty liver disease. *Prog. Lipid Res.* **2013**, *52*, 165–174. [CrossRef] [PubMed]
33. Song, S.; Zhao, W.; Lin, Q.; Pei, J.; Jin, H. Peptides from *Harpadon nehereus* Bone Ameliorate Sodium Palmitate-Induced HepG2 Lipotoxicity by Regulating Oxidative Stress and Lipid Metabolism. *Mar. Drugs* **2025**, *23*, 118. [CrossRef] [PubMed]

Disclaimer/Publisher's Note: The statements, opinions and data contained in all publications are solely those of the individual author(s) and contributor(s) and not of MDPI and/or the editor(s). MDPI and/or the editor(s) disclaim responsibility for any injury to people or property resulting from any ideas, methods, instructions or products referred to in the content.

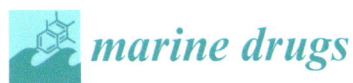

Article

The Structural Characteristics and Bioactivity Stability of *Cucumaria frondosa* Intestines and Ovum Hydrolysates Obtained by Different Proteases

Qiuting Wang [1], Gongming Wang [2], Chuyi Liu [3], Zuli Sun [4], Ruimin Li [1], Jiarun Gao [1], Mingbo Li [1] and Leilei Sun [1,*]

[1] College of Life Science, Yantai University, Yantai 264005, China; wqt1981979471@163.com (Q.W.); 17861135192@163.com (R.L.); 15863805335@163.com (J.G.); sllshd1991@163.com (M.L.)
[2] Yantai Key Laboratory of Quality and Safety Control and Deep Processing of Marine Food, Shandong Marine Resource and Environment Research Institute, Yantai 264006, China; wgmsd105@163.com
[3] Marine Biomedical Research Institute of Qingdao, Qingdao 266073, China; liucy@ouc.edu.cn
[4] College of Health, Yantai Nanshan University, Yantai 265713, China; sunzuli98@163.com
* Correspondence: leilei.198966@163.com; Tel.: +86-0535-6902638

Abstract: The study aimed to investigate the effects of alcalase, papain, flavourzyme, and neutrase on the structural characteristics and bioactivity stability of *Cucumaria frondosa* intestines and ovum hydrolysates (CFHs). The findings revealed that flavourzyme exhibited the highest hydrolysis rate (51.88% ± 1.87%). At pH 2.0, the solubility of hydrolysate was the lowest across all treatments, while the solubility at other pH levels was over 60%. The primary structures of hydrolysates of different proteases were similar, whereas the surface hydrophobicity of hydrolysates was influenced by the types of proteases used. The hydrolysates produced by different proteases were also analyzed for their absorption peaks and antioxidant activity. The hydrolysates of flavourzyme had β-fold absorption peaks (1637 cm^{-1}), while the neutrase and papain hydrolysates had N-H bending vibrations. The tertiary structure of CFHs was unfolded by different proteases, exposing the aromatic amino acids and red-shifting of the λ-peak of the hydrolysate. The alcalase hydrolysates showed better antioxidant activity in vitro and better surface hydrophobicity than the other hydrolysates. The flavourzyme hydrolysates displayed excellent antioxidant stability and pancreatic lipase inhibitory activity during gastrointestinal digestion, indicating their potential use as antioxidants in the food and pharmaceutical industries.

Keywords: *Cucumaria frondosa* intestines; ovum hydrolysate; protease; structural characteristic; bioactivity; simulated gastrointestinal digestion

1. Introduction

Sea cucumbers, a member of the phylum Echinodermata, are widely distributed in both tropical and temperate waters, ranging from intertidal zones to the colder depths of the ocean [1]. Sea cucumbers are known for their abundance of nutrients, including sea cucumber peptides, polysaccharides, saponins, vitamins, and trace elements [2]. Research has shown that these compounds have multiple activities, having antioxidant [3], antibacterial [4], anticancer, antitumor, hypoglycemic [5], hypolipidemic [6], and hypotensive effects [7]. The *Cucumaria frondosa*, also known as the Icelandic red cucumber or North Atlantic sea cucumber, is a spiny-skinned marine animal belonging to the sea cucumber family Cucumariidae. The species is the most abundant and widely distributed on the east coast of Canada [8]. *Cucumaria frondosa* is primarily grown in Iceland near the Arctic Circle. It grows at a depth of approximately 30 feet in the North Atlantic Ocean, with surface water temperatures not exceeding 4 °C. The *Cucumaria frondosa* generally reaches over 10 years of age [9]. Cucumaria frondosa is a sea cucumber variety that boasts superior quality due to its minimal pollutant content and rich nutrient accumulation [10].

However, after harvest, *Cucumaria frondosa* is commonly gutted, which involves removing all internal organs, including the respiratory tract, ovum, and intestines, accounting for approximately 50% of the total weight. Tripoteau et al. [11] demonstrated the in vitro antiviral activity of *Cucumaria frondosa*, while Senadheera et al. [9] demonstrated the antioxidant activity of hydrolyzed proteins from the body parts of the North Atlantic sea cucumber. Unfortunately, despite the presence of various bioactive compounds, the offal of *Cucumaria frondosa* is discarded entirely as waste, and the byproducts of *Cucumaria frondosa* are under-exploited in comparison to other echinoderm species, resulting in significant waste [12].

Proteins can serve as a functional substance, but studies have demonstrated that the enzymatic hydrolysates of proteins exhibit higher biological activity [13]. The physicochemical properties and biological activity of hydrolysates depend mainly on the types of proteases and the hydrolysis process [14]. However, limited research has been conducted on the effects of different enzymatic hydrolyses on the structure, physicochemical properties, and bioactivity of *Cucumaria frondosa* intestines and ovum.

The study aims to investigate the impact of different proteases on the structural characteristics and biological activities of hydrolysates. Four hydrolysates, prepared using alcalase, papain, flavourzyme, and neutrase, were selected based on their degree of hydrolysis. The hydrolysates were evaluated for their antioxidant potential and pancreatic lipase inhibitory activity. Additionally, the stability of their bioactivity was assessed after in vitro gastrointestinal digestion. The findings of this study determine the optimal protease for producing hydrolysates from the byproducts of *Cucumaria frondosa* and provide theoretical support for their industrial use.

2. Results and Discussion

2.1. Degree of Hydrolysis (DH) of Hydrolysates Obtained by Different Proteases

Figure 1A displayed the DH values of four proteases under their respective optimal conditions. The highest DH was observed in flavourzyme hydrolysates (51.88% ± 1.86%), followed by alcalase hydrolysates (36.61% ± 0.60%) and neutrase hydrolysates (21.43% ± 0.14%), while papain hydrolysates (18.33% ± 0.46%) had the lowest DH. The DH values were found to be significantly different ($p < 0.05$) among the four CFHs. Alcalase, a deep endopeptidase, primarily cleaves peptide bonds at the C-terminal polypeptide bond of hydrophobic amino acids. The DH of the hydrolysates varied depending on the types of proteases used. The DHs of the flavourzyme and alcalase hydrolysates were found to be higher compared to those of neutrase and papain. The difference can be attributed to the fact that alcalase acts as an endopeptidase with a serine active site, whereas flavourzyme is both an exopeptidase and endopeptidase of a cysteine protease with a leucine aminopeptidase [15].

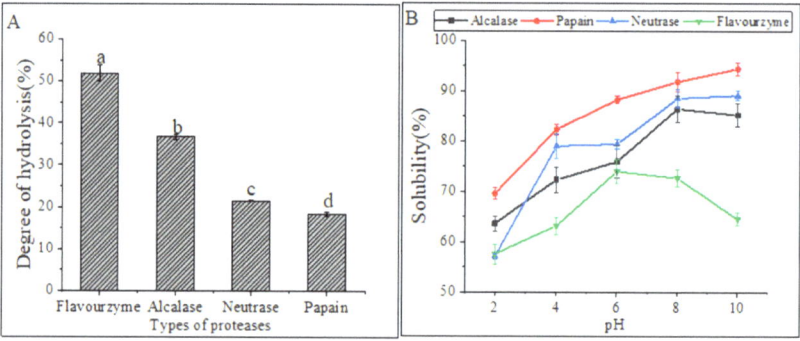

Figure 1. (**A**) Degrees of hydrolysis of different proteases. The lowercase letters indicate significant differences ($p < 0.05$) in the DHs of CFHs obtained by different proteases' hydrolysis. (**B**) Solubility of hydrolysates.

2.2. Solubility of Hydrolysates Obtained by Different Proteases

Hydrolysates' solubility is a crucial physicochemical property that significantly influences their functional properties [16]. The solubility of hydrolysates prepared at various pH levels (2.0–10.0) is shown in Figure 1B. The solubility of the hydrolysates was the lowest for all treatments at a pH of 2.0. Enzymatic digestion alters the hydrophobicity of protein hydrolysates by affecting the balance of the hydrophilic and hydrophobic groups of the hydrolysates, as well as the release of polar and ionized groups [17]. In general, the solubility improved as the pH shifted toward basic conditions. Similar solubility profiles were observed in protein hydrolysates prepared from body wall of the North Atlantic sea cucumber [9].

2.3. Structural Characteristics of Hydrolysates

2.3.1. Surface Hydrophobicity

The surface hydrophobicity of the hydrolysates is shown in Figure 2A. Gbemisola et al. [18] found that the surface hydrophobicity of a protein depended on its spatial conformations and the amount of amino acids exposed during proteolysis. Peptidases can ruin hydrophobic areas, making them more hydrophilic and thus improving the dispersibility of the hydrolysates in water. The alcalase hydrolysates had a significantly higher surface hydrophobicity compared to the other three proteases, indicating a higher concentration of aromatic amino acids. This finding was consistent with that of Zohreh et al. [13].

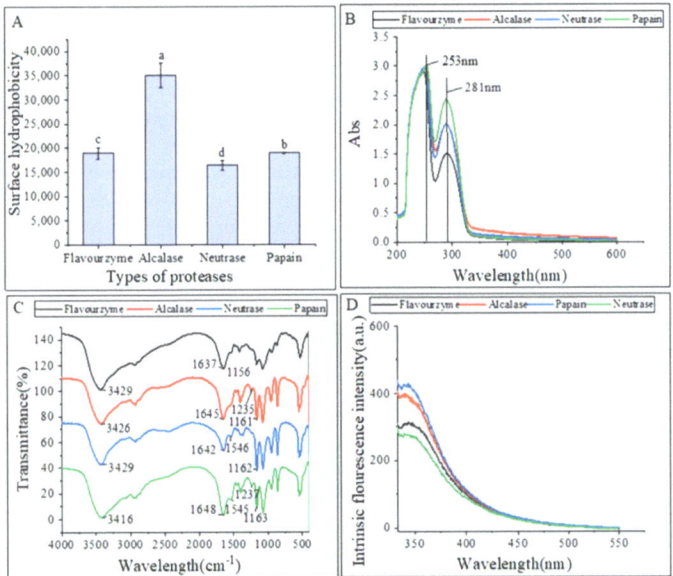

Figure 2. (**A**) Surface hydrophobicity of hydrolysates; (**B**) UV–vis spectra of hydrolysates; (**C**) FTIR spectra of hydrolysates; (**D**) intrinsic fluorescence spectroscopy of hydrolysates. The lowercase letters indicate significant differences ($p < 0.05$) in the surface hydrophobicity of CFHs obtained by different proteases' hydrolysis.

2.3.2. Ultraviolet-Visible (UV-Vis) Spectroscopy Analysis

Figure 2B displayed that the UV-Vis spectra of these hydrolysates were quite similar, with strong absorption peaks at 260 nm and 280 nm. This could be attributed to the influence of tyrosine (278 nm) and phenylalanine (257 nm). The hydrolysates exhibited a strong absorption peak around 280 nm, which is characteristic of hydrophobic amino acids such as tyrosine, phenylalanine, and tryptophan, indicating the hydrophobic property of the extracted hydrolysates [19].

2.3.3. Fourier Transform Infrared Spectroscopy (FTIR) Analysis

The differences in the secondary structures of the hydrolysates were analyzed using FTIR. The FTIR spectra of hydrolysates from different proteases are presented in Figure 2C. FTIR is commonly used to examine peptides and proteins since it can detect the amide (peptide) bonds, which exhibit distinct IR signals for folded peptides and proteins [20]. The vibrational frequency is determined by the hydrogen bonding nature between C=O and C-N in the amide-I band (1600–1700 cm^{-1}). The α-helix structure is identified by the absorption peak at 1650–1658 cm^{-1} in the amide-I band, while the β-fold structure is identified by the peak at 1610–1640 cm^{-1}. The random curl structure is identified by the peak at 1640–1650 cm^{-1}, and the β-turn structure is identified by the peak at 1660–1695 cm^{-1}. In the amide III region, the β-fold structure is identified by the peak at 1181–1248 cm^{-1}, the β-turn structure is identified by the peak at 1270–1295 cm^{-1}, and the irregular curl structure is identified by the peak at 1255–1288 cm^{-1}. The C=O stretching vibration absorption peak is located at 1630–1680 cm^{-1} in the peptide bond, while the N-H bending vibration peak is located around 1550 cm^{-1}. The N-H stretching vibrations are identified by the absorption peak around 3100–3500 cm^{-1} [21].

The FTIR spectra analysis revealed that hydrolysates treated with different proteases exhibited changes in their spectra, with only slight shifts in bands. Specifically, hydrolysates treated with alcalase, neutrase, and papain displayed irregular curls at 1645 cm^{-1}, 1642 cm^{-1}, and 1648 cm^{-1}, respectively, whereas hydrolysates treated with flavourzyme exhibited mainly β-fold absorption peaks at 1637 cm^{-1}. The α-helix structure, an ordered structure, is easily influenced by conformational changes. On the other hand, the β-sheet and β-turn structures are also ordered structures but with relative stretches, whereas the random coil structure is a disordered structure. The decrease in β-sheet structures in the hydrolysates and the increase in random coil structures indicated that the protease treatments caused the ordered structure of CFHs to become disordered. Similarly, the structure of mung bean protein enzymatic hydrolysates was analyzed, and it was found that the neutrase and papain hydrolysates showed N-H bending vibrations, while the flavourzyme and alcalase hydrolysates did not, suggesting that the N-H bending vibrations were disrupted during the enzymatic digestion of the flavourzyme and alcalase [22].

2.3.4. Intrinsic Fluorescence Spectroscopy Analysis

Intrinsic fluorescence spectroscopy is a sensitive technique used to detect conformational changes in the tertiary structure of proteins [23]. This is achieved by exciting the aromatic amino acid residues (Trp, Tyr, and Phe) with excitation light, which produces fluorescence [24]. Figure 2D shows that the fluorescence emission spectra of flavourzyme, alcalase, and neutrase hydrolysates were red-shifted as compared to those of papain. This shift might be attributed to changes in the protein structure after enzymatic hydrolysis. The side-chain groups of the aromatic amino acid residues that were originally buried in the protein were gradually exposed to the molecular surface, resulting in a change in the polar environment of the tryptophan residues and leading to the red shift of the peak.

2.4. Antioxidant Activity of Hydrolysates Obtained by Different Proteases

Examination of the DPPH radical scavenging activity is a commonly used technique for assessing the in vitro antioxidant activity of compounds. The technique is based on the principle that DPPH provides maximum absorbance at 517 nm. The antioxidant activity of the hydrolysate is expressed as a decrease in absorbance or a decrease in the pure color intensity of the sample [25]. As shown in Figure 3A, the DPPH radical scavenging capacity of all samples was concentration-dependent and exhibited stronger scavenging ability with increasing concentration. The flavourzyme hydrolysates showed significantly higher scavenging activity than the other three proteases. At a concentration of 8 mg/mL, the scavenging activity of flavourzyme hydrolysates was comparable to that of ascorbic acid. Moreover, nearly all samples treated with flavourzyme or its combination exhibited relatively high DPPH radical scavenging activity [9].

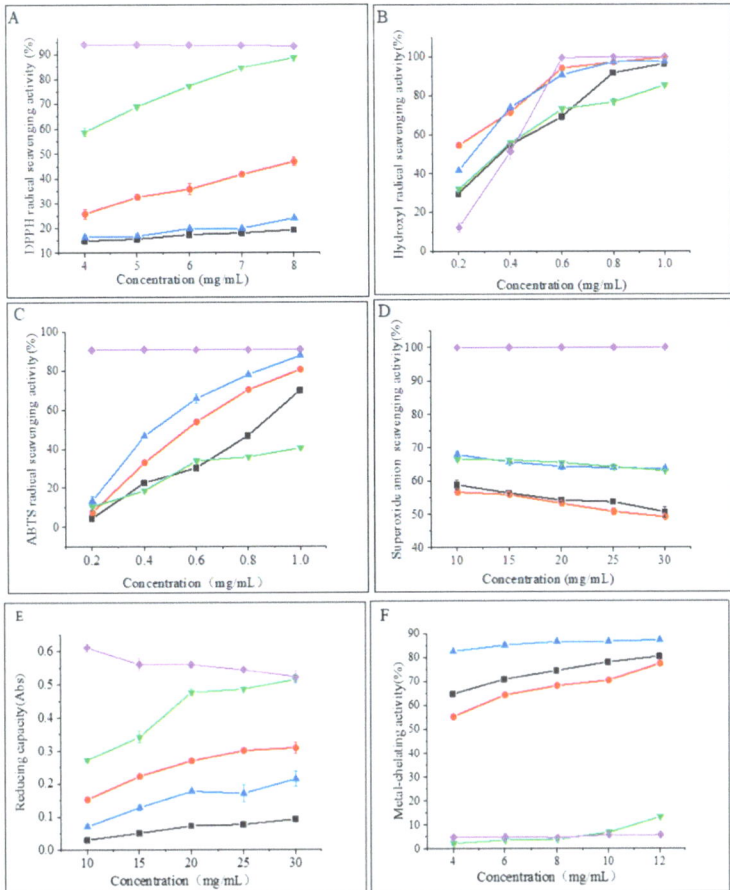

Figure 3. (**A**) DPPH radical scavenging activity of hydrolysates; (**B**) hydroxyl radical scavenging activity of hydrolysates; (**C**) ABTS radical scavenging activity of hydrolysates; (**D**) superoxide anion scavenging activity of hydrolysates; (**E**) reducing capacity of hydrolysates; and (**F**) metal-chelating activity of hydrolysates. Purple diamonds represent ascorbic acid; black boxes represent neutrase; red circles represent papain; green inverted triangles represent flavourzyme; and blue triangles represent alcalase.

Hydroxyl radicals are highly reactive free radicals found in biological tissues that can cause physiological disorders by reacting with proteins, DNA, and lipids. These radicals play an essential role in lipid peroxidation and hydrophilic oxidation [26]. Figure 3B shows that the hydroxyl radical scavenging activity increased significantly ($p < 0.05$) with increasing the sample concentration from 0.2 to 0.6 mg/mL and tended to level off at 0.6–1.0 mg/mL. The free radical scavenging activity of alcalase and papain hydrolysates at a concentration of 0.8 mg/mL was found to be similar to that of ascorbic acid. The strong hydroxyl radical scavenging activity can be attributed to the high content of hydrophobic amino acids [26]. It has been shown that the presence of a benzene ring group in aromatic amino acids acts as an oxidative chain breaker through the hydrogen-atom transfer (HAT) mechanism. In a study conducted by Kai Wang et al. [27], it was revealed that alcalase and papain hydrolysates contained higher levels of aromatic amino acids, which resulted in an increased hydroxyl radical scavenging capacity of these two hydrolysates.

The decolorization of the radical ABTS cation in the green solution (ABTS•+) is used to confirm the radical activity of the hydrolysates [28]. As depicted in Figure 3C, the ABTS radical scavenging activity of the CFHs was found to be concentration-dependent, with alcalase showing significantly higher ($p < 0.05$) activity than the other three proteases. This could be attributed to the synergistic effect of the peptides in the hydrolysate on the ABTS radical scavenging activity. The ABTS radical scavenging activity of the alcalase hydrolysate at a concentration of 1 mg/mL was found to be comparable to that of ascorbic acid. A study by Zohreh Karami et al. [13] revealed that the ABTS radical scavenging activity of hydrolysates from adzuki bean (*Vigna angularis*) and mung bean (*Vigna radiata*) protein concentrates was significantly higher ($p < 0.05$) using alcalase in comparison to using flavourzyme hydrolysates.

According to Figure 3D, the CFHs exhibited a lower superoxide anion scavenging activity ($p < 0.05$) compared to the ascorbic acid. No significant difference ($p > 0.05$) in scavenging activity between flavourzyme and alcalase was observed, but both showed higher activity than neutrase and papain. It is possible that CFHs contain inactive polypeptides, resulting in an overall lower clearance activity [21].

The potential antioxidant capacity of protein hydrolysates is often measured by their reduction capacity [29]. Figure 3E demonstrates that the reduction capacity of CFHs was concentration-dependent. The radical scavenging activity of the flavourzyme hydrolysate was significantly higher ($p < 0.05$) than the activity of the other three proteases. At 30 mg/mL, the activity of the flavourzyme hydrolysate was similar to that of the ascorbic acid. The reduction capacity was influenced by the concentration and type of proteases. This might be due to the fact that flavourzyme increased the number of free amino acids, thereby increasing the number of protons and electrons exposed and available for redox reactions [25].

As shown in Figure 3F, the metal-chelating activity of the CFHs increased as the concentration increased ($p < 0.05$). The hydrolysates of alcalase, papain, and neutrase all exhibited significantly higher chelating activity than that of the ascorbic acid, especially alcalase hydrolysates, showing the highest activity. Additionally, the flavourzyme hydrolysate demonstrated higher chelating activity than the ascorbic acid at concentrations above 0.8 mg/mL. Our findings were in agreement with those of Liu et al. [22] and Zohreh Karami et al. [13], who found that alcalase was more effective than flavourzyme, papain, and neutrase in producing metal-chelating peptides from adzuki bean (*Vigna angularis*) and mung bean (*Vigna radiata*) proteins. Alcalase is a highly effective protease with a wide range of specificity, capable of cleaving polypeptide bonds and releasing additional carboxyl and amino groups on branched chains, leading to the liberation of more acidic and basic amino acids, with a particular emphasis on Phe, Tyr, and Lys. The end result is an increase in the negative charge, which in turn facilitates the binding of Fe^{2+} radicals [13,22,30].

2.5. Effect of Different Proteases on the Pancreatic Lipase Inhibitory Activity of Hydrolysates

Pancreatic lipase is the primary enzyme responsible for breaking down triacylglycerols during fat digestion and absorption in the intestine. To limit intestinal fat absorption, pancreatic lipase inhibitors have been developed and shown to be effective in controlling hyperlipidemias, making them promising drugs for weight loss. Figure 4 displays the pancreatic lipase inhibitory activity of hydrolysates created from different proteases at 20 mg/mL. Flavourzyme hydrolysates had greater pancreatic lipase inhibitory activity (62.27% ± 0.73%) compared to those of papain (61.36% ± 2.93%), neutrase (50.18% ± 2.74%), and alcalase (47.34% ± 0.46%) hydrolysates. In a study conducted by Priti Mudgil et al. [31], it was found that the hydrolysates obtained through papain had superior pancreatic lipase inhibitory activity compared to that of those obtained through alcalase. Another recent study suggested that the pancreatic lipase inhibitory activity of CFHs was weaker than camel casein hydrolysates, which could be attributed to the longer enzymatic digestion time of CFHs [32].

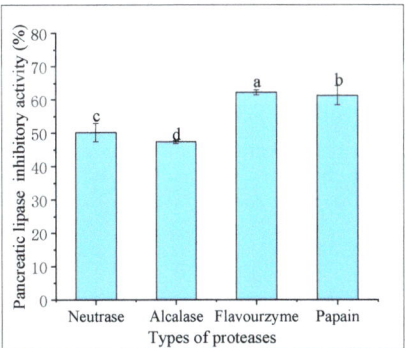

Figure 4. Pancreatic lipase inhibitory activity of hydrolysates. The lowercase letters indicate significant differences ($p < 0.05$) in the pancreatic lipase inhibitory activity of CFHs obtained by different proteases' hydrolysis.

2.6. Bioactivity Stability of CFHs after Simulated Gastrointestinal Digestion In Vitro

In recent times, in vitro digestion models have proven to be a valuable tool for comprehending the structural and chemical transformations that occur during simulated gastrointestinal conditions. These models have been widely employed to assess the digestibility, bioavailability, and physicochemical properties of peptides [33]. During digestion, the biological activity of hydrolysates can either be activated or inactivated. One of the crucial determinants of the bioactivity of peptides in vitro is their resistance to gastrointestinal digestion [15]. The study investigated the changes in the stability of antioxidant activity and pancreatic lipase inhibitory activity in CFHs obtained from different proteases during simulated gastrointestinal digestion in vitro.

2.6.1. Antioxidant Activity

According to the findings presented in Figure 5, the antioxidant activity of the CFHs persisted after simulated gastrointestinal digestion in vitro. The hydroxyl radical scavenging activity and superoxide anion scavenging activity were observed to be significantly higher ($p < 0.05$), while the DPPH radical scavenging activity, ABTS radical scavenging activity, and reduction capacity were significantly lower ($p < 0.05$). The results could be attributed to a decrease in the quantity of amino acids possessing antioxidant activity in CFHs during simulated gastrointestinal digestion in vitro [33]. The antioxidant activity of peptides is related to their structural characteristics such as hydrophobicity, sequence, and amino acid composition [33]. After simulated gastrointestinal digestion in vitro, the metal-chelating activity of hydrolysates obtained by each protease increased significantly ($p < 0.05$), except for that of the alcalase hydrolysates. The finding was consistent with a study conducted by Zhang et al. [15]. As shown in Figure 5, the flavourzyme CFHs exhibited higher gastrointestinal digestive stability than the other three proteases, indicating that the stability of the hydrolysates during gastrointestinal digestion was influenced by the protease used [15,33].

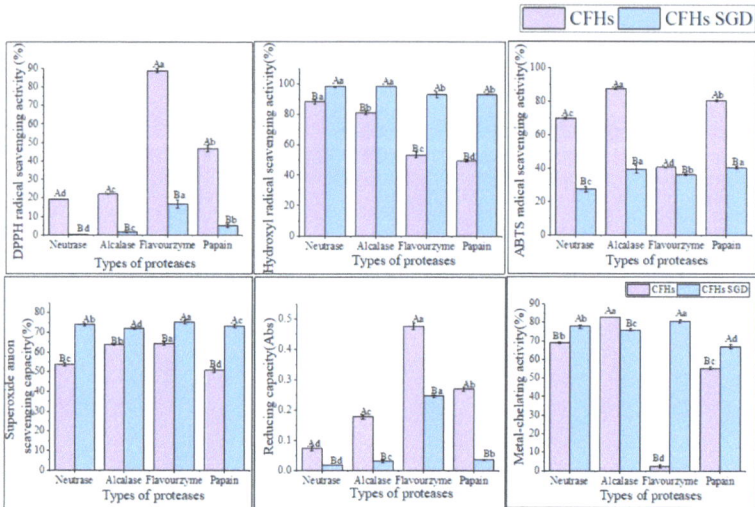

Figure 5. The antioxidant activity stability of CFHs before and after simulated gastrointestinal digestion in vitro. The uppercase letters represent significant differences ($p < 0.05$) in the activity of CFHs before and after simulated gastrointestinal digestion in vitro, while the lowercase letters indicate significant differences ($p < 0.05$) in the activity of CFHs obtained by different proteases' hydrolysis.

2.6.2. Pancreatic Lipase Inhibitory Activity

As shown in Figure 6, the pancreatic lipase inhibitory activity of the hydrolysates obtained by all proteases decreased significantly ($p < 0.05$) after simulated gastrointestinal digestion in vitro. The highest inhibitory activity was observed in the flavourzyme after digestion (44.12% ± 0.49%). The results of the antioxidant activity stability were consistent with the above findings. The interaction of the peptide with phospholipase is inhibited by lipase [34]. Peptides that can bind more binding sites are dominated by hydrophobic amino acids, such as folic acid and proline [34]. The decrease in activity after simulated gastrointestinal digestion in vitro might be attributed to a reduction in the hydrophobic amino acid content of the individual hydrolysates after digestion.

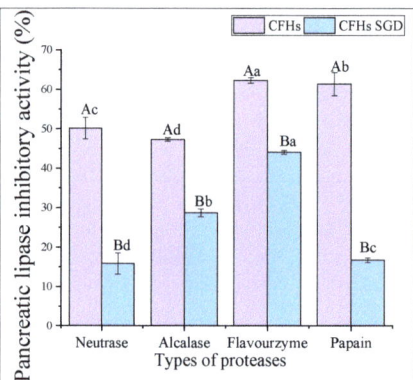

Figure 6. The pancreatic lipase inhibitory activity stability of CFHs. The uppercase letters represent significant differences ($p < 0.05$) in the activity of CFHs before and after simulated gastrointestinal digestion in vitro, while the lowercase letters indicate significant differences ($p < 0.05$) in the activity of CFHs obtained by different proteases' hydrolysis.

3. Materials and Methods

3.1. Materials and Reagents

Fresh *Cucumaria frondosa* intestines and ovum were purchased from Haizhongbao seafood trading center (Yantai, China). Neutrase (50,000 U/g), alcalase (200,000 U/g), flavourzyme (15,000 U/g), and papain (100,000 U/g) were of food grade and were purchased from Solarbio Biotechnology Co. Ltd. (Beijing, China). All other reagents and chemicals used in this study were of analytical grade and were purchased from Sinopharm Chemical Reagent Co. Ltd. (Shanghai, China).

3.2. Preparation of Hydrolysates

As shown in Table 1, CFHs were prepared by hydrolyzing *Cucumaria frondosa* intestines and ovum with proteases at optimum temperature and mild agitation at 100 rpm in an orbital shaker incubator. Once the hydrolysis was complete, the mixture was heated in a boiling water bath for 15 min to stop the hydrolysis. After cooling the mixture in ice water, it was centrifuged at 10,000× g for 15 min at 4 °C, and the resulting supernatants were lyophilized to obtain the final CFH product.

Table 1. Hydrolysis conditions of different proteases.

Proteases	Temperature (°C)	pH	Solid–Liquid Ratio (w/v)	Proteases Addition (U/g Protein)	Time (h)
Neutrase	50	7	1:20	6000	7
Alcalase	60	10.5	1:20	7000	7
Flavourzyme	35	5.5	1:15	10,000	9
Papain	60	7.5	1:8	7000	7

3.3. Determination of DH

The DH was determined using a modified ninhydrin colorimetric method [35]. A sample was taken in a test tube and 1 mL of ninhydrin solution was added. The mixture was sealed with plastic wrap and heated in a boiling water bath for 15 min. After boiling, the tube was rapidly cooled in cold water and 5 mL of 40% ethanol solution was added. The solution was shaken well until it faded to brownish-red and left at room temperature for 10 min. The solution was zeroed with distilled water and the absorbance was measured at 570 nm.

$$\text{DH (\%)} = h/h_{tot} \times 100 \tag{1}$$

where h represents the number of millimoles of peptide bonds cleaved per gram of sample (mmol), and h_{tot} represents the number of millimoles of peptide bonds per gram of sample (mmol). For this experiment, a value of 7.99 mmol/g was used based on the amino acid composition of the sample.

3.4. Solubility

The solubility of the proteins in the hydrolysates was determined according to the method described by Vásquez [36] with slight modifications. The hydrolysates were dissolved in distilled water at a concentration of 1% w/v, and the pH of the mixture was adjusted to 2.0, 4.0, 6.0, 8.0, and 10.0 using either 1 mol/L NaOH or 1 mol/L HCl. After centrifugation at 4000 rpm for 20 min, the soluble fraction (supernatant) was collected, and the protein content was determined using the Lowry and Randall [37] method. The percentage of solubility was calculated according to the following equation.

$$\text{Solubility (\%)} = (\text{Protein content of the supernatant})/(\text{Protein content of the sample}) \times 100 \tag{2}$$

3.5. Structural Characteristics of CFHs

3.5.1. Surface Hydrophobicity

The surface hydrophobicity of the samples was determined using the method developed by Zhang et al. [38]. We used 1-anilino-8-naphthalenesulfonate (ANS), a hydrophobic probe. Each sample was diluted with 0.1 M phosphate buffer (pH 7.0) to a concentration of 1 mg/mL and mixed with 20 μL of 8 mM ANS solution and 2 mL of ACH hydrolysate. The fluorescence intensity of each sample was measured at an excitation wavelength of 375 nm and a scanning (SHIMADZU, Tohoku, Japan) wavelength range of 400–650 nm.

3.5.2. UV-Vis Spectroscopy

A UV-Vis spectrum (UV-Vis Spectroscopy, METASH, Shanghai, China) was obtained by dissolving 15 mg of the CFHs in 10 mL of ultrapure water to acquire a concentration of 1.5 mg/mL and scanning in the range of 200–600 nm.

3.5.3. FTIR

Two mg samples of enzymatic hydrolysates were compressed with potassium bromide. The infrared spectrometer (Perkin Elmer, Waltham, MA, USA) was utilized for a full-spectrum scan with a resolution of 4 cm^{-1}, ranging from 4000 to 400 cm^{-1}. The Spectrum 10.4.1 software version was employed for infrared spectrum mapping and data collection.

3.5.4. Intrinsic Fluorescence Spectroscopy

The fluorescence spectra of protein hydrolysates were measured through fluorescence spectrophotometry (SHIMADZU, Tohoku, Japan), following the method outlined by Du et al. [24]. The excitation wavelength was set at 290 nm, and the emission spectrum range was set from 330–550 nm with a gap width of 5 nm. Prior to measurement, the sample was diluted to a concentration of 0.2 mg/mL in a phosphate buffer with a pH of 7.0.

3.6. Antioxidant Activity of CFHs

3.6.1. DPPH Radical Scavenging Activity

The DPPH radical scavenging activity of protein hydrolysate was determined as described by Du Mx [39] with slight modifications. The samples were prepared at different concentrations (4.0, 5.0, 6.0, 7.0, and 8.0 mg/mL) and mixed with DPPH (0.2 mM) in equal proportions. The mixture was allowed to stand in the dark for 30 min, and the absorbance was monitored at 517 nm using a microplate reader (Thermo Scientific, Pleasanton, CA, USA). Anhydrous ethanol was used as the blank control, and VC was used as the positive control. The DPPH radical scavenging activity was calculated as follows:

$$\text{DPPH radical scavenging activity (\%)} = [1 - (A_1 - A_2)/A_0] \times 100 \quad (3)$$

where A_0 represents the absorbance value of anhydrous ethanol instead of sample, A_1 represents the absorbance value of the sample group, and A_2 represents the absorbance value of anhydrous ethanol instead of DPPH.

3.6.2. Hydroxyl Radical Scavenging Activity

The hydroxyl radical scavenging activity was determined using a modified method based on Zhou et al. [40]. In short, a mixture of 1.0 mL FeSO$_4$ (2 mM), 1.0 mL salicylic acid-ethanol solution (6 mM), and 1.0 mL sample (0.2, 0.4, 0.6, 0.8, and 1.0 mg/mL) was prepared. To the mixture, 1.0 mL H$_2$O$_2$ (6 mM) was added and incubated at 37 °C for 30 min. The absorbance of the mixture was immediately measured at 510 nm using a microplate reader (Thermo Scientific, USA). The hydroxyl radical scavenging activity was calculated using the following formula:

$$\text{Hydroxyl radical scavenging activity (\%)} = [1 - (A_2 - A_1)/A_0)] \times 100 \quad (4)$$

where A_0 represents the absorbance value of distilled water instead of the sample, A_1 represents the absorbance value of distilled water instead of the hydrogen peroxide solution, and A_2 represents the absorbance value of the sample mixed with ferrous sulfate, hydrogen peroxide, and salicylic acid ethanol solution.

3.6.3. Superoxide Anion Scavenging Activity

The superoxide anion scavenging activity was measured with reference to the method developed by Xie et al. [41]. Samples of 0.5 mL each (1.8, 2.0, 2.2, 2.4, and 2.6 mg/mL) were mixed with 5.0 mL of Tris-HCl buffer solution (50 mM, pH 8.2) and incubated in a water bath at 25 °C for 20 min, followed by the addition of 0.5 mL of 3 mM pyrogallol solution pre-heated to 25 °C. The absorbance values were measured at 325 nm every 30 s for 5 min. Ascorbic acid was used as a positive control. The superoxide anion scavenging activity was calculated using the following equation:

$$\text{Superoxide anion scavenging activity (\%)} = (1 - A_1/A_0) \times 100 \qquad (5)$$

where A_1 represents the absorbance value of the sample group, and A_0 represents the absorbance value of the blank group.

3.6.4. Reduction Capacity

To determine the reduction capacity, the method of Liu et al. [42] was used with some modifications. A total of 1 mL of each CFH at different concentrations (10.0, 15.0, 20.0, 25.0, and 30.0 mg/mL) was mixed with 2.5 mL of 1% potassium ferricyanide solution and 2.5 mL of 0.2 M phosphate buffer (pH 6.6). The resulting mixture was placed in a 50 °C water bath for 20 min and cooled to room temperature, and 2.5 mL of 10% TCA was added. After centrifugation at 3000 rpm for 10 min, 2.5 mL of the supernatant was transferred into a test tube, then 2.5 mL of distilled water and 0.5 mL of 0.1% $FeCl_3$ were added. The absorbance values of the mixture were measured at 700 nm using an enzyme marker (Thermo Scientific, CA, USA). An increase in the absorbance value indicated an increase in the reduction capacity.

3.6.5. Metal-Chelating Activity

The Fe^{2+} chelating activity was determined as follows [21]: 100 µL of the sample at concentrations of 4.0, 6.0, 8.0, 10.0, and 12.0 mg/mL, along with 135 µL of distilled water and 5 µL of 2 mM $FeCl_2$, were mixed together. After 3 min, 10 µL of 5 mM iron reagent was added to the mixture. The mixture was then shaken at 25 °C and allowed to stand for 10 min. Finally, the absorbance was measured at 562 nm using a microplate reader (Thermo Scientific, USA). The absorbance of the blank was also determined using distilled water. The metal-chelating activity was determined as follows:

$$\text{Metal-chelating activity (\%)} = (1 - A_1/A_0) \times 100 \qquad (6)$$

where A_1 represents the absorbance value of the sample group and A_0 represents the absorbance value of the blank group.

3.6.6. ABTS Radical Scavenging Activity

The ABTS radical scavenging ability of the CFHs was determined using the method described by Liu et al. [42]. A solution of ABTS (7.0 mmol/L) and potassium persulfate (2.45 mmol/L) was mixed at a 1:1 ratio and left to react in the dark for 12 h. The resulting solution was diluted with ethanol to an absorbance of approximately 0.70 ± 0.05 at 734 nm and stored in a dark environment. Samples with varying concentrations (0.2, 0.4, 0.6, 0.8, and 1 mg/mL) were mixed with ABTS solution at a 1:8 ratio and incubated for 10 min at

37 °C. The absorbance was measured at A_{734} and the ABTS radical scavenging ability was calculated using the following formula:

$$\text{ABTS radical scavenging activity (\%)} = (1 - A_1/A_0) \times 100 \tag{7}$$

where A_0 represents the absorbance value of the blank group and A_1 represents the absorbance value of the sample group.

3.7. Pancreatic Lipase Inhibitory Activity

According to the method by Fisayo et al. [43], 50 µL of different CFH samples, along with 25 µL of 5 mM p-nitrophenyl butyrate and 55 µL of sodium phosphate buffer (100 mM, pH 7.4, containing 100 mM NaCl), were mixed together and added to a 96-well microplate. The mixture was preincubated at 37 °C for 5 min. The reaction was initiated by the addition of 20 µL of 50 mg/mL pancreatic lipase, and the final volume was adjusted to 150 µL with assay buffer. The reaction plate was then incubated at 37 °C for 30 min, and the absorbance of released p-nitrophenyl produced for each test sample was recorded at 405 nm using a microplate reader (Thermo Scientific, USA). The pancreatic lipase inhibitory activity was determined using the following equation:

$$\text{Pancreatic lipase inhibitory activity (\%)} = [A_1 - (A_2 - A_3)]/A_1 \times 100 \tag{8}$$

where A_1 represents the absorbance value without adding a sample, A_2 represents the absorbance value after adding the sample, and A_3 represents the absorbance value after adding the sample but without adding the substrate and enzyme solution.

3.8. Simulated Gastrointestinal Digestion In Vitro of Hydrolysates

The hydrolysates underwent digestion in vitro according to the method of Minekus et al. [44]. In brief, a 5 mL of sample was combined with 7.5 mL of simulated gastric fluid containing 1.6 mL of pepsin (2000 U/mL). The mixture was stirred for 2 h at 37 °C at a speed of 200 rpm. The gastric phase was then interrupted by adjusting the pH to 7.0 with 1 mol/L NaOH. Next, 5 mL of trypsin solution (100 U/mL) and 11 mL of simulated intestinal fluid were added to the digested sample. The mixture was then stirred for another 2 h at 37 °C at a speed of 200 rpm. After completion, the final mixture was immediately placed in ice water for precooling for 10 min, followed by refrigeration at −40 °C for 10 min to halt the trypsin reaction. The resulting hydrolysates from the gastric and gastrointestinal phases were collected, frozen, and freeze-dried for subsequent analysis.

3.9. Statistical Analysis

The experimental data were tested in triplicate, and the results are presented as the average ± standard deviation (n = 3). The ANOVA analysis was performed using SPSS 13.0 software (SPSS Inc., Chicago, IL, USA).

4. Conclusions

In this study, we investigated the structural characteristics, antioxidant activities, pancreatic lipase inhibitory activity, and stability of hydrolysates produced using four different proteases. The selection of protease types is crucial for the production of bioactive hydrolysates as it can significantly impact their biological activity. We found that the alcalase hydrolysate exhibited the highest surface hydrophobicity, which can be attributed to the exposure of numerous hydrophobic groups. As a result, the alcalase hydrolysates demonstrated superior antioxidant activity, including hydroxyl radical scavenging activity, ABTS radical scavenging activity, and metal-chelating activity compared to the other hydrolysates. Meanwhile, the flavourzyme hydrolysate had the highest DH and exhibited the highest DPPH radical scavenging activity, reduction capacity, and pancreatic lipase inhibitory activity. Papain, on the other hand, exhibited a high hydroxyl radical scavenging activity and demonstrated the highest solubility across different pH levels. Additionally, the hydrolysates of flavourzyme displayed excellent antioxidant stability and showed pancreatic lipase inhibitory activity during simulated gastrointestinal digestion in vitro. Based on these findings, the hydrolysates of *Cucumaria frondosa* intestines and ovum prepared using flavourzyme were identified as the optimal choice for the production of functional foods with biological activity. These results suggest that CFHs have the potential to be utilized as antioxidants and for their hypolipidemic activity in functional foods, dietary supplements, and nutraceuticals.

Author Contributions: Conceptualization, Q.W., R.L. and L.S.; methodology, Q.W., G.W. and L.S.; software, Q.W., C.L. and L.S.; formal analysis, Q.W. and C.L.; investigation, Z.S. and M.L.; data curation, Q.W., Z.S., J.G. and R.L.; writing—original draft preparation, Q.W.; writing—review and editing, Q.W. and L.S.; supervision, Q.W. and L.S.; funding acquisition, L.S. All authors have read and agreed to the published version of the manuscript.

Funding: This research was supported by National Natural Science Foundation of China (No. 42106111); Fund of Yantai Key Laboratory of Quality and Safety Control and Deep Processing of Marine Food (No. QSCDP202304); and Natural Science Foundation of Shandong Province (No. ZR2021QD030).

Institutional Review Board Statement: Not applicable.

Informed Consent Statement: Not applicable.

Data Availability Statement: The data that support the findings of this study are available from the corresponding author, upon reasonable request.

Conflicts of Interest: The authors declare no conflict of interest.

References

1. Li, P.H.; Lu, W.C.; Chan, Y.J.; Ko, W.C.; Jung, C.C.; Huynh, D.T.L.; Ji, Y.X. Extraction and characterization of collagen from sea cucumber (*Holothuria cinerascens*) and its potential application in moisturizing cosmetics. *Aquaculture* **2020**, *515*, 734590. [CrossRef]
2. Xu, C.; Zhang, R.; Wen, Z. Bioactive compounds and biological functions of sea cucumbers as potential functional foods. *J. Funct. Foods* **2018**, *49*, 73–84. [CrossRef]
3. Jattujan, P.; Chalorak, P.; Siangcham, T.; Sangpairoj, K.; Nobsathian, S.; Poomtong, T.; Sobhon, P.; Meemon, K. Holothuria scabra extracts possess anti-oxidant activity and promote stress resistance and lifespan extension in *Caenorhabditis elegans*. *Exp. Gerontol.* **2018**, *110*, 158–171. [CrossRef]
4. Li, X.R.; Yang, R.W.; Ju, H.P.; Wang, K.; Lin, S.Y. Identification of dominant spoilage bacteria in sea cucumber protein peptide powders (SCPPs) and methods for controlling the growth of dominant spoilage bacteria by inhibiting hygroscopicity. *LWT Food Sci. Technol.* **2021**, *136*, 110355. [CrossRef]
5. Gong, P.X.; Wang, B.K.; Wu, Y.C.; Li, Q.Y.; Qin, B.W.; Li, H.J. Release of antidiabetic peptides from *Stichopus japonicas* by simulated gastrointestinal digestion. *Food Chem.* **2020**, *315*, 126273. [CrossRef]
6. Wang, T.T.; Zheng, L.; Wang, S.G.; Zhao, M.M.; Liu, X.L. Anti-diabetic and anti-hyperlipidemic effects of sea cucumber (*Cucumaria frondosa*) gonad hydrolysates in type II diabetic rats. *Food Sci. Hum. Wellness* **2022**, *11*, 1614–1622. [CrossRef]
7. Forghani, B.; Zarei, M.; Ebrahimpour, A.; Philip, R.; Bakar, J.; Hamid, A.A.; Saari, N. Purification and characterization of angiotensin converting enzyme-inhibitory peptides derived from *Stichopus horrens*: Stability study against the ACE and inhibition kinetics. *J. Funct. Foods* **2016**, *20*, 276–290. [CrossRef]
8. Hossain, A.; Dave, D.; Shahidi, F. Northern sea cucumber (*Cucumaria frondosa*): A potential candidate for functional food, nutraceutical, and pharmaceutical sector. *Mar. Drugs* **2020**, *18*, 274. [CrossRef]
9. Senadheera, T.R.L.; Dave, D.; Shahidi, F. Antioxidant potential and physicochemical properties of protein hydrolysates from body parts of North Atlantic sea cucumber (*Cucumaria frondosa*). *Food Prod. Process. Nutr.* **2021**, *3*, 3. [CrossRef]
10. Bordbar, S.; Anwar, F.; Saari, N. High-value components and bioactives from sea cucumbers for functional foods—A review. *Mar. Drugs* **2011**, *9*, 1761–1805. [CrossRef]
11. Tripoteau, L.; Bedoux, G.; Gagnon, J.; Bourgougnon, N. In vitro antiviral activities of enzymatic hydrolysates extracted from byproducts of the Atlantic holothurian *Cucumaria frondosa*. *Process Biochem.* **2015**, *50*, 867–875. [CrossRef]
12. Mamelona, J.; Saint-Louis, R.; Pelletier, E. Proximate composition and nutritional profile of by-products from green urchin and Atlantic sea cucumber processing plants. *Int. J. Food Sci. Technol.* **2010**, *45*, 2119–2126. [CrossRef]
13. Karami, Z.; Butkinaree, C.; Yingchutrakul, Y.; Simanon, N.; Duangmal, K. Comparative study on structural, biological and functional activities of hydrolysates from Adzuki bean (*Vigna angularis*) and mung bean (*Vigna radiata*) protein concentrates using Alcalase and Flavourzyme. *Food Res. Int.* **2022**, *161*, 111797. [CrossRef] [PubMed]
14. Zheng, Z.J.; Li, J.X.; Li, J.W.; Sun, H.; Liu, Y.F. Physicochemical and antioxidative characteristics of black bean protein hydrolysates obtained from different enzymes. *Food Hydrocoll.* **2019**, *97*, 105222. [CrossRef]

15. Zhang, X.D.; Dai, Z.Y.; Zhang, Y.Q.; Dong, Y.; Hu, X.J. Structural characteristics and stability of salmon skin protein hydrolysates obtained with different proteases. *LWT Food Sci. Technol.* **2022**, *153*, 112460. [CrossRef]
16. Sharma, S.; Pradhan, R.; Manickavasagan, A.; Tsopmo, A.; Thimmanagari, M.; Dutta, A. Corn distillers solubles by two-step proteolytic hydrolysis as a new source of plant-based protein hydrolysates with ACE and DPP4 inhibition activities. *Food Chem.* **2023**, *401*, 134120. [CrossRef] [PubMed]
17. Intarasirisawat, R.; Benjakul, S.; Visessanguan, W.; Wu, H.P. Antioxidative and functional properties of protein hydrolysate from defatted skipjack (*Katsuwonous pelamis*) roe. *Food Chem.* **2012**, *135*, 3039–3048. [CrossRef]
18. Fadimu, G.J.; Gill, H.; Farahnaky, A.; Truong, T. Improving the enzymolysis efficiency of lupin protein by ultrasound pretreatment: Effect on antihypertensive, antidiabetic and antioxidant activities of the hydrolysates. *Food Chem.* **2022**, *383*, 132457. [CrossRef]
19. Abdollahi, M.; Rezaei, M.; Jafarpour, A.; Undeland, I. Dynamic rheological, microstructural and physicochemical properties of blend fish protein recovered from kilka (*Clupeonella cultriventris*) and silver carp (*Hypophthalmichthys molitrix*) by the pH-shift process or washing-based technology. *Food Chem.* **2017**, *229*, 695–709. [CrossRef]
20. Barth, A. Infrared spectroscopy of proteins. *Biochim. Biophys. Acta (BBA) Bioenerg.* **2007**, *1767*, 1073–1101. [CrossRef]
21. Xie, J.; Du, M.; Shen, M.; Wu, T.; Lin, L. Physico-chemical properties, antioxidant activities and angiotensin-I converting enzyme inhibitory of protein hydrolysates from Mung bean (*Vigna radiate*). *Food Chem.* **2019**, *270*, 243–250. [CrossRef] [PubMed]
22. Liu, F.F.; Li, Y.Q.; Wang, C.Y.; Liang, Y.; Zhao, X.Z.; He, J.X.; Mo, H.Z. Physicochemical, functional and antioxidant properties of mung bean protein enzymatic hydrolysates. *Food Chem.* **2022**, *393*, 133397. [CrossRef] [PubMed]
23. Wang, J.; Shi, S.; Li, F.; Du, X.; Kong, B.; Wang, H.; Xia, X. Physicochemical properties and antioxidant activity of polysaccharides obtained from sea cucumber gonads via ultrasound-assisted enzymatic techniques. *LWT Food Sci. Technol.* **2022**, *160*, 113307. [CrossRef]
24. Du, X.; Jing, H.; Wang, L.; Huang, X.; Wang, X.; Wang, H. Characterization of structure, physicochemical properties, and hypoglycemic activity of goat milk whey protein hydrolysate processed with different proteases. *LWT Food Sci. Technol.* **2022**, *159*, 113257. [CrossRef]
25. Wardani, D.W.; Ningrum, A.; Manikharda; Vanidia, N.; Munawaroh, H.S.H.; Susanto, E.; Show, P.-L. In silico and in vitro assessment of yellowfin tuna skin (*Thunnus albacares*) hydrolysate antioxidation effect. *Food Hydrocoll. Health* **2023**, *3*, 100126. [CrossRef]
26. Zhang, X.; Huang, Y.; Ma, R.; Tang, Y.; Li, Y.; Zhang, S. Structural properties and antioxidant activities of soybean protein hydrolysates produced by *Lactobacillus delbrueckii* subsp. bulgaricus cell envelope proteinase. *Food Chem.* **2023**, *410*, 135392. [CrossRef]
27. Wang, K.; Han, L.; Tan, Y.; Hong, H.; Luo, Y. Generation of novel antioxidant peptides from silver carp muscle hydrolysate: Gastrointestinal digestion stability and transepithelial absorption property. *Food Chem.* **2023**, *403*, 134136. [CrossRef]
28. Ahmed, S.A.; Taie, H.A.A.; Abdel Wahab, W.A. Antioxidant capacity and antitumor activity of the bioactive protein prepared from orange peel residues as a by-product using fungal protease. *Int. J. Biol. Macromol.* **2023**, *234*, 123578. [CrossRef]
29. Pv, S. Protein hydrolysate from duck egg white by Flavourzyme® digestion: Process optimisation by model design approach and evaluation of antioxidant capacity and characteristic properties. *LWT Food Sci. Technol.* **2022**, *156*, 113018. [CrossRef]
30. Liu, F.F.; Li, Y.Q.; Sun, G.J.; Wang, C.Y.; Liang, Y.; Zhao, X.Z.; He, J.X.; Mo, H.Z. Influence of ultrasound treatment on the physicochemical and antioxidant properties of mung bean protein hydrolysate. *Ultrason. Sonochem.* **2022**, *84*, 105964. [CrossRef]
31. Mudgil, P.; Kamal, H.; Yuen, G.C.; Maqsood, S. Characterization and identification of novel antidiabetic and anti-obesity peptides from camel milk protein hydrolysates. *Food Chem.* **2018**, *259*, 46–54. [CrossRef]
32. Baba, W.N.; Mudgil, P.; Baby, B.; Vijayan, R.; Gan, C.Y.; Maqsood, S. New insights into the cholesterol esterase- and lipase-inhibiting potential of bioactive peptides from camel whey hydrolysates: Identification, characterization, and molecular interaction. *J. Dairy Sci.* **2021**, *104*, 7393–7405. [CrossRef]
33. Lee, S.Y.; Lee, D.Y.; Hur, S.J. Changes in the stability and antioxidant activities of different molecular weight bioactive peptide extracts obtained from beef during in vitro human digestion by gut microbiota. *Food Res. Int.* **2021**, *141*, 110116. [CrossRef] [PubMed]
34. Wu, W.F.; Li, B.F.; Hou, H.; Zhang, H.W.; Zhao, X. Identification of iron-chelating peptides from Pacific cod skin gelatin and the possible binding mode. *J. Funct. Foods* **2017**, *35*, 418–427. [CrossRef]
35. Huang, C.; Tang, X.; Liu, Z.; Huang, W.; Ye, Y. Enzymes-dependent antioxidant activity of sweet apricot kernel protein hydrolysates. *LWT Food Sci. Technol.* **2022**, *154*, 112825. [CrossRef]
36. Vásquez, P.; Sepúlveda, C.T.; Zapata, J.E. Functional properties of rainbow trout (*Oncorhynchus mykiss*) viscera protein hydrolysates. *Biocatal. Agric. Biotechnol.* **2022**, *39*, 102268. [CrossRef]
37. Lowry, O.; Rosebrough, N.; Farr, A.L.; Randall, R. Protein measurement with the Folin phenol reagent. *J. Biol. Chem.* **1951**, *193*, 265–275. [CrossRef]
38. Zhang, Q.T.; Tu, Z.C.; Xiao, H.; Wang, H.; Huang, X.Q.; Liu, G.X.; Liu, C.M.; Shi, Y.; Fan, L.L.; Lin, D.R. Influence of ultrasonic treatment on the structure and emulsifying properties of peanut protein isolate. *Food Bioprod. Process.* **2014**, *92*, 30–37. [CrossRef]
39. Du, M.X.; Xie, J.H.; Gong, B.; Xu, X.; Tang, W.; Li, X.; Li, C.; Xie, M.Y. Extraction, physicochemical characteristics and functional properties of Mung bean protein. *Food Hydrocoll.* **2018**, *76*, 131–140. [CrossRef]
40. Zhou, C.; Mi, S.; Li, J.; Gao, J.; Wang, X.H.; Sang, Y.X. Purification, characterisation and antioxidant activities of chondroitin sulphate extracted from *Raja porosa* cartilage. *Carbohydr. Polym.* **2020**, *241*, 116306. [CrossRef]

41. Xie, J.H.; Wang, Z.J.; Shen, M.Y.; Nie, S.P.; Gong, B.; Li, H.S.; Zhao, Q.; Li, W.J.; Xie, M.Y. Sulfated modification, characterization and antioxidant activities of polysaccharide from *Cyclocarya paliurus*. *Food Hydrocoll.* **2016**, *53*, 7–15. [CrossRef]
42. Liu, J.B.; Jin, Y.; Lin, S.Y.; Jones, G.S.; Chen, F. Purification and identification of novel antioxidant peptides from egg white protein and their antioxidant activities. *Food Chem.* **2015**, *175*, 258–266. [CrossRef] [PubMed]
43. Fisayo Ajayi, F.; Mudgil, P.; Gan, C.Y.; Maqsood, S. Identification and characterization of cholesterol esterase and lipase inhibitory peptides from amaranth protein hydrolysates. *Food Chem. X* **2021**, *12*, 100165. [CrossRef] [PubMed]
44. Minekus, M.; Alminger, M.; Alvito, P.; Ballance, S.; Bohn, T.; Bourlieu, C.; Carriere, F.; Boutrou, R.; Corredig, M.; Dupont, D.; et al. A standardised static in vitro digestion method suitable for food—An international consensus. *Food Funct.* **2014**, *5*, 1113–1124. [CrossRef] [PubMed]

Disclaimer/Publisher's Note: The statements, opinions and data contained in all publications are solely those of the individual author(s) and contributor(s) and not of MDPI and/or the editor(s). MDPI and/or the editor(s) disclaim responsibility for any injury to people or property resulting from any ideas, methods, instructions or products referred to in the content.

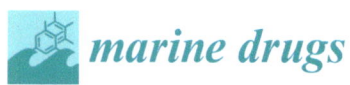

Article

Antidiabetic Effect of Collagen Peptides from *Harpadon nehereus* Bones in Streptozotocin-Induced Diabetes Mice by Regulating Oxidative Stress and Glucose Metabolism

Qianxia Lin [1,†], Yueping Guo [2,†], Jie Li [1], Shuqi He [1], Yan Chen [1,*] and Huoxi Jin [1,*]

[1] Zhejiang Provincial Engineering Technology Research Center of Marine Biomedical Products, School of Food and Pharmacy, Zhejiang Ocean University, Zhoushan 316022, China; linqianxia@zjou.edu.cn (Q.L.)
[2] Jinhua Food and Drug Inspection and Testing Institute, Jinhua 321015, China
[*] Correspondence: cyancy@zjou.edu.cn (Y.C.); jinhuoxi@163.com (H.J.)
[†] These authors contributed equally to this work.

Abstract: Oxidative stress and abnormal glucose metabolism are the important physiological mechanisms in the occurrence and development of diabetes. Antioxidant peptides have been reported to attenuate diabetes complications by regulating levels of oxidative stress, but few studies have focused on peptides from marine bone collagen. In this study, we prepared the peptides with a molecular weight of less than 1 kD (HNCP) by enzymolysis and ultrafiltration derived from *Harpadon nehereus* bone collagen. Furthermore, the effects of HNCP on blood glucose, blood lipid, liver structure and function, oxidative stress, and glucose metabolism were studied using HE staining, kit detection, and Western blotting experiment in streptozotocin-induced type 1 diabetes mice. After the 240 mg/kg HNCP treatment, the levels of blood glucose, triglyceride (TG), and low-density lipoprotein cholesterol (LDL-C) in streptozotocin-induced diabetes mice decreased by 32.8%, 42.2%, and 43.2%, respectively, while the levels of serum insulin and hepatic glycogen increased by 142.0% and 96.4%, respectively. The antioxidant enzymes levels and liver function in the diabetic mice were markedly improved after HNCP intervention. In addition, the levels of nuclear factor E2-related factor 2 (Nrf2), glucokinase (GK), and phosphorylation of glycogen synthase kinase-3 (p-GSK3β) in the liver were markedly up-regulated after HNCP treatment, but the glucose-6-phosphatase (G6Pase) and phosphoenolpyruvate carboxykinase1 (PEPCK1) were down-regulated. In conclusion, HNCP could attenuate oxidative stress, reduce blood glucose, and improve glycolipid metabolism in streptozotocin-induced type 1 diabetes mice.

Keywords: diabetes; collagen peptides; Nrf2; glucose metabolism; oxidative stress

Citation: Lin, Q.; Guo, Y.; Li, J.; He, S.; Chen, Y.; Jin, H. Antidiabetic Effect of Collagen Peptides from *Harpadon nehereus* Bones in Streptozotocin-Induced Diabetes Mice by Regulating Oxidative Stress and Glucose Metabolism. *Mar. Drugs* 2023, *21*, 518. https://doi.org/10.3390/md21100518

Academic Editor: Fernando Albericio

Received: 4 September 2023
Revised: 27 September 2023
Accepted: 28 September 2023
Published: 29 September 2023

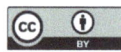

Copyright: © 2023 by the authors. Licensee MDPI, Basel, Switzerland. This article is an open access article distributed under the terms and conditions of the Creative Commons Attribution (CC BY) license (https:// creativecommons.org/licenses/by/ 4.0/).

1. Introduction

Diabetes mellitus is a syndrome characterized by the disorder of sugar and lipid metabolism. Diabetes is known as a "silent killer" due to a large number of chronic complications [1,2]. Low levels of in insulin in the body and a decline in glucose metabolism will lead to an increase in blood glucose [3]. At present, some enzymes related to glucose metabolisms, such as glucokinase (GK) [4], phosphoenolpyruvate carboxykinase1 (PEPCK1) [5], and glucose-6-phosphatase (G6Pase) [6], have been confirmed to be associated with diabetes. Under long-term high hyperglycemia, a large number of reactive oxygen species (ROS) are accumulated in the body, resulting in cell damage and tissue dysfunction. The liver is damaged due to the long-term accumulation of hyperglycemia [7], which can cause metabolic abnormalities and dysfunction, and eventually lead to non-alcoholic fatty liver and other complications [8,9]. Studies have shown that diabetes and its complications are closely related to oxidative stress and glucose metabolism caused by high glucose, but the mechanism is still unclear [10,11].

Because oxidative stress is closely related to diabetes, one of the potential strategies for preventing and treating diabetes is to reduce oxidative stress levels [12]. Studies have reported that some bioactive peptides have dual antioxidation and hypoglycemic functions, such as peptides from yeast hydrolysates [13], milk protein-derived hydrolysates [14], and egg-yolk protein hydrolysates [15]. In the past decades, bioactive peptides from marine organisms have attracted extensive attention due to their various biological properties, including antioxidant [16–18], antihypertensive [19], antidiabetic [20], immunoregulation [21], and antifatigue [22] properties. The Bombay duck (Harpadon nehereus), an important edible fish in China, is widely distributed in the coastal areas of China. The meat of Harpadon nehereus is soft, tender and smooth, and rich in protein (up to 70% of the dry weight) [23]. The bones of the Harpadon nehereus are discarded because they are not edible, but they are rich in collagen and calcium, causing a waste of resources. Therefore, the preparation of collagen peptides with nutritional or medical value from *Harpadon nehereus* bones can greatly improve the economic value of *Harpadon nehereus*.

Nuclear factor E2-related factor 2 (Nrf2) plays a backbone role in cellular antioxidant defense. Nrf2 regulates the expression of antioxidant enzyme genes by binding to anti-response elements (ARE) [24]. In addition to Nrf2, the ARE binding site is also the target gene for NAD(P)H quinone oxidoreductase 1 (NQO1) and heme-oxygenase (HO-1) [25]. The activation of the Nrf2-ARE signal pathway has been shown to reduce the production of free radicals and oxidative stress, playing a protective role in the kidney [26,27]. However, it has not been elucidated yet whether collagen peptides from Harpadon nehereus bones have preventive and therapeutic effects on streptozocin-induced diabetes. Therefore, the purpose of this study was to evaluate the therapeutic effect and explore the potential mechanism of collagen peptides from Harpadon nehereus in streptozocin-induced diabetic mice, laying a theoretical foundation for the application of collagen peptides in diabetes prevention.

2. Results

2.1. Preparation of HNCP and Its Antioxidative Activity

The hydrolysates of bone collagen from *Harpadon nehereus* were analyzed by high-performance liquid chromatography (HPLC) with chromatographic column TSK-GEL 2000SWXL. The ribonuclease A, aprotinin, bacitracin, and glycine-glycine-glycine were used as the standard substances. As shown in Figure 1A, all the standard substances were eluted within 20 min. According to the relationship between the logarithm of relative molecular mass (lg Mw) and retention time (t) of each standard, the standard curve was obtained: lg Mw = $-0.4105t + 7.3036$, $R2 = 0.997$. The molecular weight logarithm showed a good correlation with the retention time under the chromatographic conditions. Thus, the standard curve was used to evaluate the molecular weight distribution of peptides in the hydrolysates of the bone collagen from *Harpadon nehereus*. Figure 1B shows that the molecular weight (Mw) of the hydrolysates by protease was mostly distributed below 3 kDa. According to the range of the molecular weight, the peptides were divided into five components, which were respectively named HNCP (Mw < 1 kDa), HNCP 1 (1~3 kDa), HNCP 2 (3~5 kDa), HNCP 3 (5~10 kDa), and HNCP 4 (Mw > 10 kDa). The content and DPPH• scavenging rate of HNCP were 37.3% and 44.1%, respectively, both of which were the highest among all components (Figure 1C,D). The amino acid analysis (Table 1) showed that HNCP was rich in glycine (Gly, 336.2 residues), alanine (Ala, 117.3 residues), and proline (Pro, 116.0 residues) but low in hydrophobic amino acids such as phenylalanine (Phe, 12.3 residues), isoleucine (Ile, 12.3 residues), and tyrosine (Tyr, 4.2 residues). In addition, the contents of hydroxyproline (Hyp) and glutamic acid (Glu) were more than 70 residues/1000 residues.

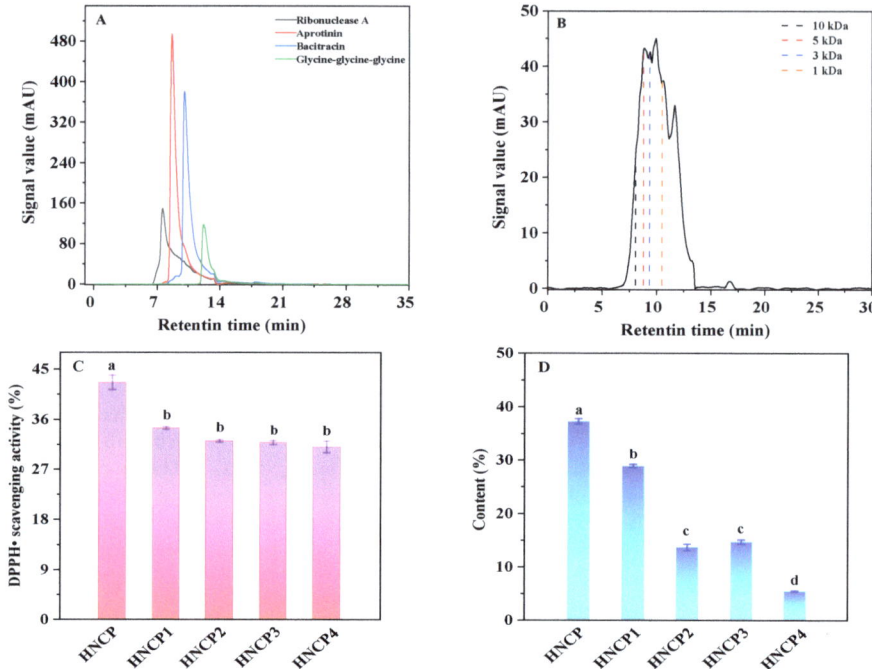

Figure 1. The HPLC diagram of standards (**A**) and hydrolysates of bone collagen from *Harpadon nehereus* (**B**); The DPPH• scavenging activity (**C**) and content (**D**) of each component in the hydrolysates. Values with different letters (a–d) indicate significant differences between groups ($p < 0.05$).

Table 1. Amino acid composition of HNCP.

Amino Acid	Residues/1000 Residues
Aspartic acid (Asp)	47.4
Threonine (Thr)	29.2
Serine (Ser)	34.8
Glutamic acid (Glu)	71.4
Glycine (Gly)	336.2
Alanine (Ala)	117.3
Valine (Val)	26.1
Methionine (Met)	11.6
Isoleucine (Ile)	12.3
Leucine (Leu)	27.8
Tyrosine (Tyr)	4.2
Phenylalanine (Phe)	12.3
Lysine (Lys)	22.0
Histidine (His)	6.0
Arginine (Arg)	37.3
Proline (Pro)	116.0
Hydroxyproline (Hyp)	76.5
Hydroxylysine (Hyl)	11.9

2.2. Effects of HNCP on Glucose Metabolism in Diabetic Mice

The intervention effect of HNCP on glucose metabolism in STZ-induced type 1 diabetic mice was investigated. The blood glucose of mice in the Con group (the normal mice group) remained at a normal level all the time and was markedly lower than that of diabetic mice. After intervention with HNCP as shown in Figure 2A, the blood glucose levels gradually decreased and were significantly lower than those in the DM group (STZ-induced model group). Compared with that in the Con group, the serum insulin content in the DM group was significantly decreased ($p < 0.05$). Remarkably, the serum insulin levels of diabetic mice after HNCP intervention increased significantly to the level of the Con group (Figure 2B), but there was no significant difference between the 80 mg/kg and 240 mg/kg HNCP groups.

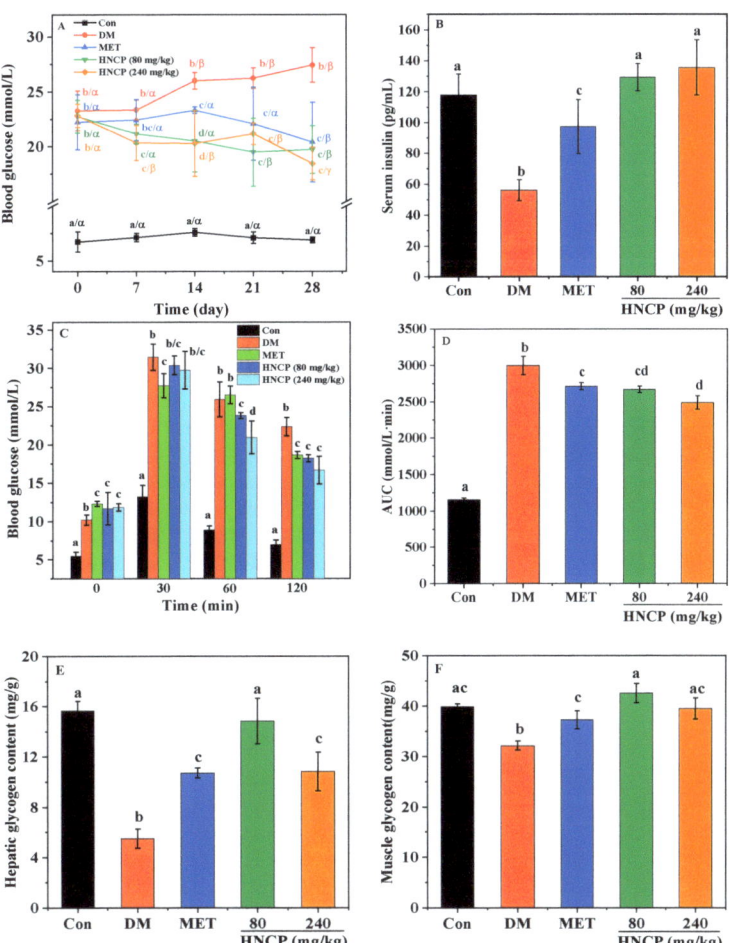

Figure 2. Effects of HNCP treatments on blood glucose (**A**), serum insulin (**B**), glucose tolerance (**C,D**), and glycogen levels (**E,F**) in STZ-induced type 1 diabetic mice. Values with different letters (a–d) indicate significant differences between groups at the same time ($p < 0.05$); Values with different letters (α–γ) indicate significant differences between different times in the same group ($p < 0.05$).

The oral glucose tolerance test was used to measure glucose tolerance in the diabetic mice, which can evaluate the secretory function of pancreatic β cells and reflect the ability to regulate blood glucose. After glucose intragastric administration, blood glucose rose rapidly to the highest levels in all groups and then declined (Figure 2C). At 120 min, the blood glucose levels in the Con group returned to normal but remained at a high level in the diabetic mice. However, high levels of blood glucose in the diabetic mice were significantly decreased by the HNCP intervention. Compared with the Con group, AUC increased significantly in the DM group (Figure 2D). The AUC value of the HNCP group was significantly lower than that of the DM group ($p < 0.05$). However, there was no significant difference in the AUC values of different doses of HNCP.

Glucose is mainly stored in the body as glycogen, which maintains the stability of blood glucose by synthesis or decomposition. Glycogen contents in diabetic mice were analyzed, and the results are shown in Figure 2E,F. Lower levels of liver and muscle glycogen were observed in the DM group relative to that of the Con group ($p < 0.05$). It was observed that the glycogen levels of two organs were significantly increased ($p < 0.05$) after metformin (MET) and HNCP treatments. However, the high-dose HNCP (240 mg/kg) group did not show higher glycogen levels than the low-dose (80 mg/kg) HNCP group. These results indicate that HNCP can promote glycogen synthesis in diabetic mice and increase the ability of glucose uptake in the blood.

2.3. Effects of HNCP on Blood Lipids in Diabetic Mice

The liver plays an important role in all stages of lipid metabolism, synthesis, and transport. Diabetes often leads to impaired liver function, which leads to dyslipidemia and accelerates liver damage. To investigate the improvement effects of HNCP on dyslipidemia, the contents of triglyceride (TG), total cholesterol (TC), high-density lipoprotein cholesterol (HDL-C), and low-density lipoprotein cholesterol (LDL-C) in serum were measured. As depicted in Figure 3A–D, serum TG, TC, and LDL-C contents in the DM group were significantly increased compared with the Con group ($p < 0.05$), while HDL-C content was significantly decreased ($p < 0.05$). HNCP intervention reversed the change trends of serum TG, TC, LDL-C, and HDL-C in the diabetic mice. In particular, the levels of TC, LDL-C, and HDL-C in the high-dose (240 mg/kg) HNCP group returned to the same levels as those in the Con group. There were significant differences in LDL-C and HDL-C levels between the two concentrations of HNCP groups, showing a concentration-dependent relationship, but no such relationship was observed for TC and TG levels. These results suggest that HNCP can effectively mitigate dyslipidemia in diabetic mice.

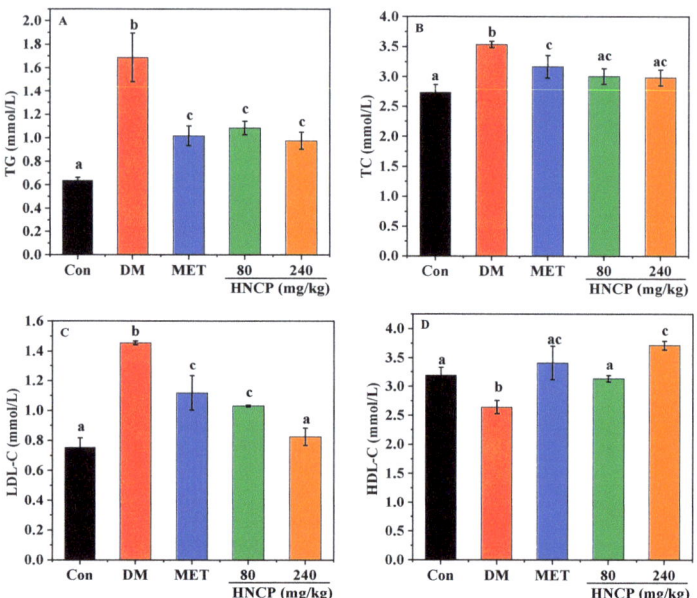

Figure 3. Effects of HNCP treatments on the contents of TG (**A**), TC (**B**), LDL-C (**C**), and HDL-C (**D**) in serum of STZ-induced type 1 diabetic mice. Values with different letters (a–c) represent significant differences between groups ($p < 0.05$).

2.4. Improvement of HNCP on Liver and Pancreas Injury in Diabetes Mice

H&E staining in the liver and pancreas was performed to investigate the effects of HNCP treatment on the histological alterations of the liver and pancreas. As shown in Figure 4A, cells in the Con group were of a regular shape with clear boundaries, but more serious necrosis was observed in the DM group relative to that of the Con group. Meanwhile, hepatocytes were swollen and disordered, and some hepatocytes around the central vein were vacuolated in the DM group. However, it was observed that the adipose vacuoles and swelling of hepatocytes were significantly alleviated after MET and HNCP administration. Pancreatic islets (black arrow in Figure 4B) in the pancreas of mice in the Con group were normal in shape, clear in outline, and abundant in quantity. In the DM group, the volume and morphology of pancreatic islets were clearly changed. Blurred outlines, scattered structures, and a reduced number of pancreatic islets were observed. After the intervention of HNCP, the shape of pancreatic islets changed regularly, and the outline became clearer relative to that in the DM group.

Aspartate aminotransferase (AST) and alanine aminotransferase (ALT) are important indicators of liver function. To determine the improvement effects of HNCP treatment on liver function in the diabetic mice, the levels of plasma AST and ALT were measured (Figure 4C,D). AST and ALT levels in the DM group were observed to be higher than those of the Con group ($p < 0.05$). The high levels of ALT and AST were markedly decreased after MET and HNCP treatments, but there was no significant difference between the groups. It can be seen from the above results that HNCP can alleviate the liver injury of STZ-induced diabetic mice.

2.5. Effects of HNCP on Hepatic Oxidative Damage in Diabetic Mice

According to the above experiments, HNCP has a free-radical scavenging ability in vitro. The effects of HNCP on the activities of catalase (CAT), superoxide dismutase (SOD), and glutathione peroxidase (GSH-Px), as well as the content of malondialdehyde (MDA), were determined to investigate whether HNCP can alleviate the oxidative stress level in diabetic mice. As shown in Figure 5A–D, the activities of CAT, SOD, and GSH-Px in the DM group were significantly lower than those in the Con group ($p < 0.05$), while the content of MDA was significantly higher ($p < 0.05$). Meanwhile, the activities of CAT, SOD, and GSH-Px were remarkedly increased in the HNCP groups in comparison with the DM group. The levels of CAT, SOD, GSH-Px, and MDA in the 240 mg/kg HNCP group were similar to those in the Con group. These results suggested that HNCP could effectively alleviate oxidative stress in the liver of STZ-induced type 1 diabetic mice.

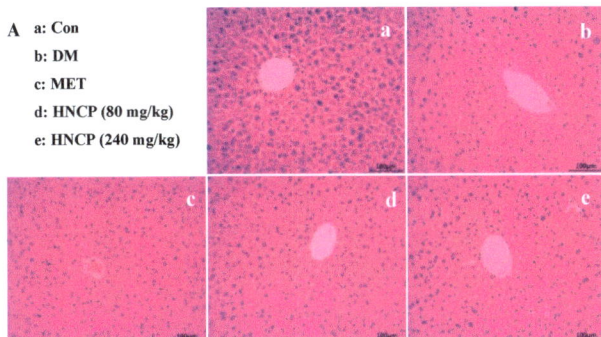

Figure 4. Cont.

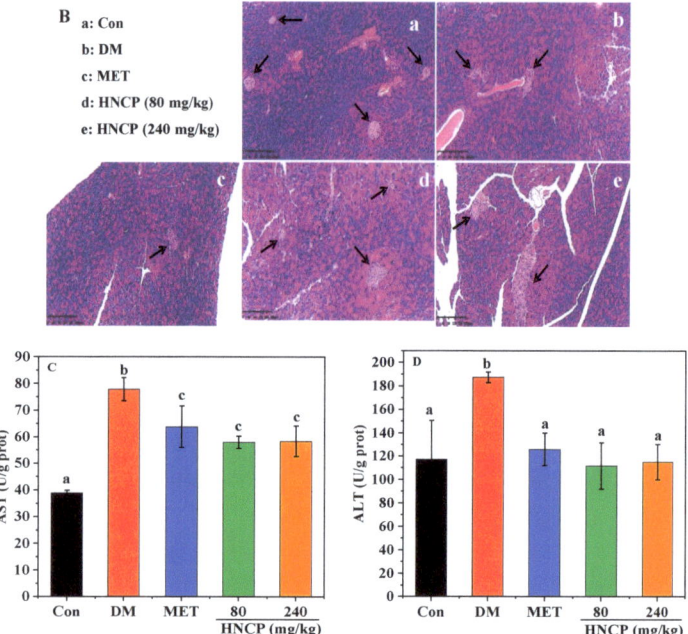

Figure 4. Effects of HNCP treatments on the liver structure (**A**, 200×), pancreas structure (**B**, 100×), and the levels of AST (**C**) and ALT (**D**) in STZ-induced type 1 diabetic mice. Different lowercase English letters (a–c) in (**C**,**D**) represent significant differences between groups ($p < 0.05$).

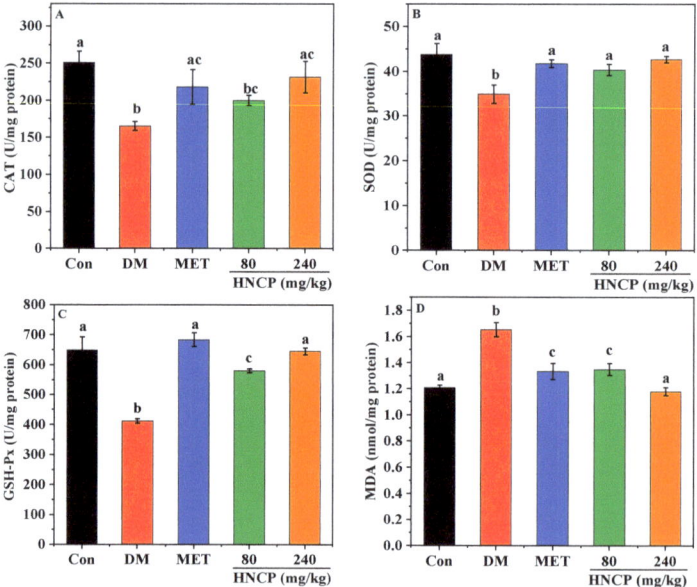

Figure 5. Effects of HNCP treatments on the levels of CAT (**A**), SOD (**B**), GSH-Px (**C**), and MDA (**D**) in the liver of STZ-induced type 1 diabetic mice. Values with different letters (a–c) represent significant differences between groups ($p < 0.05$).

2.6. Effects of HNCP on Nrf2 Signaling Pathway

Nrf2 is an important endogenous transcription factor for cells to resist oxidative stress, which can regulate the expression levels of antioxidant genes such as heme oxygenase (HO-1) and NAD(P)H: quinone oxidoreductase 1 (NQO1). To elucidate the potential mechanism underlying HNCP-mediated alleviation of oxidative stress, the levels of Nrf2 and its related proteins (NQO1 and HO-1) expressions in the liver of STZ-induced diabetic mice were assessed by Western blot. As shown in Figure 6A–E, the levels of nuclear Nrf2 (n-Nrf2) in the DM group had no significant difference compared with the Con group, but the 240 mg/kg HNCP treatment significantly enhanced n-Nrf2 expression relative to that in the DM group ($p < 0.05$). Furthermore, the level of total Nrf2 (t-Nrf2) in the 240 mg/kg HNCP group was significantly higher than that in the DM group. The expression levels of downstream target proteins HO-1 and NQO1 in the 240 mg/kg HNCP group were significantly higher than those in the DM group, which was consistent with the n-Nrf2 level. These results indicated that HNCP might promote the transcription of Nrf2 into the nucleus to activate the Nrf2 signaling pathway, thereby increasing the expression of antioxidant enzymes such as HO-1 and NQO1.

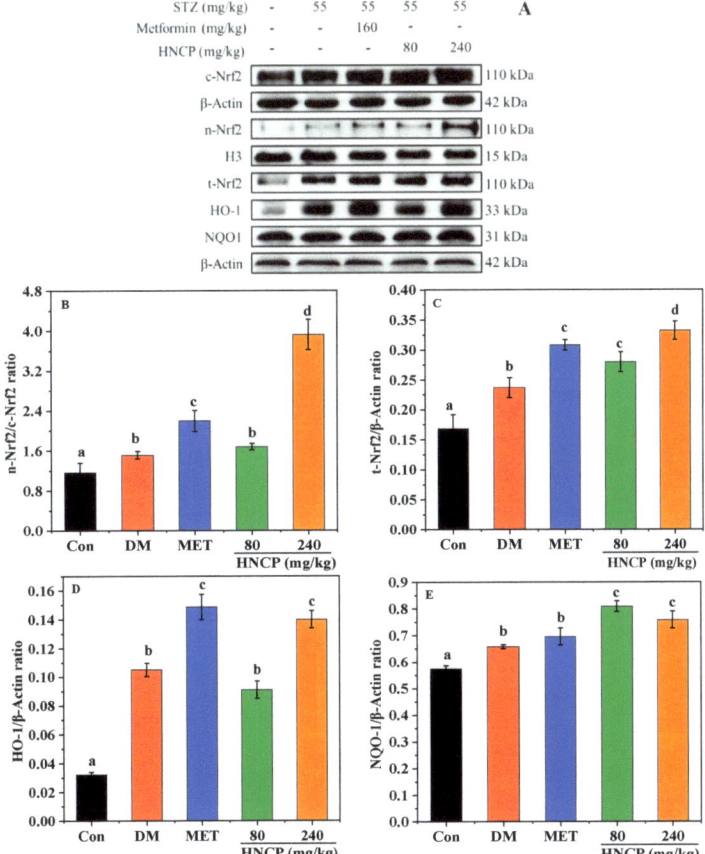

Figure 6. Effects of HNCP treatments on the expression of Nrf2 signaling pathway-related proteins in the liver of the STZ-induced diabetic mice (**A**). Analysis of protein expression levels of n-Nrf2/c-Nrf2 (**B**), t-Nrf2 (**C**), HO-1 (**D**), and NQO1 (**E**). Values with different letters (a–d) represent significant differences between groups ($p < 0.05$).

2.7. Effects of HNCP on the Expression of Glucometabolic-Related Proteins

Glucokinase (GK), phosphoenolpyruvate carboxykinase1 (PEPCK1), and glucose-6-phosphatase (G6Pase) are key enzymes in glucose metabolism and play an important role in regulating blood glucose. Glycogen synthase kinase-3 (GSK-3β) can regulate the activity of glycogen synthase (GS) in the insulin signaling pathway. To evaluate the effects of HNCP on glycometabolism in STZ-induced type 1 diabetic mice, the protein expressions of GK, PEPCK1, G6Pase, and GSK-3β in liver tissues were assessed. As shown in Figure 7, the expression levels of G6Pase and PEPCK1 were significantly up-regulated in the DM group relative to that in the Con group, while the GK and phosphorylation of GSK-3β were significantly down-regulated. After HNCP intervention, the expression levels of G6Pase and PEPCK1 in the liver of the diabetic mice were decreased, while the GK and phosphorylation of GSK-3β were increased. The results indicated that HNCP treatment could significantly improve glucose metabolism disorder in STZ-induced diabetes mice.

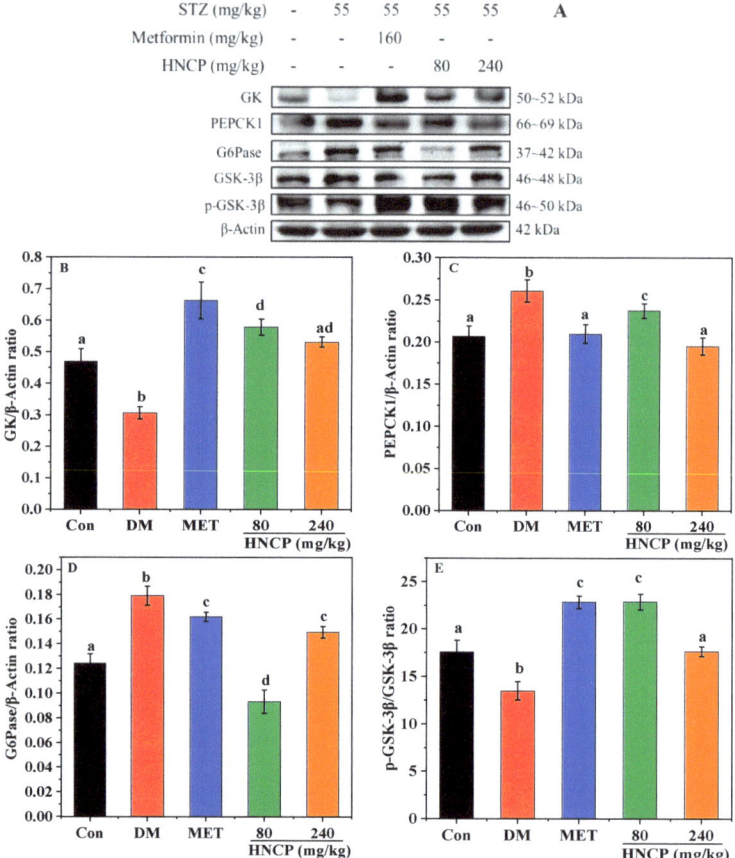

Figure 7. Effects of HNCP treatments on the expression of glucose metabolism-related proteins in STZ-induced type 1 diabetic mice (**A**). Analysis of GK (**B**), PEPCK1 (**C**), G6Pase (**D**), and p-GSK-3β (**E**) levels. Different letters (a–d) represent significant differences between groups ($p < 0.05$).

3. Discussion

Marine by-products such as skin and bone of fish are rich sources of collagen. Marine collagen hydrolysates have demonstrated antioxidant and anti-diabetic activities [28,29]. The amino acid composition and molecular weight of peptides in the hydrolysate were found to be the key factors for antioxidant activity. It was reported that small molecular peptides with 2–20 amino acid residues from marine by-products had the most potent antioxidant activities [30]. Thus, we compared the antioxidant activities of different-molecular-weight components of collagen hydrolysates from *Harpadon nehereus* bones. As expected, the small molecular (Mw < 1 kDa, HNCP) had the highest content and DPPH scavenging activity (42.0% at 5 mg/mL) among all the components with different molecular weights. The peptide fractions < 3 kDa from brown *Lens culinaris* protein hydrolysates showed about 23% of DPPH scavenging rate at a 5 mg/mL concentration, which was significantly lower than that of HNCP [31]. Moreover, the total amino acid compositions showed that HNCP is rich in Gly, Ala, and Pro but low in Phe, Ile, and Tyr. Several studies have shown that peptides containing hydrophobic amino acids such as Phe, Tyrosine, Iso, and Pro exert a higher antioxidant activity [32]. Therefore, the antioxidant activity of HNCP might be predominantly due to the high contents of Pro.

Diabetes is a metabolic disease characterized by high blood glucose levels and metabolic disorders. According to statistics, there were 529 million people living with diabetes worldwide in 2021 [33]. Accumulating evidence shows that the pathological and functional damage of organs induced by diabetes is an important cause of death, while the high level of oxidative stress is closely related to organ damage and dysfunction [34,35]. Thus, antioxidant peptides from marine collagen have gained widespread interest as a potential drug to combat oxidative stress in diabetes patients. In this study, high-dose STZ-induced type 1 diabetes mice were used to study the effect of HNCP on diabetes and the underlying mechanisms. It was observed that a 240 mg/kg HNCP administration decreased the blood glucose levels by 44.5% after 120 min and increased insulin secretion by 142.0% in STZ-induced diabetes mice, which were significantly higher than those by peptides from red deer antlers (about 30%) [36]. In addition to regulating insulin secretion, glycogen synthesis and decomposition are also important ways to regulate blood glucose levels. Our study found that HNCP treatment could increase the synthesis of liver glycogen and muscle glycogen in STZ-induced diabetes mice, indicating that HNCP might improve the glucose tolerance of diabetic mice. This speculation was supported by glucose tolerance tests as shown in Figure 2C. These results indicated that HNCP had a significant therapeutic effect on STZ-induced diabetes mice by improving the insulin level and synthesis of glycogen.

Diabetes often affects liver function, which in turn leads to abnormal lipid metabolism. The study on lipid metabolism showed a higher serum lipid concentration including TG, TC, and LDL-C in STZ-induced diabetes mice than those in the Con group. The levels of TG, TC, and LDL-C were significantly lower in the HNCP-treated mice, whereas the HDL-C levels were higher. In particular, TG decreased by 42.2% after the 240 mg/kg HNCP treatment, while no significant decrease in TG levels was observed in diabetic mice treated with peptides from red deer antlers [36]. These findings suggested that HNCP administration could improve the lipid metabolism disorder of STZ-induced diabetes mice. Similar results were reported in collagen peptides from skate (*Raja kenojei*) skin [37]. We assumed that the blood glucose-lowering effects of HNCP might positively contribute to the lipid levels. The liver is the major organ responsible for glucose and lipid metabolism. Abnormal blood glucose and lipid levels indicate the presence of liver damage. In addition, the insulin level is an important indicator of pancreatic function. Our previous study demonstrated that abnormal blood glucose, insulin, and lipid levels were present in STZ-induced type 1 diabetes mice, and HNCP ameliorated the abnormality of these indicators. Thus, the effects of HNCP on liver and pancreatic damage were evaluated. H&E staining showed that HNCP treatment attenuated the cell swelling and apoptosis in the liver and pancreas. In addition, HNCP supplementation significantly reduced the serum ALT and AST levels in the STZ-induced diabetes mice. ALT and AST are biological indicators of liver pathological changes [38]. High levels of ALT and AST in serum are often accompanied by liver damage [39]. Therefore, these results indicated that HNCP treatment could alleviate hepatic damage in diabetic mice.

In the process of diabetes, hyperglycemia causes a surge of free radicals in the body, which contributes to liver damage. Therefore, oxidative stress is one of the typical pathophysiological features of diabetes. In the present study, lower levels of antioxidant enzymes (SOD, CAT, and GSH-Px) and higher levels of lipid peroxidation product (MDA) were observed in the DM group compared with those in the Con group. However, HNCP administration markedly decreased the MDA level and increased the levels of SOD, CAT, and GSH-Px in STZ-induced diabetes mice. These results indicated that HNCP significantly reduced oxidative stress by increasing the expression of antioxidant enzymes in diabetes mice, thus alleviating liver damage as shown in Figure 4. Our results are consistent with the previous studies wherein the marine peptides mitigated oxidative stress by increasing the levels of antioxidant enzymes such as CAT, SOD, and GSH-Px [40–42]. It has been reported that peptides with a high proportion of hydrophobic amino acids tend to have strong ability to enhance antioxidant enzyme activities [43]. Therefore, the reason that HNCP improves the activities of antioxidant enzymes may be related to its high proportion of Pro.

The increase in the expression of antioxidant enzymes can enhance the antioxidant capacity of the body to remove excess free radicals, which are regulated by the upstream signaling molecule Nrf2. Under the intervention of some substances, Nrf2 is dissociated from Keap1 into the nucleus and binds to the antioxidant response elements, resulting in the transcription of antioxidant enzymes. Thus, the level of nuclear Nrf2 (n-Nrf2) is positively correlated with the antioxidant capacity of the body. A large number of studies have reported that Nrf2 activation can effectively suppress intracellular oxidative stress in diabetes and mitigate its complications [44–46]. In our study, HNCP treatment significantly increased the n-Nrf2 expression and downstream proteins HO-1 and NQO1 in STZ-induced diabetes mice. Accordingly, we assumed that the attenuating effects of HNCP on oxidative damage in diabetic mice might positively contribute to the activation of Nrf2-mediated antioxidant pathways.

Glucose metabolism is directly related to blood glucose concentration. The above experiments confirm that HNCP can reduce the blood glucose of diabetic mice by increasing the content of liver and muscle glycogen. To further explore the hypoglycemic mechanism of HNCP, the effects of HNCP on the expression of proteins related to glucose metabolisms such as GK, G6Pase, PEPCK1, and GSK-3β were investigated. Numerous studies have shown that GK expression and GSK-3β phosphorylation are generally significantly reduced in the liver of diabetic patients [47], while G6Pase and PEPCK1 are usually significantly increased [48]. Our results showed that the expression levels of G6Pase and PEPCK1 in hepatocytes were significantly increased, but GK and GSK-3β phosphorylation were significantly decreased in STZ-induced diabetic mice. However, HNCP administration significantly improved this phenomenon. This result indicated that HNCP could improve the expression levels of glycogenesis and gluconeogenesis enzymes in diabetic mice, which might be attributed to improvements in blood glucose levels and insulin secretion.

To date, many compounds have been reported to improve diabetes symptoms or complications by mediating oxidative stress and glucose metabolism. Peptides derived from seaweed protein revealed antioxidant and antidiabetic properties [20]. The collagen peptides from *Oreochromis niloticus* skin have also been reported to exhibit antioxidant and hypoglycemic effects [49]. In this study, HNCP, the small peptides (Mw < 1 kDa) derived from the collagen hydrolysate of *Harpadon nehereus* bones, exhibited the antioxidant effect by activating an Nrf2/ARE pathway and a hypoglycemic effect by improving the glucose metabolism in STZ-induced diabetic mice. Further studies are needed to isolate the peptides and identify those sequences, and subsequently, verify the activities of these peptides.

4. Materials and Methods

4.1. Chemicals and Reagents

Harpadon nehereus were purchased from Zhoushan aquatic products market. Papain was purchased from Aladdin Reagent Co., LTD (Shanghai, China). The antioxidant enzymes kits were from Nanjing Jiancheng Bioengineering Institute (Nanjing, China). Streptozocin (STZ) was purchased from Sigma Company (Saint Louis, Missouri, USA). Citrate-sodium citrate buffer and 4% paraformaldehyde were purchased from Ranger Technology Co., LTD (Beijing, China). The insulin ELISA kit was purchased from Wuhan Illarite Biotechnology Co., LTD (Wuhan, China). RIPA lysate was purchased from Biyuntian Biotechnology Research Institute (Shanghai, China). The antibody of β-Actin and horseradish peroxidase (HRP) were purchased from Biyuntian Biotechnology Co., LTD (Shanghai, China). The remaining antibodies were purchased from Proteintech Group, Inc (Wuhan, China). The reagents used in the Western blot were purchased from the reagent supplier Ningbo Hangjing Biotechnology Co., LTD (Ningbo, China).

4.2. Preparation of Collagen Peptides from Harpadon nehereus Bone

Under the conditions of pH 8, 55 °C, enzyme dosage of 5500 U/g, and enzymolysis time of 4 h, papain was selected for the enzymolysis of the bone collagen of Harpadon nehereus. The molecular weight (Mw) distribution of polypeptides in the hydrolysate was analyzed by HPLC. Ultrafiltration membranes with interception diameters of 10, 5, 3, and 1 kDa were used sequentially. The filtrate of each part was collected and freeze-dried for the determination of the DPPH free-radical scavenging rate according to the method by Abdelmawgood [50]. Based on the DPPH scavenging rate and content, peptides with Mw < 1 kD (HNCP) were calculated for animal experiments.

4.3. Laboratory Animals

Male C57BL/6J mice weighing 18 ± 2 g were fed in the SPF animal laboratory of Zhejiang Ocean University for 7 days under a 12 h dark/light cycle, with free access to food and water. The mice were randomly divided into a control group (Con) and an experimental group according to body weight. Mice in the experimental group were intraperitoneally injected with STZ (55 mg/kg/d) for 5 days to establish the type 1 diabetes model. The fasting blood glucose level of the mice was continuously monitored on the 7th day after the injection. Excluding 2 mice with failed modeling, the remaining mice with successful modeling were randomly divided into 4 groups: diabetic model group (DM, $n = 8$), positive drug group (MET, $n = 8$), low-dose HNCP group ($n = 7$), and high-dose HNCP group ($n = 7$). They were given sufficient drinking water and food, and the bedding material was changed in time. The Con group and the DM group were fed the same amount of distilled water every day. The MET group was given a metformin solution by gavage at a dose of 160 mg/kg, and the low-dose HNCP and high-dose HNCP groups were fed the HNCP solution by gavage at a dose of 80 mg/kg and 240 mg/kg, respectively. Excluding one dead mouse in the DM group, all the mice were euthanized by cervical dislocation after 4 weeks of feeding [51]. Blood was collected from the eyeballs, and tissues such as liver, kidney, epididymis fat, and pancreas were quickly extracted and stored at -80 °C. All animal experiments were carried out in accordance with the guidelines of the Animal Protection and Utilization Committee of the China Animal Protection Commission (No. 2021029).

4.4. Measurement of Blood Glucose, Insulin, and Glycogen

Water and fasting were prohibited 8 h before blood glucose measurement. Blood was collected with a disposable needle tail vein for measurement of blood glucose using a blood glucose test paper and blood glucose meter (Bayanjin flagship store). The obtained blood was immediately centrifuged at 4 °C and 8000 r/min for 5 min. Insulin content in the upper serum and glycogen content in the liver/muscle were measured using the mouse insulin enzyme-linked immunosorbent assay kit (NanJing JianCheng Bioengineering Institute, Nanjing, China) and the anthracenone method, respectively [52].

4.5. Oral Glucose Tolerance Test (OGTT)

The oral glucose tolerance test (OGTT) was performed according to the method of Wang et al. [53] with minor modifications. After four weeks of administration, the mice fasted overnight during the fifth week. Each mouse was given a 40% glucose solution by gavage at a dose of 2 g/kg. After feeding the glucose, the blood was collected and measured for blood glucose at 0, 30, 60, and 120 min using a blood glucose test paper (Bayanjin flagship store). The blood glucose time curve was drawn, and the area under the curve of blood glucose response (AUC) was calculated.

4.6. Determination of Lipid-Related Indexes in Mice

The contents of TG, TC, HDL-C, and LDL-C in the serum were measured using an enzymatic method [54] provided by the kits (TG, TC, HDL-C, and LDL-C kits) (NanJing JianCheng Bioengineering Institute, Nanjing, China).

4.7. Histological Evaluation of Liver and Pancreas

Liver and pancreas tissues were fixed with 4% paraformaldehyde for 24–48 h and dehydrated using anhydrous ethanol. The fixed tissues were embedded with paraffin and cut into 3 μM thick sections. The sections were stained with standard hematoxylin-eosin (H&E), and then the morphological changes of the liver and pancreas were captured by a light microscope [55].

4.8. Detection of ALT, AST, MDA, CAT, SOD, and GSH-Px Levels in Liver

The liver tissue was ground into homogenate in cold saline and centrifuged at 12,000 r/min for 10 min. The levels of ALT, AST, MDA, CAT, SOD, and GSH-Px in the supernatant were determined by the kits from NanJing JianCheng Bioengineering Institute (ALT, AST, MDA, CAT, SOD, and GSH-Px kits) [56]. The protein concentration in the tissue homogenate was measured using the BAC protein detection kit (NanJing JianCheng Bioengineering Institute, Nanjing, China).

4.9. Western Blot

The liver tissue (0.1 g) that had been ground into a fine powder was mixed with the lysate (RIPA lysis buffer: protease inhibitor mixture: phosphatase inhibitor = 50:1:1) and incubated on ice for 30 min with agitation every 6 min. After centrifugation at 12,000 rpm for 10 min, protein was extracted from the cytoplasm and nucleus using a protein extraction kit from NanJing JianCheng Bioengineering Institute (Nanjing, China) [57]. After extraction, the total proteins concentrations in the liver were measured with a BCA protein assay kit (NanJing JianCheng Bioengineering Institute, Nanjing, China). The protein sample was diluted to a suitable concentration with a buffer at a ratio of 1:4. The mixture was boiled in the water bath for 10 min and then centrifuged at 12,000 r/min for 10 min. The supernatant was collected and stored at $-80\ °C$ as a standby.

A PVDF membrane was immersed in 5% BSA solution prepared using TBST (containing 0.1% Tween-80) and closed at room temperature for at least 1 h. They were then incubated overnight with the corresponding primary antibody against Nrf2 (1:2000), β-Actin (1:1000), H3 (1:8000), HO-1 (1:2000), NQO1 (1:20,000), GK (1:2000), PEPCK1 (1:10,000), G6Pase (1:2000), GSK-3β (1:20,000), and p-GSK-3β (1:5000) at 4 °C. The membrane was then incubated with horseradish peroxidase (HRP) (1:500)-labeled secondary antibody at room temperature for 1 h. An enhanced chemiluminescence (ECL) kit (NanJing JianCheng Bioengineering Institute, Nanjing, China) was used to detect the strength of specific bands.

4.10. Statistical Analysis

All experiments were conducted in parallel 3 times. The software GraphPad Prism8.0 was used for one-way ANOVA. The comparison between groups was performed using the Tukey method, and the results were expressed as Mean $\pm$ SD.

5. Conclusions

In this study, small-molecule peptides (Mw < 1 kD) were prepared from the bone collagen of *Harpadon nehereus* (HNCP). HNCP showed a remarkable antioxidant activity by activating the Nrf2 pathway to increase the level of antioxidant enzymes such as SOD, CAT, HO-1, GSH-Px, and NQO1. In addition, HNCP significantly increased glucose tolerance and insulin secretion in STZ-induced type 1 diabetic mice, thereby reducing blood glucose levels. HNCP can also improve glucose metabolism in STZ-induced type 1 diabetic mice by regulating the expression levels of glycosynthesis- and gluconeogenesis-related enzymes such as GK, PEPCK1, G6Pase, and GSK-3β. This is the first time of preparing antioxidant and hypoglycemic peptides from marine bone collagen. Our results indicated that HNCP may be a potential diabetes treatment. However, further research into the sequences of peptides with these effects is required.

Author Contributions: Methodology, J.L. and S.H.; software, Q.L. and J.L.; investigation, Q.L. and J.L.; resources, Y.G.; data curation, J.L. and S.H.; writing—original draft preparation, Q.L.; writing—review and editing, Y.G., Y.C. and H.J.; project administration, Y.G., Y.C. and H.J.; funding acquisition, Y.G. and Y.C. All authors have read and agreed to the published version of the manuscript.

Funding: This research was funded by the Zhoushan Science and Technology Program (No. 2023C41009) and Jinhua Science and Technology Bureau (2022-3-070).

Institutional Review Board Statement: The study was conducted according to the guidelines of the Declaration of Helsinki, and approved by the Animal Protection and Utilization Committee of the China Animal Protection Commission (No. 2021029, 2021-09-01).

Data Availability Statement: The data presented in this study are available on request from the corresponding author.

Conflicts of Interest: The authors declare no conflict of interest.

References

1. Zheng, G.; Mo, F.; Ling, C.; Peng, H.; Gu, W.; Li, M.; Chen, Z. Portulaca oleracea L. alleviates liver injury in streptozotocin-induced diabetic mice. *Drug Des. Devel Ther.* **2018**, *12*, 47–55. [CrossRef] [PubMed]
2. Al-Attar, A.M.; Alsalmi, F.A. Influence of olive leaves extract on hepatorenal injury in streptozotocin diabetic rats. *Saudi J. Biol. Sci.* **2019**, *26*, 1865–1874. [CrossRef] [PubMed]
3. Bergmann, K.; Sypniewska, G. Diabetes as a complication of adipose tissue dysfunction. Is there a role for potential new biomarkers? *Clin. Chem. Lab. Med.* **2013**, *51*, 177–185. [CrossRef] [PubMed]
4. Wang, P.; Liu, H.; Chen, L.; Duan, Y.; Chen, Q.; Xi, S. Effects of a Novel Glucokinase Activator, HMS5552, on Glucose Metabolism in a Rat Model of Type 2 Diabetes Mellitus. *J. Diabetes Res.* **2017**, *2017*, 5812607. [CrossRef] [PubMed]
5. Ren, Y.R.; Ye, Y.L.; Feng, Y.; Xu, T.F.; Shen, Y.; Liu, J.; Huang, S.L.; Shen, J.H.; Leng, Y. SL010110, a lead compound, inhibits gluconeogenesis via SIRT2-p300-mediated PEPCK1 degradation and improves glucose homeostasis in diabetic mice. *Acta Pharmacol. Sin.* **2021**, *42*, 1834–1846. [CrossRef]
6. Gurumayum, S.; Bharadwaj, S.; Sheikh, Y.; Barge, S.R.; Saikia, K.; Swargiary, D.; Ahmed, S.A.; Thakur, D.; Borah, J.C. Taxifolin-3-O-glucoside from Osbeckia nepalensis mediates antihyperglycemic activity in CC1 hepatocytes and in diabetic Wistar rats via regulating AMPK/G6Pase/PEPCK signaling axis. *J. Ethnopharmacol.* **2023**, *303*, 115936. [CrossRef]
7. Desai, S.M.; Sanap, A.P.; Bhonde, R.R. Treat liver to beat diabetes. *Med. Hypotheses* **2020**, *144*, 110034. [CrossRef]
8. Loguercio, C.; Federico, A. Oxidative stress in viral and alcoholic hepatitis. *Free Radic. Biol. Med.* **2003**, *34*, 1–10. [CrossRef]
9. Bedi, O.; Aggarwal, S.; Trehanpati, N.; Ramakrishna, G.; Krishan, P. Molecular and Pathological Events Involved in the Pathogenesis of Diabetes-Associated Nonalcoholic Fatty Liver Disease. *J. Clin. Exp. Hepatol.* **2019**, *9*, 607–618. [CrossRef]
10. Leo, E.E.M.; Fernandez, J.J.A.; Campos, M.R.S. Biopeptides with antioxidant and anti-inflammatory potential in the prevention and treatment of diabesity disease. *Biomed. Pharmacother.* **2016**, *83*, 816–826.
11. Halim, M.; Halim, A. The effects of inflammation, aging and oxidative stress on the pathogenesis of diabetes mellitus (type 2 diabetes). *Diabetes Metab. Syndr. Clin. Res. Rev.* **2019**, *13*, 1165–1172. [CrossRef] [PubMed]
12. Sottero, B.; Gargiulo, S.; Russo, I.; Barale, C.; Poli, G.; Cavalot, F. Postprandial Dysmetabolism and Oxidative Stress in Type 2 Diabetes: Pathogenetic Mechanisms and Therapeutic Strategies. *Med. Res. Rev.* **2015**, *35*, 968–1031. [CrossRef]
13. Jung, E.Y.; Lee, H.-S.; Choi, J.W.; Ra, K.S.; Kim, M.-R.; Suh, H.J. Glucose tolerance and antioxidant activity of spent brewer's yeast hydrolysate with a high content of cyclo-His-Pro (CHP). *J. Food Sci. Technol.* **2011**, *76*, C272–C278. [CrossRef] [PubMed]
14. Nongonierma, A.B.; Fitzgerald, R.J. Dipeptidyl peptidase IV inhibitory and antioxidative properties of milk protein-derived dipeptides and hydrolysates. *Peptides* **2013**, *39*, 157–163. [CrossRef] [PubMed]

15. Zambrowicz, A.; Pokora, M.; Setner, B.; Dabrowska, A.; Szoltysik, M.; Babij, K.; Szewczuk, Z.; Trziszka, T.; Lubec, G.; Chrzanowska, J. Multifunctional peptides derived from an egg yolk protein hydrolysate: Isolation and characterization. *Amino Acids* 2015, *47*, 369–380. [CrossRef]
16. Unnikrishnan, P.; Kizhakkethil, B.P.; George, J.C.; Abubacker, Z.A.; Ninan, G.; Nagarajarao, R.C. Antioxidant Peptides from Dark Meat of Yellowfin Tuna (*Thunnus albacares*): Process Optimization and Characterization. *Waste Biomass Valorization* 2021, *12*, 1845–1860. [CrossRef]
17. Sheng, Y.; Qiu, Y.T.; Wang, Y.M.; Chi, C.F.; Wang, B. Novel Antioxidant Collagen Peptides of Siberian Sturgeon (*Acipenser baerii*) Cartilages: The Preparation, Characterization, and Cytoprotection of H2O2-Damaged Human Umbilical Vein Endothelial Cells (HUVECs). *Mar. Drugs* 2022, *20*, 325. [CrossRef]
18. Wang, Y.M.; Li, X.Y.; Wang, J.; He, Y.; Chi, C.F.; Wang, B. Antioxidant peptides from protein hydrolysate of skipjack tuna milt: Purification, identification, and cytoprotection on H2O2 damaged human umbilical vein endothelial cells. *Process Biochem.* 2022, *113*, 258–269. [CrossRef]
19. Gaikwad, S.B.; More, P.R.; Sonawane, S.K. Antioxidant and Anti-hypertensive Bioactive Peptides from Indian Mackerel Fish Waste. *J. Int. J. Pept. Res. Ther.* 2021, *27*, 2671–2684. [CrossRef]
20. Admassu, H.; Gasmalla, M.A.A.; Yang, R.J.; Zhao, W. Bioactive Peptides Derived from Seaweed Protein and Their Health Benefits: Antihypertensive, Antioxidant, and Antidiabetic Properties. *J. Food Sci.* 2018, *83*, 6–16. [CrossRef]
21. Abachi, S.; Offret, C.; Fliss, I.; Marette, A.; Bazinet, L.; Beaulieu, L. Isolation of Immunomodulatory Biopeptides from Atlantic Mackerel (*Scomber scombrus*) Protein Hydrolysate based on Molecular Weight, Charge, and Hydrophobicity. *Food Bioprocess. Technol.* 2022, *15*, 852–874. [CrossRef]
22. Ye, J.; Shen, C.; Huang, Y.; Zhang, X.; Xiao, M. Anti-fatigue activity of sea cucumber peptides prepared from Stichopus japonicus in an endurance swimming rat model. *J. Sci. Food Agric.* 2017, *97*, 4548–4556. [CrossRef] [PubMed]
23. Chakraborty, P.; Sahoo, S.; Bhattacharyya, D.K.; Ghosh, M. Marine lizardfish (*Harpadon nehereus*) meal concentrate in preparation of ready-to-eat protein and calcium rich extruded snacks. *J. Food Sci. Technol.* 2020, *57*, 338–349. [CrossRef] [PubMed]
24. Bardallo, R.G.; Panisello-Rosello, A.; Sanchez-Nuno, S.; Alva, N.; Rosello-Catafau, J.; Carbonell, T. Nrf2 and oxidative stress in liver ischemia/reperfusion injury. *Febs. J.* 2022, *289*, 5463–5479. [CrossRef]
25. Paul, N.; Truyen, N.; Sherratt Philip, J.; Pickett Cecil, B. The Carboxy-Terminal Neh3 Domain of Nrf2 Is Required for Transcriptional Activation. *Mol. Cell. Biol.* 2005, *25*, 10895–10906.
26. He, S.; Zhao, W.; Chen, X.; Li, J.; Zhang, L.; Jin, H. Ameliorative Effects of Peptide Phe-Leu-Ala-Pro on Acute Liver and Kidney Injury Caused by CCl4 via Attenuation of Oxidative Stress and Inflammation. *ACS Omega* 2022, *7*, 44796–44803. [CrossRef]
27. Wu, H.; Kong, L.; Tan, Y.; Epstein, P.N.; Zeng, J.; Gu, J.; Liang, G.; Kong, M.; Chen, X.; Miao, L. C66 ameliorates diabetic nephropathy in mice by both upregulating NRF2 function via increase in miR-200a and inhibiting miR-21. *Diabetologia* 2016, *59*, 1558–1568. [CrossRef]
28. Wang, J.B.; Xie, Y.; Pei, X.R.; Yang, R.Y.; Zhang, Z.F.; Li, Y. The lipid-lowering and antioxidative effects of marine collagen peptides. *Zhonghua Yu Fang Yi Xue Za Zhi* 2008, *42*, 226–230.
29. Zhu, C.F.; Li, G.Z.; Peng, H.B.; Zhang, F.; Chen, Y.; Li, Y. Treatment with marine collagen peptides modulates glucose and lipid metabolism in Chinese patients with type 2 diabetes mellitus. *Appl. Physiol. Nutr. Metab.* 2010, *35*, 797–804. [CrossRef]
30. Castellano, P.; Mora, L.; Escudero, E.; Vignolo, G.; Aznar, R.; Toldra, F. Antilisterial peptides from Spanish dry-cured hams: Purification and identification. *Food Microbiol.* 2016, *59*, 133–141. [CrossRef]
31. Kuerban, A.; Al-Malki, A.L.; Kumosani, T.A.; Sheikh, R.A.; Al-Abbasi, F.A.M.; Alshubaily, F.A.; Abulnaja, K.O.; Moselhy, S.S. Identification, protein antiglycation, antioxidant, antiproliferative, and molecular docking of novel bioactive peptides produced from hydrolysis of Lens culinaris. *J. Food Biochem.* 2020, *44*, e13494. [CrossRef] [PubMed]
32. Gao, D.; Cao, Y.; Li, H. Antioxidant activity of peptide fractions derived from cottonseed protein hydrolysate. *J. Sci. Food Agric.* 2010, *90*, 1855–1860. [CrossRef] [PubMed]
33. Collaborators, G.D. Global, regional, and national burden of diabetes from 1990 to 2021, with projections of prevalence to 2050: A systematic analysis for the Global Burden of Disease Study 2021. *Lancet* 2023, *402*, 203–234.
34. Droge, W. Free radicals in the physiological control of cell function. *Physiol. Rev.* 2002, *82*, 47–95. [CrossRef] [PubMed]
35. Garcia-Compean, D.; Jaquez-Quintana, J.O.; Gonzalez-Gonzalez, J.A.; Maldonado-Garza, H. Liver cirrhosis and diabetes: Risk factors, pathophysiology, clinical implications and management. *World J. Gastroenterol.* 2009, *15*, 280–288. [CrossRef]
36. Jiang, N.; Zhang, S.J.; Zhu, J.; Shang, J.; Gao, X.D. Hypoglycemic, Hypolipidemic and Antioxidant Effects of Peptides from Red Deer Antlers in Streptozotocin-Induced Diabetic Mice. *Tohoku J. Exp. Med.* 2015, *236*, 71–79. [CrossRef]
37. Woo, M.; Seol, B.G.; Kang, K.H.; Choi, Y.H.; Cho, E.J.; Noh, J.S. Effects of collagen peptides from skate (*Raja kenojei*) skin on improvements of the insulin signaling pathway via attenuation of oxidative stress and inflammation. *Food Funct.* 2020, *11*, 2017–2025. [CrossRef]
38. Zhao, W.; Fang, H.-H.; Liu, Z.-Z.; Huang, M.-Q.; Su, M.; Zhang, C.-W.; Gao, B.-Y.; Niu, J. A newly isolated strain of Haematococcus pluvialis JNU35 improves the growth, antioxidation, immunity and liver function of golden pompano (*Trachinotus ovatus*). *Aquac. Nutr.* 2021, *27*, 342–354. [CrossRef]
39. Najmeh, S.; Hossein, T.-N.; Ali, K.O.; Hamed, N.E.M. Effects of Haematococcus pluvialis supplementation on antioxidant system and metabolism in rainbow trout (*Oncorhynchus mykiss*). *Fish Physiol. Biochem.* 2011, *38*, 413–419.

40. Zhu, C.F.; Peng, H.B.; Liu, G.Q.; Zhang, F.; Li, Y. Beneficial effects of oligopeptides from marine salmon skin in a rat model of type 2 diabetes. *Nutrition* **2010**, *26*, 1014–1020. [CrossRef]
41. Zhu, C.; Zhang, W.; Mu, B.; Zhang, F.; Lai, N.; Zhou, J.; Xu, A.; Liu, J.; Li, Y. Effects of marine collagen peptides on glucose metabolism and insulin resistance in type 2 diabetic rats. *J. Food Sci. Technol.* **2017**, *54*, 2260–2269. [CrossRef] [PubMed]
42. Lu, Z.; Xu, X.; Li, D.; Sun, N.; Lin, S. Sea Cucumber Peptides Attenuated the Scopolamine-Induced Memory Impairment in Mice and Rats and the Underlying Mechanism. *J. Agric. Food Chem.* **2022**, *70*, 157–170. [CrossRef] [PubMed]
43. He, S.; Xu, Z.; Li, J.; Guo, Y.; Lin, Q.; Jin, H. Peptides from Harpadon nehereus protect against hyperglycemia-induced HepG2 via oxidative stress and glycolipid metabolism regulation. *J. Funct. Foods* **2023**, *108*, 105723. [CrossRef]
44. Kumar, A.; Mittal, R. Nrf2: A potential therapeutic target for diabetic neuropathy. *Inflammopharmacology* **2017**, *25*, 393–402. [CrossRef]
45. Wu, J.; Sun, X.; Jiang, Z.; Jiang, J.; Xu, L.; Tian, A.; Sun, X.; Meng, H.; Li, Y.; Huang, W.; et al. Protective role of NRF2 in macrovascular complications of diabetes. *J. Cell Mol. Med.* **2020**, *24*, 8903–8917. [CrossRef] [PubMed]
46. Albert-Garay, J.S.; Riesgo-Escovar, J.R.; Sanchez-Chavez, G.; Salceda, R. Retinal Nrf2 expression in normal and early streptozotocin-diabetic rats. *Neurochem. Int.* **2021**, *145*, 105007. [CrossRef] [PubMed]
47. Hao, Q.; Zheng, A.; Zhang, H.; Cao, H. Down-regulation of betatrophin enhances insulin sensitivity in type 2 diabetes mellitus through activation of the GSK-3beta/PGC-1alpha signaling pathway. *J. Endocrinol. Investig.* **2021**, *44*, 1857–1868. [CrossRef] [PubMed]
48. Zheng, H.; Wan, J.; Shan, Y.; Song, X.; Jin, J.; Su, Q.; Chen, S.; Lu, X.; Yang, J.; Li, Q.; et al. MicroRNA-185-5p inhibits hepatic gluconeogenesis and reduces fasting blood glucose levels by suppressing G6Pase. *Theranostics* **2021**, *11*, 7829–7843. [CrossRef]
49. Zhang, R.; Chen, J.; Jiang, X.; Yin, L.; Zhang, X. Antioxidant and hypoglycaemic effects of tilapia skin collagen peptide in mice. *Int. J. Food Sci. Technol.* **2016**, *51*, 2157–2163. [CrossRef]
50. Abdelmawgood, I.A.; Mahana, N.A.; Badr, A.M.; Mohamed, A.S.; Al Shawoush, A.M.; Atia, T.; Abdelrazak, A.E.; Sakr, H.I. Echinochrome Ameliorates Physiological, Immunological, and Histopathological Alterations Induced by Ovalbumin in Asthmatic Mice by Modulating the Keap1/Nrf2 Signaling Pathway. *Mar. Drugs* **2023**, *21*, 455. [CrossRef]
51. Okan, A.; Doganyigit, Z.; Eroglu, E.; Akyuz, E.; Demir, N. Immunoreactive definition of TNF- alpha, HIF-1 alpha, Kir6.2, Kir3.1 and M2 muscarinic receptor for cardiac and pancreatic tissues in a mouse model for type 1 diabetes. *Life Sci.* **2021**, *284*, 119886. [CrossRef]
52. Wu, Z.Q.; Lu, J.; Chen, H.H.; Chen, W.S.; Xu, H.G. Individualized correction of insulin measurement in hemolyzed serum samples. *Immunol. Res.* **2017**, *65*, 605–608. [CrossRef] [PubMed]
53. Wang, H.Y.; Li, Q.M.; Yu, N.J.; Chen, W.D.; Zha, X.Q.; Wu, D.L.; Pan, L.H.; Duan, J.; Luo, J.P. Dendrobium huoshanense polysaccharide regulates hepatic glucose homeostasis and pancreatic ss-cell function in type 2 diabetic mice. *Carbohyd Polym.* **2019**, *211*, 39–48. [CrossRef] [PubMed]
54. Liu, Y.L.; Gao, Z.Z.; Guo, Q.T.; Wang, T.; Lu, C.E.; Chen, Y.; Sheng, Q.; Chen, J.; Nie, Z.M.; Zhang, Y.Z.; et al. Anti-Diabetic Effects of CTB-APSL Fusion Protein in Type 2 Diabetic Mice. *Mar. Drugs* **2014**, *12*, 1512–1529. [CrossRef] [PubMed]
55. Tang, Y.P.; Zhao, R.; Pu, Q.Y.; Jiang, S.; Yu, F.M.; Yang, Z.S.; Han, T. Investigation of nephrotoxicity on mice exposed to polystyrene nanoplastics and the potential amelioration effects of DHA-enriched phosphatidylserine. *Sci. Total Environ.* **2023**, *892*, 164808. [CrossRef]
56. Park, S.Y.; Fernando, I.P.S.; Han, E.J.; Kim, M.J.; Jung, K.; Kang, D.S.; Ahn, C.B.; Ahn, G. In Vivo Hepatoprotective Effects of a Peptide Fraction from Krill Protein Hydrolysates against Alcohol-Induced Oxidative Damage. *Mar. Drugs* **2019**, *17*, 690. [CrossRef]
57. Jiang, Q.J.; Chen, Q.; Li, C.P.; Gong, Z.G.; Li, Z.G.; Ding, S.F. ox-LDL-Induced Endothelial Progenitor Cell Oxidative Stress via p38/Keap1/Nrf2 Pathway. *Stem Cells Int.* **2022**, *2022*, 5897194. [CrossRef]

Disclaimer/Publisher's Note: The statements, opinions and data contained in all publications are solely those of the individual author(s) and contributor(s) and not of MDPI and/or the editor(s). MDPI and/or the editor(s) disclaim responsibility for any injury to people or property resulting from any ideas, methods, instructions or products referred to in the content.

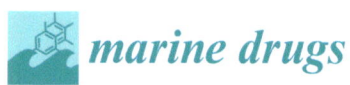

Article

Novel Ca-Chelating Peptides from Protein Hydrolysate of Antarctic Krill (*Euphausia superba*): Preparation, Characterization, and Calcium Absorption Efficiency in Caco-2 Cell Monolayer Model

Ming-Xue Ge [1,†], Ru-Ping Chen [1,†], Lun Zhang [2], Yu-Mei Wang [1,*], Chang-Feng Chi [2] and Bin Wang [1,*]

1. Zhejiang Provincial Engineering Technology Research Center of Marine Biomedical Products, School of Food and Pharmacy, Zhejiang Ocean University, Zhoushan 316022, China; gmx8670@163.com (M.-X.G.); 15157780517@163.com (R.-P.C.)
2. National and Provincial Joint Laboratory of Exploration and Utilization of Marine Aquatic Genetic Resources, National Engineering Research Center of Marine Facilities Aquaculture, School of Marine Science and Technology, Zhejiang Ocean University, Zhoushan 316022, China; zl15525864652@163.com (L.Z.)
* Correspondence: wangyumei731@163.com (Y.-M.W.); wangbin@zjou.edu.cn (B.W.); Tel./Fax: +86-580-2554818 (Y.-M.W. & B.W.)
† These authors contributed equally to this work.

Abstract: Antarctic krill (*Euphausia superba*) is the world's largest resource of animal proteins and is thought to be a high-quality resource for future marine healthy foods and functional products. Therefore, Antarctic krill was degreased and separately hydrolyzed using flavourzyme, pepsin, papain, and alcalase. Protein hydrolysate (AKH) of Antarctic krill prepared by trypsin showed the highest Ca-chelating rate under the optimized chelating conditions: a pH of 8.0, reaction time of 50 min, temperature of 50 °C, and material/calcium ratio of 1:15. Subsequently, fourteen Ca-chelating peptides were isolated from APK by ultrafiltration and a series of chromatographic methods and identified as AK, EAR, AEA, VERG, VAS, GPK, SP, GPKG, APRGH, GVPG, LEPGP, LEKGA, FPPGR, and GEPG with molecular weights of 217.27, 374.40, 289.29, 459.50, 275.30, 300.36, 202.21, 357.41, 536.59, 328.37, 511.58, 516.60, 572.66, and 358.35 Da, respectively. Among fourteen Ca-chelating peptides, VERG presented the highest Ca-chelating ability. Ultraviolet spectrum (UV), Fourier Transform Infrared (FTIR), and scanning electron microscope (SEM) analysis indicated that the VERG-Ca chelate had a dense granular structure because the N-H, C=O and -COOH groups of VERG combined with Ca^{2+}. Moreover, the VERG-Ca chelate is stable in gastrointestinal digestion and can significantly improve Ca transport in Caco-2 cell monolayer experiments, but phytate could significantly reduce the absorption of Ca derived from the VERG-Ca chelate. Therefore, Ca-chelating peptides from protein hydrolysate of Antarctic krill possess the potential to serve as a Ca supplement in developing healthy foods.

Keywords: Antarctic krill (*Euphausia superba*); Ca-chelating peptide; VERG; property analysis; absorption efficiency; Caco-2 cell model

Citation: Ge, M.-X.; Chen, R.-P.; Zhang, L.; Wang, Y.-M.; Chi, C.-F.; Wang, B. Novel Ca-Chelating Peptides from Protein Hydrolysate of Antarctic Krill (*Euphausia superba*): Preparation, Characterization, and Calcium Absorption Efficiency in Caco-2 Cell Monolayer Model. *Mar. Drugs* **2023**, *21*, 579. https://doi.org/10.3390/md21110579

Academic Editor: Jae-Young Je

Received: 13 October 2023
Revised: 31 October 2023
Accepted: 3 November 2023
Published: 5 November 2023

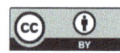

Copyright: © 2023 by the authors. Licensee MDPI, Basel, Switzerland. This article is an open access article distributed under the terms and conditions of the Creative Commons Attribution (CC BY) license (https://creativecommons.org/licenses/by/4.0/).

1. Introduction

Dietary minerals as micronutrients have an extremely crucial impact on human health, but some factors, such as diet, lifestyle, habits, living environment, and genetics, can make people subjected to mineral deficiency and lead to many types of illness [1]. For instance, zinc deficiency influences about 2 billion people and results in immune dysfunction, delayed wound healing, growth retardation, hypogonadism, hair loss, and brain atrophy and dysfunction; iron and copper deficiency may result in impaired hematopoiesis function, iron deficiency anemia, and neurological disorders [2]. The human body contains about 700–1400 g of calcium (Ca), which is the richest inorganic element and is involved in a variety of physiological activities, including bone strength, neurotransmission, blood coagulation, enzyme activation, cellular proliferation, and muscle contraction [3]. In addition, Ca also takes part in regulating neural activity and the permeability of cell membranes. Ca-deficiency can lead to osteoporosis, metabolic disorders, rickets, intestine cancer, osteomalacia, and hypertension [4,5]. Compared with the recommended daily allowance of Ca (700–1200 mg), Ca intake for people from 74 countries, especially from Asia, Africa, and South America, was lower than 700 mg/day [6]. Moreover, Ca deficiency is also common in older women and often causes other diseases.

Ca deficiency is often caused by insufficient Ca intake and poor bioavailability. However, dietary intake alone may not be sufficient to meet the Ca levels required by the body's physiology. Therefore, adequate Ca intake and high bioavailability are profoundly important to maintain health benefits. Presently, various types of oral Ca supplements have been developed to resolve the problem of Ca deficiency, such as Ca gluconate, Ca lactate, and Ca carbonate [7]. Unfortunately, most Ca supplements have low bioavailability in vivo and poor effects in clinical practice due to their relatively low absorption rate, poor solubility, gastrointestinal irritation, and strong side effects [1].

In the past decades, protein hydrolysates and bioactive peptides (BPs) have been widely produced using different animal and plant proteins and engaged in human nutrition applications [8–10]. Upon proteolysis, the generated BPs with 2–20 amino acids have been regarded as high-quality nutritional supplements because of their low molecular weights (MW), resulting in easy absorption and high nutrition characteristics [11–13]. Moreover, BPs showed multifarious significant pharmacological functions, including antioxidant, antifatigue, antihypertensive, anti-aging, lipid-lowering, antimicrobial, and immunomodulatory activities [14–16]. In order to overcome the defects of Ca supplements in the current market, Ca-chelating peptides serving as a novel kind of Ca supplement have become the hot research theme [1]. Literature studies reported that Ca-chelating peptides could improve Ca absorbability and bioavailability by weakening the formation of insoluble Ca complexes and giving assistance to Ca transport into the blood. In addition, Ca-chelating peptides have the advantages of excellent stability and high safety [17,18]. Therefore, Ca-chelating peptides were produced using diverse animal and plant proteins, such as casein [19], tilapia [2], cattle bone [5], cucumber seed [4], mung bean [20], Pacific cod bone [21], oyster [22], Crimson snapper scales [18], and soy and pea [23].

Antarctic krill (*Euphausia superba*) is considered the world's largest resource of animal proteins due to its huge biomass (342–356 million tons) and high biological value [24,25]. Therefore, Antarctic krill proteins are thought of as a high-quality resource for future marine healthy foods and functional products, and the studies on the preparation and activity of BPs from Antarctic krill proteins have gathered wide attention [26,27]. For example, phosphorylated peptides from Antarctic krill could ameliorate osteoporosis and alleviate liver fibrosis [25,28]; Antioxidant peptides, such as EYEA, SNVFDMF, QYPPMQY, AMVDAIAR, and LQP, could scavenge radical, protect liver cells, and liver organism against oxidative stress [29–31]; VLGYIQIR and LVDDHFL could be appropriate for novel mineral supplements [32,33]; SSDAFFPFR and SNVFDMF could ameliorate the memory impairment of mice induced by scopolamine [34]; WF, FAS, KVEPLP, and PAL presented strong ACE and/or DPP-IV inhibitory ability [35,36]. However, there are relatively few research studies on the preparation of metal-chelated peptides from Antarctic krill proteins. Therefore, the purposes of this work were to isolate and characterize the Ca-chelating peptides from the hydrolysate of Antarctic krill proteins. Furthermore, the chelating mechanism and absorption efficiency of prepared Ca-chelating peptides were studied using the Caco-2 cell monolayer model.

2. Results and Discussion

2.1. Preparation of Protein Hydrolysate of Antarctic Krill

2.1.1. Screening of Protease Species

Antarctic krill proteins were hydrolyzed separately by five proteases, and the Ca-chelating rates of produced hydrolysates were presented in Table 1. The data indicated that the Ca-chelating rate of hydrolysate generated by trypsin was 37.91 ± 2.958%, which was remarkably greater than the rates of hydrolysates produced using flavourzyme (30.93 ± 1.37%), pepsin (24.11 ± 2.16%), papain (23.69 ± 1.98%), and alcalase (32.24 ± 2.31%), respectively ($p < 0.05$).

Table 1. Effects of different proteases on Ca-chelating rate (%) of protein hydrolysates from Antarctic krill.

Protease	Enzymolysis Condition				Ca-Chelating Rate (%)
	Temperature (°C)	Time (h)	Enzyme Dose (%)	pH	
Flavourzyme	50	4	2.0	7.0	30.93 ± 1.37 [b]
Pepsin	37.5	4	2.0	2.0	24.11 ± 2.16 [c]
Trypsin	37.5	4	2.0	7.8	37.91 ± 2.96 [a]
Papain	55	4	2.0	7.0	23.69 ± 1.98 [c]
Alcalase	55	4	2.0	9.5	32.24 ± 2.31 [b]

[a–c] Values with different letters indicate significant difference ($p < 0.05$).

Enzymatic hydrolysis is the most applied process to generate Ca-chelating peptides on account of mild reaction conditions, high safety, and environmentally friendly features [1,36]. Therefore, some proteases, including prolyve enzyme [37], neutrase [3,22], protamex [38], alcalase [23], and bromelain [39], have been screened for the production of different mineral-chelating peptides. The present results further supported the opinion that the specificity of proteases remarkably influenced the Ca-chelating rates of hydrolysates. Therefore, the hydrolysate of Antarctic krill proteins produced using trypsin was prepared and named AKH.

2.1.2. Optimized the Chelating Conditions of Ca with AKH

As shown in Figure 1, the effects of chelating conditions, including chelating time (30, 40, 50, and 60 min), temperature (30, 40, 50, and 60 °C), pH (6, 7, 8, and 9), and peptide/Ca ratio (1:5, 1:10, 1:15, and 1:20) on the Ca-chelating rate (%) of AKH were optimized by a single-factor experiment. Figure 1A illustrated that the Ca-chelating rate of AKH significantly ($p < 0.05$) increased when the chelating time increased from 30 to 50 min and achieved the highest value (38.68 ± 0.8%) at 50 min. Additionally, the Ca-chelating rate of AKH was markedly decreased when the chelating time ranged from 50 to 60 min. Figure 1B illustrated that the Ca-chelating rate of AKH significantly ($p < 0.05$) increased when the peptide/Ca ratio changed from 1:5 to 1:10 and achieved the highest value (44.57 ± 2.16%) at peptide/Ca ratio of 1:10. In addition, the Ca-chelating rate of AKH was markedly descent when the chelating time ranged from 50 to 60 min ($p > 0.05$). Figure 1C showed that the Ca-chelating rate of AKH was dramatically affected by the chelating pH, and the Ca-chelating rate (45.37 ± 0.96%) of AKH at pH 8.0 was remarkably higher than those of AKH at other pH ($p < 0.05$). Additionally, the Ca-chelating rate of AKH was a gradual decline when the pH value was higher than 8.0. Figure 1D indicated that chelating temperature significantly influenced the Ca-chelating rate of AKH, and the Ca-chelating rate (47.11 ± 1.31%) of AKH prepared at 50 °C was prominently stronger than that of hydrolysate prepared at other chelating temperatures ($p < 0.05$). Therefore, the range of chelating conditions for Ca with AKH was narrowed to chelating time (40, 50, and 60 min), temperature (40, 50, and 60 °C), pH (7, 8, and 9), and peptide/Ca ratio (1:5, 1:10, and 1:15), respectively.

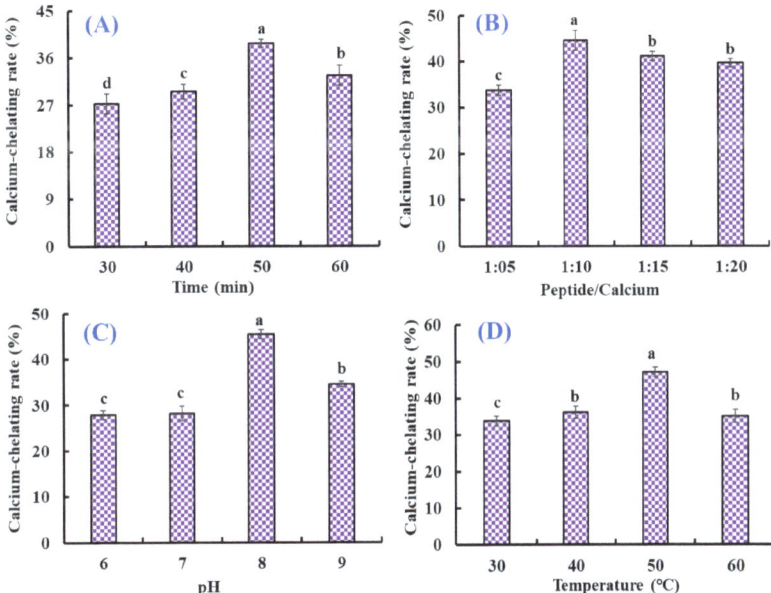

Figure 1. Effects of chelating time (**A**), peptide/Ca ratio (**B**), pH (**C**), and temperature (**D**) on the Ca-chelating rate of the hydrolysate of Antarctic krill proteins (AKH). [a–d] Values with the same letters indicate no significant difference ($p > 0.05$).

Furthermore, the orthogonal test $L_9(3)^4$ was designed to optimize the chelating conditions for Ca with AKH (Table 2). Following the R values, the conditions interfering with the Ca-chelating rate of AKH were listed in decreasing order: A (chelating pH) > B (chelating time) > C (chelating temperature) > D (peptide/Ca ratio). The chelating pH was proved to be the most important condition influencing the Ca-chelating rate of AKH, and the optimal chelating level was $A_2B_2C_3D_3$; that is to say, the optimum chelating conditions of Ca with AKH were a chelating pH of 8.0, time of 50 min, temperature of 50 °C, and peptide/Ca ratio of 1:15.

Table 2. Results of the $L_9(3)^4$ orthogonal experiment for optimizing the chelating conditions of Ca with AKH.

No.	pH	Time (min)	Temperature (°C)	Peptide/Ca Ratio	Ca-Chelating Rate (%)
1	7	40	40	1:5	42.38
2	7	50	50	1:10	47.11
3	7	60	60	1:15	46.29
4	8	40	50	1:15	51.95
5	8	50	60	1:5	53.71
6	8	60	40	1:10	49.17
7	9	40	60	1:10	47.35
8	9	50	40	1:15	49.15
9	9	60	50	1:5	47.86
K1	135.78	141.68	140.7	143.95	
K2	154.83	149.97	146.92	143.63	
K3	144.36	143.32	147.35	147.39	
Best level	A2	B2	C3	D3	
R	19.05	8.29	6.65	3.72	
R order		A > B > C > D			

2.2. Preparation of Ca-Chelating Peptides from AKH

2.2.1. Ultrafiltration

Dietary Ca forms Ca phosphate deposition in the gastrointestinal system, inducing poor absorbance [4]. However, peptides shape a peptide-Ca chelate with Ca^{2+}, which increases the solubility and bioavailability of Ca in the intestine. The Ca absorption was influenced by the structure and Ca-chelating capability of peptides, so evaluating the Ca-chelating capability of different peptide components was necessary. In the experiment, five components, including AKH-1 (MW > 10 kDa), AKH-2 (5–10 kDa), AKH-3 (3.5–5 kDa), AKH-4 (1–3.5 kDa), and AKH-5 (MW < 1 kDa), were obtained from AKH. Figure 2 showed that the Ca-chelating rate of AKH-5 was observably higher than those of AKH and the other four fractions ($p < 0.05$). Ultrafiltration is a popular technique to concentrate target fractions from protein hydrolysates according to their molecular size [40,41]. After ultrafiltration, AKH-5 collected more low MW peptides, exposing more binding sites for Ca^{2+}. Huang et al. reported that peptide fraction (<1 kDa) separated from the hydrolysate of shrimp byproducts exhibited greater affinity to Ca^{2+} [42]. In addition, low MW peptides are easier to digest and absorb in the body. Therefore, AKH-5 was chosen for further study.

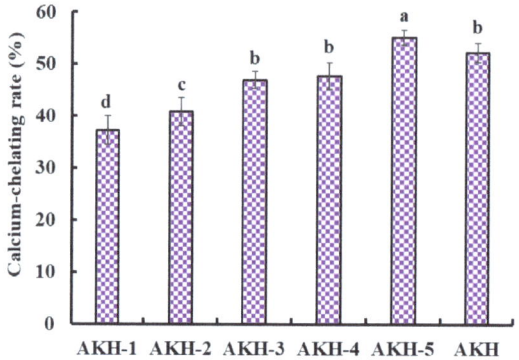

Figure 2. Ca-chelating rate of AKH and its fractions (AKH-1~AKH-5) by ultrafiltration. [a-d] Values with same letters indicate no significant difference ($p > 0.05$).

2.2.2. Anion-Exchange Chromatography of AKH-5

Ion-exchange chromatography is popularly applied to separate polar molecules (such as proteins and peptides) from crude extraction and protolysate according to their affinities to ion exchangers. As shown in Figure 3A, AKH-5 was divided into three fractions (AKH-5a, AKH-5b, and AKH-5c) by a DEAE-52 cellulose column. The Ca-chelating rate of AKH-5a was 58.74 ± 1.64%, which was observably higher than those of AKH-5, AKH-5b, and AKH-5c ($p < 0.05$) (Figure 3B). Peptides usually have polar amino acid residues, which are easier to bind to the cation or anion exchange resins, such as XK 26 DEAE, SP-Sephadex C-25, DEAE-52 cellulose, AG 50W-X2, Q Sepharose FF, etc. [43]. Reddy and Mahoney [44] reported that peptides could exhibit stronger Ca-chelating activity if they contain more groups with more negative charges. In addition, Zhao et al. [45] found that other properties of peptides, such as MW and hydrophilicity/hydrophobicity, also have significant effects on the adsorption capacity between peptides and Ca. The Ca-chelating ability of AKH-5a should be the result of multiple effects, including negative charges, molecular size, and hydrophilicity/hydrophobicity. Therefore, AKH-5a was selected for further purification.

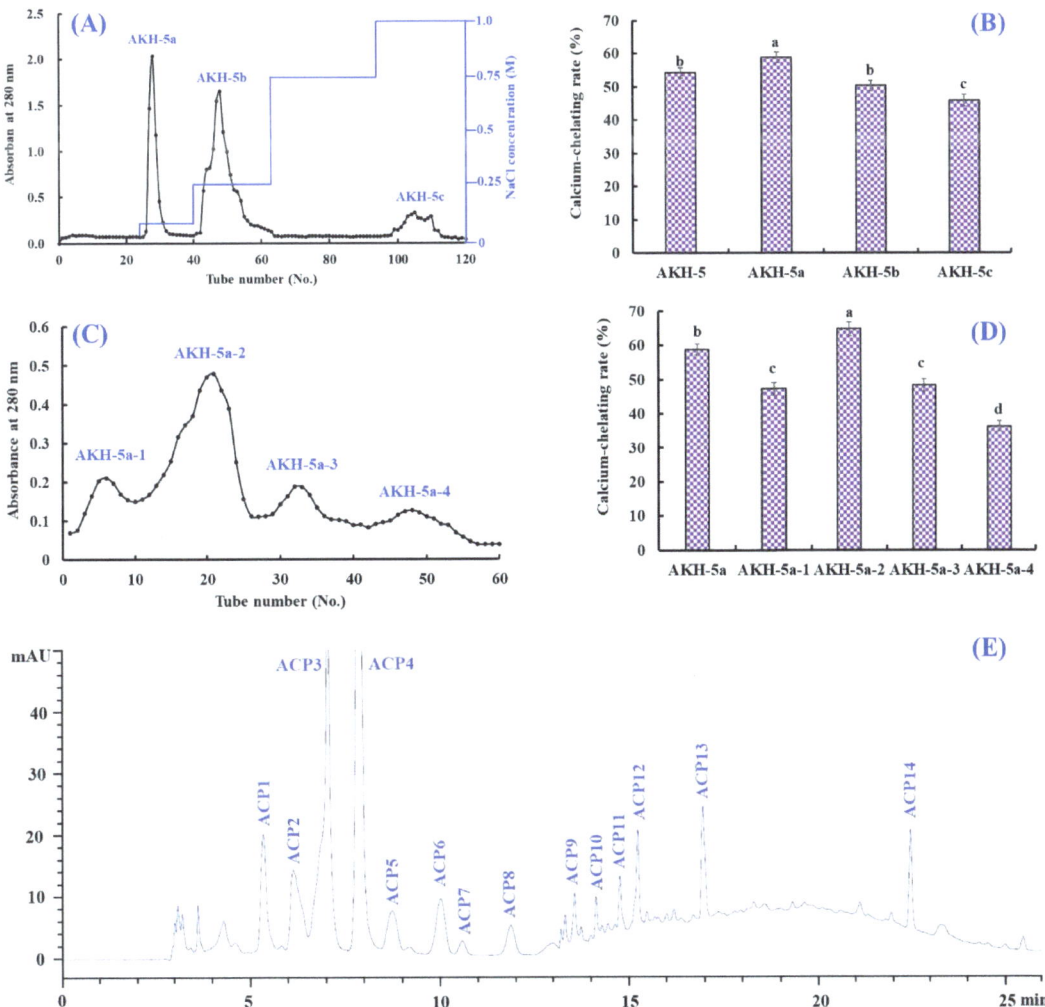

Figure 3. Isolation of Ca-chelating peptides from the ultrafiltration fraction AKH-5. (**A**) Elution profiles of AKH-5 in DEAE-52 cellulose chromatograph; (**B**) Ca-chelating ability of fractions from AKH-5. (**C**) elution profile of AKH-5a in Sephadex G-25 chromatography; (**D**) Ca-chelating ability of fractions from AKH-5a; and (**E**) elution profiles of AKH-5a-2 by RP-HPLC. [a–d] Values with same letters indicate no significant difference ($p > 0.05$).

2.2.3. Gel Permeation Chromatography (GPC) of AKH-5a

Molecular size is one of the key factors to consider in the purification of BPs [46,47]. Thus, AKH-5a was further divided into four fractions (AKH-5a-1, AKH-5a-2, AKH-5a-3, and AKH-5a-4) by a Sephadex G-25 column (Figure 3C). The Ca-chelating rate of AKH-5b-2 was 64.74 ± 1.98%, which was observably higher than those of AKH-5a, AKH-5a-1, AKH-5a-3, and AKH-5a-4, respectively ($p < 0.05$) (Figure 3D). Gel filtration is an efficient method to separate bioactive substances with different MW ranges and is widely applied for BP purification from different protein hydrolysates, such as whey [45], shrimp byproducts [42], Alaska pollock [48], monkfish [13], tilapia (*Oreochromis niloticus*) [49], *Mytilus edulis* [50], peanut [51], *Cyclina sinensis* [52,53], etc. Although AKH-5b-2 presented the best

Ca-chelating ability, its MW was not the lowest among the four peptide fractions. These findings illustrated that other factors besides MW, such as amino acid composition and hydrophilicity/hydrophobicity, also greatly influence the Ca-chelating ability of peptides. Then, AKH-5a-2 was chosen for HPLC isolation.

2.2.4. RP-HPLC Purification of AKH-5a-2

AKH-5a-2 was finally purified by RP-HPLC (Figure 3E). According to the elution profiles of AKH-5a-2 at 280 nm, fourteen Ca-chelating peptides with retention times (RTs) of 5.29 (ACP1), 6.18 (ACP2), 7.02 (ACP3), 7.95 (ACP4), 8.76 (ACP5), 10.01 (ACP6), 10.58 (ACP7), 11.91 (ACP8), 13.60 (ACP9), 14.11 (ACP10), 14.85 (ACP11), 15.22 (ACP12), 16.98 (ACP13), and 22.46 min (ACP14) were isolated and collected (Table 3). RP-HPLC is an extremely effective technology for purifying BPs according to their RT, and the RT of separated BPs can be modulated by adjusting the ratio of polar solvent (methanol and acetonitrile) in the mobile phase [50]. Therefore, RP-HPLC has been used to purify Ca-chelating peptides from protein hydrolysates of whey [45], casein [54], Alaska pollock [48], *Mytilus edulis* [50], phosvitin [55], miiuy croaker [46], tilapia (*Oreochromis niloticus*) [49], peanut [51], *Harpadon nehereus* [56], *Stolephorus chinensis* [57], etc.

Table 3. Retention time, amino acid sequence, and molecular weight of 14 peptides (ACP1–ACP14) from AKH-5b-2.

No.	Retention Time (min)	Amino Acid Sequence	Observed/Theoretical MW (Da)
ACP1	5.29	Ala-Lys (AK)	217.27/217.27
ACP2	6.18	Glu-Ala-Arg (EAR)	374.40/374.39
ACP3	7.02	Ala-Glu-Ala (AEA)	289.29/289.29
ACP4	7.95	Val-Glu-Arg-Gly (VERG)	459.50/459.50
ACP5	8.76	Val-Ala-Ser (VAS)	275.30/275.30
ACP6	10.01	Gly-Pro-Lys (GPK)	300.36/300.35
ACP7	10.58	Ser-Pro (SP)	202.21/202.21
ACP8	11.91	Gly-Pro-Lys-Gly (GPKG)	357.41/357.41
ACP9	13.60	Ala-Pro-Arg-Gly-His (APRGH)	536.59/536.58
ACP10	14.11	Gly-Val-Pro-Gly (GVPG)	328.37/328.36
ACP11	14.85	Leu-Glu-Pro-Gly-Pro (LEPGP)	511.58/511.57
ACP12	15.22	Leu-Glu-Lys-Gly-Ala (LEKGA)	516.60/516.59
ACP13	16.98	Phe-Pro-Pro-Gly-Arg (FPPGR)	572.66/572.66
ACP14	22.46	Gly-Glu-Pro-Gly (GEPG)	358.35/358.35

2.3. Determination of Sequences and MWs of Ca-Chelating Peptides (ACP1–ACP14)

By Protein/Peptide Sequencer, the fourteen Ca-chelating peptide (ACP1–ACP14) sequences were identified as Ala-Lys (AK, ACP1), Glu-Ala-Arg (EAR, ACP2), Ala-Glu-Ala (AEA, ACP3), Val-Glu-Arg-Gly (VERG, ACP4), Val-Ala-ESr (VAS, ACP5), Gly-Pro-Lys (GPK, ACP6), Ser-Pro (SP, ACP7), Gly-Pro-Lys-Gly (GPKG, ACP8), Ala-Pro-Arg-Gly-His (APRGH, ACP9), Gly-Val-Pro-Gly (GVPG, ACP10), Leu-Glu-Pro-Gly-Pro (LEPGP, ACP11), Leu-Glu-Lys-Gly-Ala (LEKGA, ACP12), Phe-Pro-Pro-Gly-Arg (FPPGR, ACP13), and Gly-Glu-Pro-Gly (GEPG, ACP14), and their MWs were determined as 217.27, 374.40, 289.29, 459.50, 275.30, 300.36, 202.21, 357.41, 536.59, 328.37, 511.58, 516.60, 572.66, and 358.35 Da, respectively, which were in good agreement with their theoretical MWs (Table 3).

2.4. Ca-Chelating Ability of Fourteen Isolated Peptides (ACP1–ACP14)

Figure 4 presents the Ca-chelating ability of fourteen isolated peptides (ACP1–ACP14). ACP4 (VERG) (70.05 ± 1.91%) showed the highest Ca-chelating ability among fourteen isolated peptides (ACP1–ACP14), and other peptides with higher Ca-chelating ability were followed by ACP8 (GPKG) and ACP9 (APRGH), respectively.

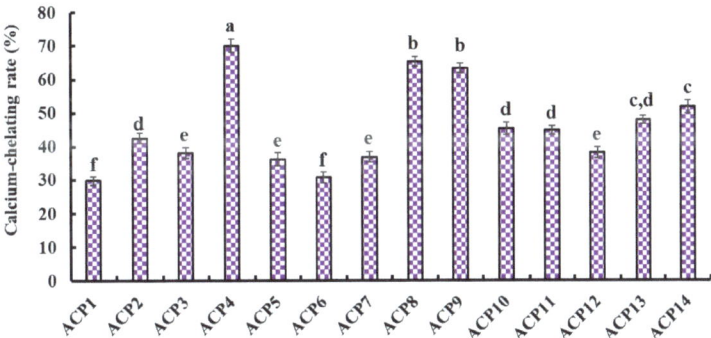

Figure 4. Ca-chelating ability of fourteen isolated peptides (ACP1-ACP14) by RP-HPLC. [a-f] Values with same letters indicate no significant difference ($p > 0.05$).

Amino acid composition and molecular size are two key factors affecting the Ca-chelating ability of peptides [19]. Peptides with short amino acid sequences, such as TCH, YDT, VLPVPQK, LLLGI, AIVIL, HADAD, YGTGL, LVFL, and LPEPV, were proved to contribute more to their Ca-chelating ability [19,41,44,48,50,52]. Guo et al. also reported that the Ca-chelating activity of tripeptides (SAC and SCH) was higher than those of SGSTGH, GPAGPR, and GPAGPHGPPG [48]. The MW of ACP4 (VERG) was 459.50 Da, which helped it easily interact with Ca^{2+} to form peptide-Ca chelate.

Amino acid composition is another widely recognized key factor that significantly influences the Ca-chelating ability of peptides. For example, Asp, Glu, and Gly residues were considered the major amino acid residues contributing to the Ca-chelating ability of peptides from porcine blood plasma [58]. Asp, Glu, Cys, and His residues are favorable for the metal-chelating activity of GPAGPHGPPG from Alaska pollock skin [48]. Liao et al. [54] indicated that Val, Pro, and Gln could significantly contribute to the high Ca-chelating ability of VLPVPQK. In general, the carboxyl group of Glu and Asp are favorable to bind Ca^{2+} because the carboxylic acid group can create an environment conducive to the chelating reaction of peptide and Ca by increasing the charge density [22]. The contents of hydrophobic amino acids, such as Val, Pro, and Leu, were also proved to be associated with the amount of Ca bound [59]. Gly residue could maintain the strong flexibility of the peptide skeleton to easily access and bind to Ca^{2+} [9]. In addition, Liu et al. [59] found that Arg was one of the main amino acid residues for the Ca-chelating peptides from wheat germ. Therefore, Val, Glu, Arg, and Gly residues should be very helpful in improving the Ca-chelating ability of ACP4 (VERG). Therefore, ACP4 (VERG) was selected to chelate with Ca and used for the next experiment.

2.5. Characterization of VERG-Ca Chelate

2.5.1. UV Absorption Spectroscopy

UV spectrum is a popular method to study the structural characteristics of substances and their derivatives. The appearance of new absorbance peaks or the changes in the pre-existing peaks in the UV spectrum indicate the formation of chelates consisting of organic ligands and metal ions [55]. Figure 5A indicated that the maximum absorption band of ACP4 (VERG) was found near 230 nm, caused by the n→π * transition of C=O in peptide bonds. The maximum absorption peak of the VERG-Ca chelate was 210 nm, suggesting that ACP4 binding with Ca^{2+} induced the absorption peak to shift towards the short wavelength. N and O in ACP4 (VERG) form a complex bond with Ca^{2+}, which influences the electronic transition of C=O and $-NH_2$ of the peptide bond. Our result is similar to the research results of peptide-Ca chelates from phosvitin [55], egg white [60], cucumber seed [4], whey [45], and sheep bone [61]. This present finding indicated that ACP4 (VERG) interacting with Ca^{2+} finally formed a new VERG-Ca chelate.

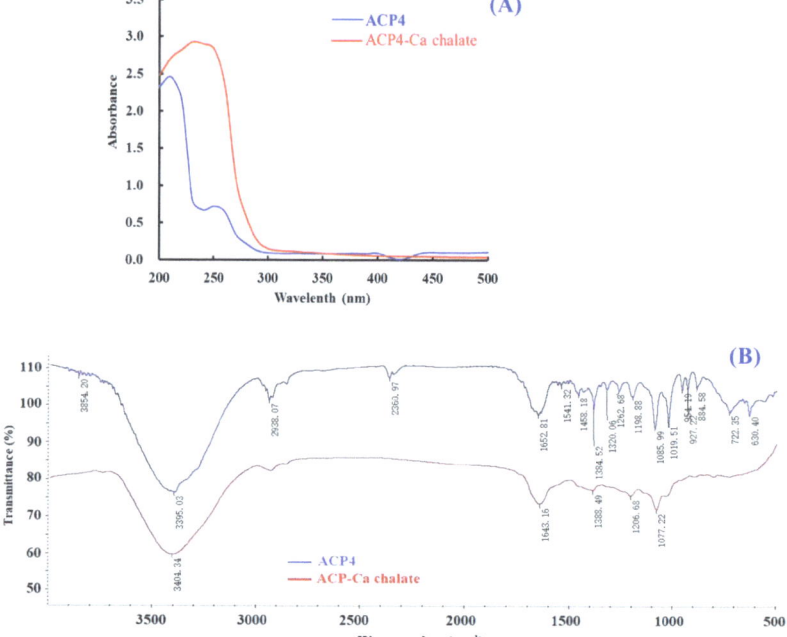

Figure 5. Characterizations of ACP4 (VERG) and VERG-Ca chelate. (**A**) UV spectra of ACP4 (VERG) and VERG-Ca chelate in the regions from 200 to 500 nm. (**B**) FTIR spectra of ACP4 (VERG) and VERG-Ca in the 4000 to 500 cm^{-1}.

2.5.2. FTIR Spectroscopy

FTIR spectroscopy is a crucial method for the research of the structural features of peptide-Ca chelates and can effectively reflect the mutual effect between peptides' ligands and Ca^{2+} during the chelating process [51]. The peptides' chelating sites with Ca^{2+} are primarily amide bonds (-CONH-) between amino acid residues and carboxyl (-COOH) and amino (-NH$_2$) groups [55]. Then, the absorption peaks, such as stretching vibration of -NH$_2$ and –COOH, are sure to shift if peptides chelate with Ca. The amide A band was attributed to the stretching vibration of the N-H bond. Figure 5B showed that the wavenumber moved from 3395.03 to 3404.34 cm^{-1} probably because of the stretching and substitution of hydrogen bonds in the VERG-Ca chelate, which manifested the participation of N–H bonds in the formation of chelate. The wavenumber (1700–1600 cm^{-1}) of the amide-I band caused by C=O stretching vibration was moved from 1643.16 to 1652.81 cm^{-1}, which indicates infrared absorption of the C=O caused by the antisymmetric stretching vibration of carboxylic acid ions. The wavenumber (1384.52 cm^{-1}) for –COO– moved to a lower frequency (1388.49 cm^{-1}) in the spectrum of the bound peptide and showed that –COOH probably bound Ca^{2+} and turned into –COO–Ca. These results were in line with the report of [55]. Based on these findings, we hypothesized that the N–H, C=O, and –COOH took responsibility for the chelation between ACP4 (VERG) and Ca^{2+}.

2.5.3. Scanning Electron Microscope (SEM)

The microstructures of ACP4 (A) and the VERG-Ca chelate (B) are displayed in Figure 6. The surface of ACP4 (VERG) is smooth. However, the surface of the VERG-Ca chelate was rougher and looser and had many irregular strips and granular aggregates. The significant difference in microstructure between ACP4 (VERG) and the VERG-Ca chelate might be caused by the interactions that ACP4 (VERG) reacted with Ca^{2+}, leading to damage to the smooth structure of the ACP4 (VERG) surface. Additionally, –COOH and –NH$_2$ in ACP4 (VERG) bound to Ca^{2+} and formed a "bridging role", which could also change the physicochemical characteristics of ACP4 (VERG) [51].

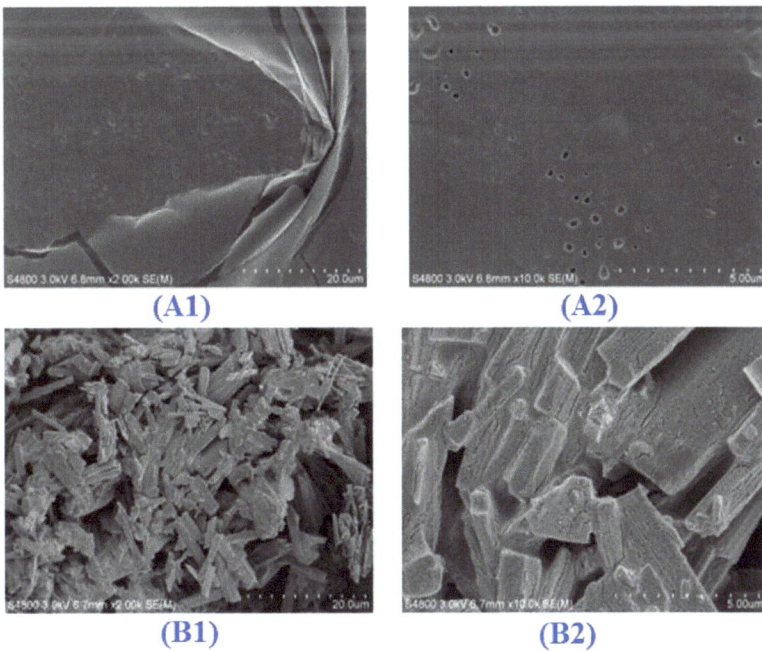

Figure 6. Scanning electron microscopy analysis of ACP4 (VERG) and VERG-Ca chelate. (**A1**) ACP4 ($\times$500); (**A2**) ($\times$2000); (**B1**) VERG-Ca ($\times$500); and (**B2**) VERG-Ca ($\times$2000).

2.6. Stability Analysis of VERG-Ca Chelate

The acid environment and protease in the gastrointestinal system could cause Ca release to generate Ca(OH)$_2$ and insoluble precipitation, leading to low bioavailability of Ca. Therefore, we studied the stability of the VERG-Ca chelate in a simulated digestive tract environment (Figure 7). Compared with the control, the Ca-retention rates of the VERG-Ca chelate in gastric juice, intestinal juice, and gastric+intestinal juice decrease to 18.72 $\pm$ 1.25% ($p < 0.001$), 95.67 $\pm$ 3.26% ($p > 0.05$), and 87.21 $\pm$ 2.73% ($p < 0.05$), respectively. In addition, the Ca-retention rate of the VERG-Ca chelate in intestinal juice is significantly higher than that of gastric juice ($p < 0.001$). The finding indicated that the gastric environment significantly reduced the stability of the VERG-Ca chelate. It is worth noting that the Ca-retention rate of the VERG-Ca chelate in gastric+intestinal juice is significantly higher than that of gastric juice ($p < 0.001$) but was not much different from that of the intestinal group. The result indicated that pepsin could lead to the partial degradation of the chelate, except for the effect of pH. Cui et al. [62] and Zhang et al. [31] reported that the main reason for Ca^{2+} release in the gastrointestinal system was pH change, and the weak alkaline environment of the intestines could induce the rechelation of peptides with Ca^{2+}. Our present finding in the gastric + intestinal juice group was in agreement with these literature studies. Therefore, gastric digestion is the key reason causing Ca to be released from the VERG-Ca chelate, but intestinal digestion had no remarkable effect on the stability of the VERG-Ca chelate. In general, most VERG-Ca chelates can remain stable in gastrointestinal digestion, which might prominently improve the bioavailability of Ca in the digestive tract environment.

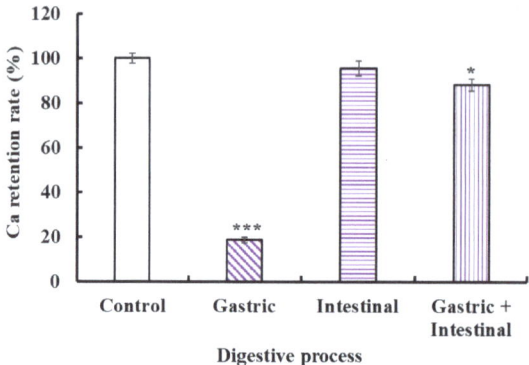

Figure 7. Stability of VERG-Ca chelate in simulated digestive tract environment. * $p < 0.05$ and *** $p < 0.001$ vs. Control.

2.7. Transport of VERG-Ca Chelate across the Caco-2 Cell Monolayer

Human intestinal epithelial cells modeled in vitro using Caco-2 cells have been applied to study the simulative absorption of minerals, medicines, and peptides [46]. In this study, the effects of the VERG-Ca chelate on the viability of Caco-2 cells were measured by the MTT assay (Figure 8A). Compared with the control group, ACP4 (VERG) and the VERG-Ca chelate had no significant effect on cell viability at 50–200 μM, but they could significantly decrease the viability of Caco-2 cells at 250 μM ($p < 0.05$). The finding manifested that ACP4 (VERG) and the VERG-Ca chelate were nontoxic at concentrations of 50–200 μM. Therefore, the following experiment can be carried out in the concentration range of 0–200 μM.

Figure 8B shows the activity changes in alkaline phosphatase of Caco-2 cells' monolayer membrane at 0–21 days. When Caco-2 cells were cultured to day 21, the activity of alkaline phosphatase on the apical side was 25.02 ± 1.32 U/L, which was 3.48-fold of that on the basolateral side (7.18 ± 0.63 U/L), indicating that Caco-2 cells completed the polar differentiation of the monolayer membrane. In addition, the change in TEER values of the Caco-2 cell monolayer within incubation time (1–21 days) was measured to create monolayers of Caco-2 cells with enterocyte architecture (Figure 8C). The results indicated that the TEER value gradually increased with the extension of incubation time, and the TEER exceeded 300 Ω cm^2 at 21 days. Therefore, the Caco-2 cell monolayer model was applied to evaluate the influence of the VERG-Ca chelate on Ca transport activity.

The effect of the VERG-Ca chelate on Ca transport in Caco-2 cell monolayers is presented in Figure 8D. The Ca transport of the VERG-Ca chelate increased with the incubation time. Compared with the CaCl$_2$ group, VERG-Ca chelate-treated groups did not display remarkable Ca transport capability in Caco-2 cell monolayers from 30 to 60 min ($p < 0.05$). However, the Ca transport improved dramatically in the presence of the VERG-Ca chelate at 120 and 180 min, and the quantity of Ca of transport reached 3.63 ± 0.27 and 5.11 ± 0.26 μg/mg protein at 120 and 180 min, which were 1.70 and 1.72 times of the CaCl$_2$ group, respectively. Previous literature studies indicated that Ca-chelating peptides, including VLPVPQK [54], EYG [42], and FPPDVA [51], could greatly improve the Ca transport across Caco-2 cell monolayers. The present findings demonstrated that the Ca transport and absorption in Caco-2 cell monolayers could be increased by the VERG-Ca chelate.

Plant-based diets are rich in bioactive compounds, but some compounds, such as vitamins, tannins, phytates, and dietary fibers (DFs), can significantly influence the bioavailability of some minerals, especially Ca [63]. Therefore, the effects of vitamin D and phytate on the absorption of Ca derived from CaCl$_2$ and VERG-Ca chelates were evaluated. Figure 8E indicated that the absorption amount of Ca significantly increased from 0 to 180 min after adding CaCl$_2$ and vitamin D3 together, and the absorption amount of Ca increased from 2.96 ± 0.28 to 5.14 ± 0.23 µg/mg protein at 180 min, indicating that vitamin D3 can promote Ca uptake by regulating the transcellular pathway of Ca^{2+}. In addition, the absorption amount of Ca significantly increased from 4.03 ± 0.27 to 4.44 ± 0.29 µg/mg protein at 120 min after adding VERG-Ca chelates and vitamin D3 together, and the absorption amount of Ca only increased from 5.11 ± 0.36 to 5.43 ± 0.43 µg/mg protein at 180 min, and no significant difference was observed. Therefore, it could be speculated that the vitamin D3 in food has no significant effect on intestinal absorption of Ca derived from VERG-Ca chelates but can significantly promote the absorption of inorganic Ca.

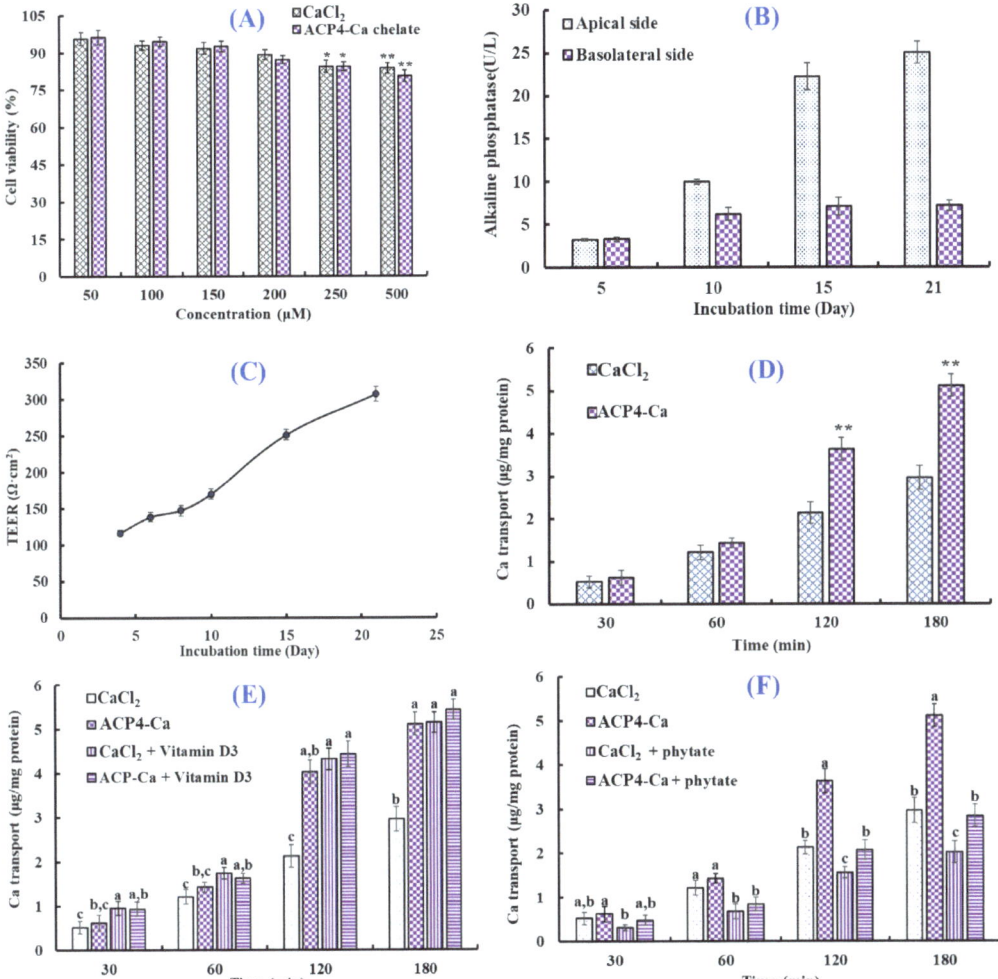

Figure 8. Transport of VERG-Ca chelate. (**A**) Cytotoxicity of VERG-Ca chelate in Caco-2 cells evaluated by the MTT assay. * $p < 0.0$ and ** $p < 0.01$ vs. control group. (**B**) Alkaline phosphatase activities on the apical and basolateral sides of the Caco-2 cell monolayer. (**C**) Transepithelial electrical resistance (TEER) of the Caco-2 cell monolayer. (**D**) Ca transport activity of VERG-Ca chelate. ** $p < 0.01$ vs. $CaCl_2$ group at same concentration. (**E**) Effects of vitamin D3 on the transmembrane transport of $CaCl_2$ and VERG-Ca chelate. (**F**) Effects of phytate on the transmembrane transport of $CaCl_2$ and VERG-Ca chelate. a–c Values with same letters at same time indicate no significant difference ($p > 0.05$).

Figure 8F showed that the absorption amount of Ca decreased significantly at 0~180 min after adding phytate with $CaCl_2$ or a VERG-Ca chelate. At 180 min, the absorption amount of Ca derived from $CaCl_2$ decreased from 2.96 ± 0.28 to 2.02 ± 0.24 µg/mg protein. The absorption amount of Ca derived from the VERG-Ca chelate decreased from 3.63 ± 0.35% to 2.842 ± 0.348 µg/mg protein. The data indicated that phytate could significantly reduce the absorption amount of Ca derived from $CaCl_2$ or the VERG-Ca chelate in Caco-2 cells, which was in agreement with the report by Amalraj and Pius [63] that Ca bioavailability in green leafy vegetables was negatively correlated with those anti-nutritional factors, such as dietary fiber, phytate, oxalate, and tannin.

3. Materials and Methods

3.1. Chemicals and Reagents

Antarctic krill was provided by Zhejiang Hailisheng Biotechnology Co., Ltd. (Zhoushan, China). Triethanolamine, trypsin, and Hanks' Balanced Salt Solution (HBSS) were purchased from Sigma-Aldrich (Shanghai) Co., Ltd. (Shanghai, China). Methanol, potassium hydroxide, hydrochloric acid, sodium chloride, ferrous sulfate, calcium indicator, and sodium cyanide were purchased from Sinopharm Chemical Reagent Co., Ltd. (Shanghai, China). The peptides (ACP1-ACP14) with purity higher than 98% were synthesized by Shanghai Apeptide Co., Ltd. (Shanghai, China).

3.2. Preparation of Protein Hydrolysate of Antarctic Krill

3.2.1. Screening of Protease Species

The degreasing process of Antarctic krill was performed using the described method by Zhao et al. [46]. Defatted Antarctic krill powders were dispersed in distilled water (DW) (10%, w/v) and separately hydrolyzed using different proteases (Table 1). After that, the hydrolysis reaction was stopped at 95 °C for 15 min and centrifuged at $9000 \times g$ at −4 °C for 20 min. The resulting supernatants were lyophilized and stored at −20 °C. The hydrolysate prepared by trypsin displayed the strongest Ca-chelating rate and was named AKH.

3.2.2. Optimization of the Chelating Conditions of Ca with AKH

Firstly, the chelating conditions of Ca with AKH were optimized by a single-factor experiment using Ca-chelating rate as the indicator. The chelating time (30, 40, 50, and 60 min), temperature (30, 40, 50, and 60 °C), pH (6, 7, 8, and 9), and peptide/Ca ratio (1:5, 1:10, 1:15 and 1:20) were chosen for the present investigation.

According to the results of single-factor experiment, orthogonal experiment was employed to estimate the influence of chelating time (40, 50, and 60 min), temperature (40, 50, and 60 °C), pH (7, 8, and 9), and peptide/Ca ratio (1:5, 1:10 and 1:15) on the Ca-chelating rate of AKH.

3.2.3. Preparation of Peptide-Ca Chelates and Determination of Ca-Chelating Rate

Peptide-Ca chelates were prepared in accordance with the previous method [5]. The lyophilized AKH, AKH fractions, and peptides were separately dissolved in DW, and $CaCl_2$ was added to the prepared solution (50 mg/mL) with designed peptide/$CaCl_2$ ratios of 1:5–1:25 (w/w). The pH of the reaction mixtures was adjusted to pH 8.0. Then, the solution was put in a water bath shaker to incubate at 50 °C and 80 r/min for 50 min. Finally, the chelates were precipitated for 4 h by adding 5 times the volume of the solution of anhydrous ethanol. After that, the solution was centrifuged at $6000 \times g$ for 15 min, and the precipitation was collected, lyophilized, and stored at −20 °C. The Ca content in the supernatant was measured by EDTA complexion titration (ECT) [59], which was denoted as C2 (g/mL). The total Ca content in mixed solution was measured by ECT assay, which was denoted as C1 (g/mL). The Ca-chelating rate was calculated as follows:

$$\text{Ca-chelating rate (\%)} = (C1 - C2/C1) \times 100\%.$$

3.2.4. Separation Process of Ca-Chelating Peptides from AKH

AKH was ultra-filtrated by 4 kinds of ultrafiltration membranes, including 1, 3.5, 5, and 10 kDa. Then, five peptide components, including AKH-1 (MW > 10 kDa), AKH-2 (5–10 kDa), AKH-3 (3.5–5 kDa), AKH-4 (1–3.5 kDa), and AKH-5 (MW < 1 kDa), were collected, concentrated, and freeze-dried, and their Ca-chelating rates were measured using the above method in Section 3.2.3.

AKH-5 (10 mL, 50.0 mg/mL) was added into a pre-equilibrated DEAE-52 cellulose column (3.8 × 150 cm) and eluted by DW, 0.10, 0.25, 0.50, 0.75, and 1.0 M NaCl solution, respectively. The flow rate of eluate was set as 3.0 mL/min. Then, three fractions (AKH-5a, AKH-5b, and AKH-5c) were separated according to the DEAE-52 cellulose chromatography of eluted peptide fractions (9 mL) at 280 nm.

AKH-5a (5 mL, 50.0 mg/mL) was loaded into a Sephadex G-25 column (2.6 cm × 120 cm) and eluted using DW. The flow rate of eluate was set as 0.6 mL/min, and the eluent was collected every 3 min. Finally, four fractions (AKH-5a-1 to AKH-5a-4) were isolated from AKH-5a and collected in accordance with the chromatographic peaks at 280 nm.

AKH-5a-2 solution was decontaminated through a 0.22 μM microporous membrane and further isolated by an RP-HPLC column of Zorbax, SB C-18 (4.6 × 250 mm, 5 μm). In brief, AKH-5a-2 was loaded into the RP-HPLC column and eluted by a linear gradient of acetonitrile with a flow rate of 1.0 mL/min. The concentration ranged from 0 to 50% in 0 to 25 min, and the eluent was monitored at 280 nm. Finally, fourteen Ca-chelating peptides (ACP1 to ACP14) were prepared according to their chromatographic peaks. The flow diagram of separation process of Ca-chelating peptides from AKH is presented in Figure 9.

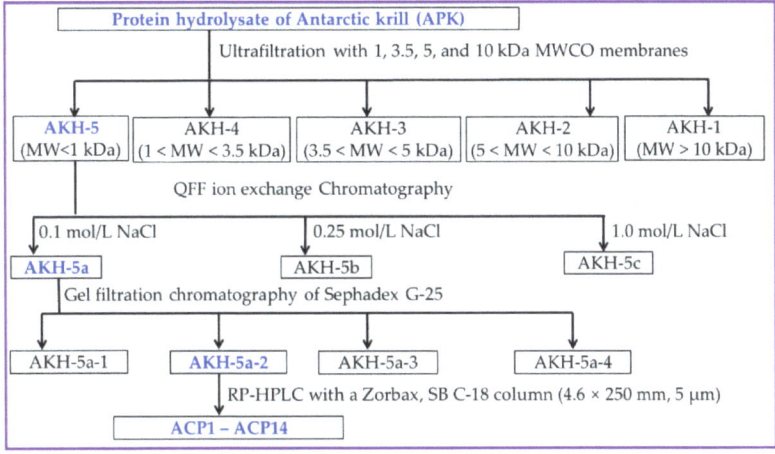

Figure 9. The flow diagram of separation process of Ca-chelating peptides from AKH.

3.3. Identification of Peptides (ACP1 to ACP14) from AKH

The amino acid sequence and molecular weight of EP1-EP6 were determined according to previous methods described by Chi et al. [64]. The amino acid sequences of ACP1 to ACP14 were measured by a 494 protein sequencer from Applied Biosystems (Perkin Elmer Co. Ltd. Foster City, CA, USA), and Edman degradation was performed according to the standard program supplied by Applied Biosystems. The MWs of ACP1 to ACP14 were determined by a Q-TOF mass spectrometer with an ESI source (Micromass, Waters, Milford, MA, USA).

3.4. Characterization of VERG-Ca Chelate

The preparation of a hydrolysate of PSC-M was carried out in accordance with the previous method [34,42]. The dispersions (1%, w/v) of ASC-M and PSC-M were separately degraded with alcalase (55 °C, pH 8.5, 4 h), neutrase (55 °C, pH 7.0, 4 H), and a double-enzyme system (alcalase (2 h) + neutrase (2 h)). The enzyme dose was designed as 2% (w/w). After the hydrolysis reaction, the proteases in the hydrolysate solution were inactivated in boiling water for 10 min. The prepared hydrolysates were centrifuged at 9000× g for 25 min, and the supernatants were freeze-dried and had their ACEi abilities detected. The hydrolysate of PSC-M generated via the double-enzyme system displayed the highest ACEi ability value and was named PSC-MH.

3.4.1. UV Absorption Spectroscopy Analysis

The UV spectra of ACP4 and VERG-Ca chelate at 1.0 mg/mL were recorded in the wavelength range of 200–500 nm by a UV-1800 spectrophotometer (Mapada Instruments Co., Ltd., Shanghai, China).

3.4.2. FTIR Spectroscopy Analysis

The FTIR spectra (4000 to 400 cm^{-1}) of ACP4 and VERG-Ca chelate were recorded in KBr disks using a Nicolet 6700 FTIR spectrophotometer [65]. Dry ACP4 or VERG-Ca chelate was uniformly ground with dry KBr at a sample/KBr ratio of 1:100 (w/w) and extruded into a transparent sheet for spectrum recording.

3.4.3. Scanning Electron Microscopy (SEM) Analysis

A suitable amount of ACP4 and VERG-Ca chelate was uniformly applied to the sample plate and sprayed with a gold plating film. Finally, the samples with a gold plating film were observed and photographed by a scanning electron microscope of JEOL JSM-6390LV (Tokyo, Japan).

3.5. Stability Analysis of VERG-Ca Chelate against Simulated Gastrointestinal Digestion

The stability of VERG-Ca chelate against simulated gastrointestinal digestion was assessed using the method described by Zhang et al. [31]. The VERG-Ca chelate solution (10 mg/mL) dissolved in DW was used in the assay. The pH values of the artificial simulation of gastric juice and intestinal juice were adjusted to 2.0 and 7.5, respectively. The stability of VERG-Ca chelate against in vitro gastric juice (2 h), intestinal juice (2 h), and gastric juice (2 h) + intestinal juice (2 h) were determined at 37 °C, respectively. Finally, the solution was heated at 100 °C for 15 min to terminate the reaction. The stability was expressed as Ca-retention rate of VERG-Ca chelate after in vitro digestion.

Ca-retention rate (%) = (Ca content in treatment group/Ca content in control group) × 100

3.6. Ca Transport Effect of VERG-Ca Chelate in Caco-2 Cell Monolayers

3.6.1. Culture of Caco-2 Cells and Establishment of Caco-2 Cell Monolayer Model

Caco-2 cells were obtained from the Shanghai Institute of Cell Biology (Shanghai, China) and cultured in EMEM with 10% fetal bovine serum, 1% antibiotic, and 1% nonessential amino acids in a humidified incubator at 37 °C with 5% CO_2. The cell culture medium was replaced every two days with a new medium of equal volume. The Caco-2 cells were dispersed using trypsin-EDTA when they covered approximately 90% of the flask and were seeded on 6-well transwell culture plates with polyester membranes. The medium was replaced every other day with a new medium of equal volume. After being cultured for 21 days, the transepithelial electrical resistance (TEER) was determined to confirm the integrity of the Caco-2 cell monolayers. The Caco-2 cell monolayers were used for Ca transport experiments when the TEER exceeded 300 Ω·cm^2 [60,66].

In addition, the alkaline phosphatase activity was determined using assay kits in accordance with the instructions of Nanjing Jiancheng Bioengineering Institute (Nanjing, China).

3.6.2. Cytotoxicity Assay

Cell cytotoxicity was determined using the MTT assay [60]. After being cultured for 24 h, the Caco-2 cells were further treated for 24 h using a 100 µL medium containing VERG-Ca chelate with concentrations of 50, 100, 150, 200, and 500 µM, respectively. Then, MTT solution (100 µL) was added per well and incubated for an additional 4 h. The MTT solution per well was replaced by an equal volume of DMSO solution to solubilize. Finally, the absorbance of the sample solution at 570 nm was measured.

3.6.3. Ca Transport Analysis

The Ca transport in the Caco-2 cell monolayer model was analyzed using previous methods [51,60]. After 21 days of incubation, the culture medium of Caco-2 cells was discarded from each well, and monolayers were immediately washed with HBSS buffer (without Ca and magnesium) two times. The Caco-2 cell monolayers were transferred to a new 6-well culture plate containing 2 mL of HBSS buffer, and 2 mL of HBSS buffer was also added to the apical side. After incubating for 30 min, the HBSS on the apical side was replaced with 2 mL of HBSS containing VERG-Ca chelate (200 µM) or Ca (150 µg/mL), and the HBSS on the basolateral side was replaced with an equal volume of fresh HBSS buffer. After incubation for 2 h, 1 mL of HBSS in the basolateral side was removed to determine Ca content at the designed time (30, 60,120, and 180 min). At the same time, fresh HBSS buffer (1 mL) was added to the basolateral side to maintain a constant volume. The content of Ca was determined by atomic absorption spectrometry using HNO_3 and $HClO_4$ as the oxidizers.

In the experiments on the effects of vitamin D3 and phytate on Ca absorption, dietary factors (vitamin D3 and phytate) were first premixed with VERG-Ca chelate or $CaCl_2$, respectively, at a mass ratio of 1:1. The experiment conditions and operation method were as described in the Ca transport analysis above.

3.7. Statistical Analysis

The experimental data were represented by the mean ± standard deviation (SD, $n = 3$). GraphPad Prism (version 8.02) was used for one-way analysis of variance, and Tukey's multiple comparison tests were used to test for differences between groups ($p < 0.05$).

4. Conclusions

In brief, fourteen Ca-chelating peptides were purified and identified from the trypsin hydrolysate of Antarctic krill proteins, and ACP4 (VERG) presented the highest Ca-chelating ability among isolated Ca-chelating peptides. UV, FTIR, and SEM analysis showed N-H, C=O, and -COOH in ACP4 (VERG) should take responsibility for the chelation of ACP4 (VERG) with Ca^{2+}. Moreover, VERG-Ca chelate is stable in gastrointestinal digestion and could significantly improve Ca transport in Caco-2 cell monolayer experiments, but phytate could significantly reduce the absorption of Ca derived from VERG-Ca chelate. The present results suggested that Ca-chelating peptides derived from Antarctic krill proteins could serve as functional ingredients in healthy food to promote Ca bioavailability. However, the absorption and transport mechanisms of VERG-Ca chelate in vivo need to be further elucidated.

Author Contributions: M.-X.G. and R.-P.C.: data curation, validation, and writing—original draft. Y.-M.W. and L.Z.: investigation, methodology, and writing—original draft. C.-F.C.: funding acquisition, resources, supervision, and writing—review and editing. B.W.: conceptualization, funding acquisition, resources, supervision, and writing—review and editing. All authors have read and agreed to the published version of the manuscript.

Funding: This work was funded by the National Natural Science Foundation of China (No. 82073764), the Ten-thousand Talents Plan of Zhejiang Province (No. 2019R52026), and the Innovation and Entrepreneurship Training Program for College Students of China (No. 202210340034).

Institutional Review Board Statement: Not applicable.

Informed Consent Statement: Not applicable.

Data Availability Statement: Data are contained within the article.

Acknowledgments: The authors thank Zhao-Hui Li at the Beijing Agricultural Biological Testing Center for his technical support on the amino acid sequence and observed mass of antioxidant peptides from Antarctic Krill.

Conflicts of Interest: The authors declare no conflict of interest.

References

1. Tian, Q.J.; Fan, Y.; Hao, L.; Wang, J.; Xia, C.S.; Hou, H. A comprehensive review of calcium and ferrous ions chelating peptides: Preparation, structure and transport pathways. *Crit. Rev. Food Sci. Nutr.* **2023**, *63*, 4418–4430. [CrossRef]
2. Luo, J.Q.; Zhou, Z.S.; Yao, X.T.; Fu, Y. Mineral-chelating peptides derived from fish collagen: Preparation, bioactivity and bioavailability. *LWT* **2020**, *134*, 110209. [CrossRef]
3. Qu, W.J.; Li, Y.H.; Xiong, T.; Feng, Y.H.; Ma, H.L.; Akpabli-Tsigbe, N.D.K. Calcium-chelating improved zein peptide stability, cellular uptake, and bioactivity by influencing the structural characterization. *Food Res. Int.* **2022**, *162*, 112033. [CrossRef] [PubMed]
4. Wang, X.; Gao, A.; Chen, Y.; Zhang, X.Y.; Li, S.H.; Chen, Y. Preparation of cucumber seed peptide-calcium chelate by liquid state fermentation and its characterization. *Food Chem.* **2017**, *229*, 487–494. [CrossRef]
5. Zhang, H.R.; Zhao, L.Y.; Shen, Q.S.; Qi, L.W.; Jiang, S.; Richel, A. Preparation of cattle bone collagen peptides-calcium chelate and its structural characterization and stability. *LWT* **2021**, *144*, 111264. [CrossRef]
6. Balk, E.M.; Adam, G.P.; Langberg, V.N.; Earley, A.; Clark, P.; Ebeling, P.R. Global dietary calcium intake among adults: A systematic review. *Osteoporos. Int.* **2017**, *28*, 3315–3324. [CrossRef]
7. Wang, G.; Liu, L.J.; Wang, Z.P.; Pei, X.; Tao, W.J.; Ao, T.Y. Comparison of inorganic and organically bound trace minerals on tissue mineral deposition and fecal excretion in broiler breeders. *Biol. Trace Elem. Res.* **2019**, *189*, 224–232. [CrossRef] [PubMed]
8. Caetano-Silva, M.E.; Netto, F.M.; Bertoldo-Pacheco, M.T.; Alegria, A.; Cilla, A. Peptide-metal complexes: Obtention and role in increasing bioavailability and decreasing the pro-oxidant effect of minerals. *Crit. Rev. Food Sci. Nutr.* **2020**, *61*, 1470–1489. [CrossRef] [PubMed]
9. He, S.; Zhao, W.; Chen, X.; Li, J.; Zhang, L.; Jin, H. Ameliorative Effects of Peptide Phe-Leu-Ala-Pro on Acute Liver and Kidney Injury Caused by CCl4 via Attenuation of Oxidative Stress and Inflammation. *ACS Omega* **2022**, *7*, 44796–44803. [CrossRef] [PubMed]
10. Zhang, S.Y.; Zhao, Y.Q.; Wang, Y.M.; Yang, X.R.; Chi, C.F.; Wang, B. Gelatins and antioxidant peptides from Skipjack tuna (*Katsuwonus pelamis*) skins: Purification, characterization, and cytoprotection on ultraviolet-A injured human skin fibroblasts. *Food Biosci.* **2022**, *50*, 102138. [CrossRef]
11. López-Medina, J.A.; López-Rodriguez, C.; Estornell-Gualde, M.A.; Rey-Fernández, L.; Gómez-Senent, S.; Ballesteros-Pomar, M.D. Relationship between nutritional treatment compliance and nutritional status improvements in patients with gastrointestinal impairment taking an oral peptide-based supplement. *Nutrition* **2022**, *102*, 111734. [CrossRef] [PubMed]
12. Rivero-Pino, F. Bioactive food-derived peptides for functional nutrition: Effect of fortification, processing and storage on peptide stability and bioactivity within food matrices. *Food Chem.* **2023**, *406*, 135046. [CrossRef] [PubMed]
13. Li, J.; Li, Y.; Lin, S.; Zhao, W.; Chen, Y.; Jin, H. Collagen peptides from Acaudina molpadioides prevent CCl4-induced liver injury via Keap1/Nrf2-ARE, PI3K/AKT, and MAPKs pathways. *J. Food Sci.* **2022**, *87*, 2185–2196. [CrossRef] [PubMed]
14. Zheng, S.L.; Wang, Y.Z.; Zhao, Y.Q.; Chi, C.F.; Zhu, W.Y.; Wang, B. High Fischer ratio oligopeptides from hard-shelled mussel: Preparation and hepatoprotective effect against acetaminophen-induced liver injury in mice. *Food Biosci.* **2023**, *53*, 102638. [CrossRef]
15. Wu, M.-F.; Xi, Q.-H.; Sheng, Y.; Wang, Y.-M.; Wang, W.-Y.; Chi, C.-F.; Wang, B. Antioxidant peptides from monkfish swim bladders: Ameliorating NAFLD in vitro by suppressing lipid accumulation and oxidative stress via regulating AMPK/Nrf2 pathway. *Mar. Drugs* **2023**, *21*, 360. [CrossRef]
16. Ren, Z.; Yang, F.; Yao, S.; Bi, L.; Jiang, G.; Huang, J.; Tang, Y. Effects of low molecular weight peptides from monkfish (Lophius litulon) roe on immune response in immunosuppressed mice. *Front. Nutr.* **2022**, *9*, 929105. [CrossRef] [PubMed]
17. Kong, J.; Hu, X.-M.; Cai, W.-W.; Wang, Y.-M.; Chi, C.-F.; Wang, B. Bioactive Peptides from Skipjack Tuna Cardiac Arterial Bulbs (II): Protective Function on UVB-Irradiated HaCaT Cells through Antioxidant and Anti-Apoptotic Mechanisms. *Mar. Drugs* **2023**, *21*, 105. [CrossRef]
18. Wu, X.P.; Wang, F.F.; Cai, X.X.; Wang, S.Y. Characteristics and osteogenic mechanism of glycosylated peptides-calcium chelate. *Curr. Res. Food Sci.* **2022**, *5*, 1965–1975. [CrossRef]
19. Miao, J.Y.; Liao, W.W.; Pan, Z.Y.; Wang, Q.; Duan, S.; Cao, Y. Isolation and identification of iron-chelating peptides from casein hydrolysates. *Food Funct.* **2019**, *10*, 2372–2381. [CrossRef]
20. Budseekoad, S.; Yupanqui, C.T.; Sirinupong, N.; Alashi, A.M.; Aluko, R.E.; Youravong, W. Structural and functional characterization of calcium and iron-binding peptides from mung bean protein hydrolysate. *J. Funct. Foods* **2018**, *49*, 333–341. [CrossRef]

21. Zhang, K.; Li, J.W.; Hou, H.; Zhang, H.W.; Li, B.F. Purification and characterization of a novel calcium-biding decapeptide from Pacific cod (*Gadus Macrocephalus*) bone: Molecular properties and calcium chelating modes. *J. Funct. Foods* **2019**, *52*, 670–679. [CrossRef]
22. Ke, H.L.; Ma, R.J.; Liu, X.U.; Xie, Y.P.; Chen, J.F. Highly effective peptide-calcium chelate prepared from aquatic products processing wastes: Stickwater and oyster shells. *LWT* **2022**, *168*, 113947. [CrossRef]
23. El Hajj, S.; Irankunda, R.; Camaño Echavarría, J.A.; Arnoux, P.; Paris, C.; Canabady-Rochelle, L. Metal-chelating activity of soy and pea protein hydrolysates obtained after different enzymatic treatments from protein isolates. *Food Chem.* **2023**, *405 Pt A*, 134788. [CrossRef]
24. Lan, C.; Zhao, Y.Q.; Li, X.R.; Wang, B. High Fischer ratio oligopeptides determination from Antartic krill: Preparation, peptides profiles, and in vitro antioxidant activity. *J. Food Biochem.* **2019**, *43*, e12827. [CrossRef] [PubMed]
25. Yue, H.; Li, Y.Q.; Cai, W.Z.; Bai, X.L.; Dong, P.; Wang, J.F. Antarctic krill peptide alleviates liver fibrosis via downregulating the secondary bile acid mediated NLRP3 signaling pathway. *Food Funct.* **2022**, *13*, 7740–7749. [CrossRef]
26. Ding, J.; Zhu, C.Y.; Jiang, P.F.; Qi, L.B.; Sun, N.K.; Lin, S.Y. Antarctic krill antioxidant peptides show inferior IgE-binding ability and RBL-2H3 cell degranulation. *Food Sci. Hum. Well.* **2023**, *12*, 1772–1778. [CrossRef]
27. Yao, M.K.; Gai, X.L.; Zhang, M.S.; Liu, X.; Cui, T.T.; Jia, A.R. Two proteins prepared from defatted Antarctic krill (*Euphausia superba*) powder: Composition, structure and functional properties. *Food Hydrocoll.* **2023**, *145*, 109009. [CrossRef]
28. Han, L.H.; Mao, X.Z.; Wang, K.; Li, Y.Y.; Zhao, M.H.; Xue, C.H. Phosphorylated peptides from Antarctic krill (*Euphausia superba*) ameliorated osteoporosis by activation of osteogenesis-related MAPKs and PI3K/AKT/GSK-3β pathways in dexamethasone-treated mice. *J. Funct. Foods* **2018**, *47*, 447–456. [CrossRef]
29. Fernando, I.P.S.; Park, S.Y.; Han, E.J.; Kim, H.S.; Kang, D.S.; Ahn, G. Isolation of an antioxidant peptide from krill protein hydrolysates as a novel agent with potential hepatoprotective effects. *J. Funct. Foods* **2020**, *67*, 103889. [CrossRef]
30. Wang, Y.Z.; Zhao, Y.Q.; Wang, Y.M.; Zhao, W.H.; Wang, P.; Wang, B. Antioxidant peptides from Antarctic krill (*Euphausia superba*) hydrolysate: Preparation, identification and cytoprotection on H_2O_2-induced oxidative stress. *J. Funct Foods* **2021**, *86*, 104701. [CrossRef]
31. Wang, M.; Zhang, L.; Yue, H.; Cai, W.; Yin, H.; Tian, Y.; Dong, P.; Wang, J. Peptides from Antarctic krill (Euphausia superba) ameliorate acute liver injury in mice induced by carbon tetrachloride via activating the Nrf2/HO-1 pathway. *Food Funct.* **2023**, *14*, 3526–3537. [CrossRef]
32. Hou, H.; Wang, S.K.; Zhu, X.; Li, Q.K.; Fan, Y.; Cheng, D.; Li, B.F. A novel calcium-binding peptide from Antarctic krill protein hydrolysates and identification of binding sites of calcium-peptide complex. *Food Chem.* **2018**, *243*, 389–395. [CrossRef]
33. Hu, S.; Lin, S.; Liu, Y.; He, X.; Zhang, S.; Sun, N. Exploration of iron-binding mode, digestion Kinetics, and iron absorption behavior of Antarctic Krill-derived heptapeptide-iron complex. *Food Res. Int.* **2022**, *154*, 110996. [CrossRef]
34. Zheng, J.R.; Gao, Y.H.; Ding, J.; Sun, N.; Lin, S.Y. Antarctic krill peptides improve scopolamine-induced memory impairment in mice. *Food Biosci.* **2022**, *49*, 101987. [CrossRef]
35. Ji, W.; Zhang, C.H.; Ji, H.W. Two novel bioactive peptides from Antarctic krill with dual angiotensin converting enzyme and dipeptidyl peptidase IV inhibitory activities. *J. Food Sci.* **2017**, *82*, 1742–1749. [CrossRef]
36. Qiao, Q.Q.; Luo, Q.B.; Suo, S.K.; Zhao, Y.Q.; Chi, C.F.; Wang, B. Preparation, characterization, and cytoprotective effects on HUVECs of fourteen novel angiotensin-I-converting enzyme inhibitory peptides from protein hydrolysate of tuna processing by-products. *Front. Nutr.* **2022**, *9*, 868681. [CrossRef]
37. Beaubier, S.; Durand, E.; Lenclume, C.; Fine, F.; Aymes, A.; Framboisier, X.; Kapel, R.; Villeneuve, P. Chelating peptides from rapeseed meal protein hydrolysates: Identification and evaluation of their capacity to inhibit lipid oxidation. *Food Chem.* **2023**, *422*, 136187. [CrossRef]
38. Hou, T.; Liu, Y.S.; Guo, D.J.; Li, B.; He, H. Collagen peptides from crucian skin improve calcium bioavailability and structural characterization by HPLC-ESI-MS/MS. *J. Agric. Food Chem.* **2017**, *65*, 8847–8854. [CrossRef]
39. Fan, C.Z.; Ge, X.F.; Hao, J.Y.; Wu, T.; Liu, R.; Zhang, M. Identification of high iron-chelating peptides with unusual antioxidant effect from sea cucumbers and the possible binding mode. *Food Chem.* **2023**, *399*, 133912. [CrossRef]
40. Sheng, Y.; Qiu, Y.T.; Wang, Y.M.; Chi, C.F.; Wang, B. Novel antioxidant collagen peptides of Siberian sturgeon (*Acipenserbaerii*) cartilages: The preparation, characterization, and cytoprotection of H_2O_2-damaged human umbilical vein endothelial cells (HUVECs). *Mar. Drugs* **2022**, *20*, 325. [CrossRef] [PubMed]
41. Hu, Y.-D.; Xi, Q.-H.; Kong, J.; Zhao, Y.-Q.; Chi, C.-F.; Wang, B. Angiotensin-I-converting enzyme (ACE)-inhibitory peptides from the collagens of monkfish (*Lophius litulon*) swim bladders: Isolation, characterization, molecular docking analysis and activity evaluation. *Mar. Drugs* **2023**, *21*, 516. [CrossRef]
42. Huang, G.R.; Ren, L.; Jiang, J.X. Purification of a histidine-containing peptide with calcium binding activity from shrimp processing byproducts hydrolysate. *Eur. Food Res. Technol.* **2011**, *232*, 281–287. [CrossRef]
43. Chi, C.F.; Wang, B.; Wang, Y.M.; Zhang, B.; Deng, S.G. Isolation and characterization of three antioxidant peptides from protein hydrolysate of bluefin leatherjacket (*Navodon septentrionalis*) heads. *J. Funct. Foods* **2015**, *12*, 1–10. [CrossRef]
44. Reddy, I.M.; Mahoney, A.W. Solution visible difference spectral properties of Fe^{3+}-L-amino acid complexes at pH 6.70. *J. Agric. Food Chem.* **1995**, *43*, 1436–1443. [CrossRef]
45. Zhao, L.N.; Cai, X.X.; Huang, S.L.; Wang, S.Y.; Huang, Y.F.; Rao, P.F. Isolation and identification of a whey protein-sourced calcium-binding tripeptide Tyr-Asp-Thr. *Int. Dairy J.* **2015**, *40*, 16–23. [CrossRef]

46. Jin, H.X.; Xu, H.P.; Li, Y.; Zhang, Q.W.; Xie, H. Preparation and evaluation of peptides with potential antioxidant activity by microwave assisted enzymatic hydrolysis of collagen from sea cucumber Acaudina molpadioides obtained from Zhejiang Province in China. *Mar. Drugs.* **2019**, *17*, 169. [CrossRef] [PubMed]
47. Cai, W.-W.; Hu, X.-M.; Wang, Y.-M.; Chi, C.-F.; Wang, B. Bioactive peptides from Skipjack tuna cardiac arterial bulbs: Preparation, identification, antioxidant activity, and stability against thermal, pH, and simulated gastrointestinal digestion treatments. *Mar. Drugs* **2022**, *20*, 626. [CrossRef] [PubMed]
48. Guo, L.; Harnedy, P.A.; O'Keeffe, M.B.; Zhang, L.; Li, B.; FitzGerald, R.J. Fractionation and identification of Alaska pollock skin collagen-derived mineral chelating peptides. *Food Chem.* **2015**, *173*, 536–542. [CrossRef]
49. Liu, B.T.; Zhuang, Y.L.; Sun, L.P. Identification and characterization of the peptides with calcium-binding capacity from tilapia (*Oreochromis niloticus*) skin gelatin enzymatic hydrolysates. *J. Food. Sci.* **2020**, *85*, 114–122.
50. Suo, S.K.; Zhao, Y.Q.; Wang, Y.M.; Pan, X.Y.; Chi, C.F.; Wang, B. Seventeen novel angiotensin converting enzyme (ACE) inhibitory peptides from the protein hydrolysate of *Mytilus edulis*: Isolation, identification, molecular docking study, and protective function on HUVECs. *Food Funct.* **2022**, *13*, 7831–7846. [CrossRef]
51. Wang, J.; Zhang, Y.X.; Huai, H.P.; Hou, W.Y.; Qi, Y.; Min, W.H. Purification, identification, chelation mechanism, and calcium absorption activity of a novel calcium-binding peptide from peanut (*Arachis hypogaea*) protein hydrolysate. *J. Agric. Food Chem.* **2023**, *71*, 11970–11981. [CrossRef]
52. Li, W.; Ye, S.; Zhang, Z.; Tang, J.; Jin, H.; Huang, F.; Yang, Z.; Tang, Y.; Chen, Y.; Ding, G.; et al. Purification and characterization of a novel pentadecapeptide from protein hydrolysates of *Cyclina sinensis* and its immunomodulatory effects on RAW264.7 cells. *Mar. Drugs* **2019**, *17*, 30. [CrossRef] [PubMed]
53. Yu, F.; Zhang, Z.; Luo, L.; Zhu, J.; Huang, F.; Yang, Z.; Tang, Y.; Ding, G. Identification and molecular docking study of a novel angiotensin-I converting enzyme inhibitory peptide derived from enzymatic hydrolysates of *Cyclina sinensis*. *Mar. Drugs* **2018**, *16*, 411. [CrossRef]
54. Liao, W.W.; Liu, S.J.; Liu, X.R.; Duan, S.; Xiao, S.Y.; Miao, J.Y. The purification, identification and bioactivity study of a novel calcium-binding peptide from casein hydrolysate. *Food Funct.* **2019**, *10*, 7724–7732. [CrossRef]
55. Zhang, X.W.; Jia, Q.; Li, M.Y.; Liu, H.P.; Wang, Q.; Liu, Z.T. Isolation of a novel calcium-binding peptide from phosvitin hydrolysates and the study of its calcium chelation mechanism. *Food Res. Int.* **2021**, *141*, 110169. [CrossRef]
56. He, S.; Xu, Z.; Li, J.; Guo, Y.; Lin, Q.; Jin, H. Peptides from *Harpadon nehereus* protect against hyperglycemia-induced HepG2 via oxidative stress and glycolipid metabolism regulation. *J. Funct. Foods* **2023**, *108*, 105723. [CrossRef]
57. Xu, B.; Ye, L.; Tang, Y.; Zheng, J.; Tian, X.; Yang, Y.; Yang, Z. Preparation and purification of an immunoregulatory peptide from Stolephorus chinensis of the East Sea of China. *Process Biochem.* **2020**, *98*, 151–159. [CrossRef]
58. Lee, S.; Song, K. Isolation of a calcium-binding peptide from enzymatic hydrolysates of porcine blood plasma protein. *J. Korean Soc. Appl. Biol. Chem.* **2009**, *52*, 290–294. [CrossRef]
59. Liu, F.R.; Wang, L.; Wang, R.; Chen, Z.X. Calcium-binding capacity of wheat germ protein hydrolysate and characterization of peptide-calcium complex. *J. Agric. Food Chem.* **2013**, *61*, 7537–7544. [CrossRef]
60. Huang, W.; Lan, Y.; Liao, W.; Lin, L.; Liu, G.; Miao, J. Preparation, characterization and biological activities of egg white peptides-calcium chelate. *LWT* **2021**, *149*, 112035. [CrossRef]
61. Wang, X.Q.; Zhang, Z.; Xu, H.Y.; Li, X.Y.; Hao, X.D. Preparation of sheep bone collagen peptide-calcium chelate using enzymolysis-fermentation methodology and its structural characterization and stability analysis. *RSC Adv.* **2020**, *10*, 11624–11633. [CrossRef] [PubMed]
62. Cui, P.; Lin, S.; Han, W.; Jiang, P.; Zhu, B.; Sun, N. Calcium delivery system assembled by a nanostructured peptide derived from the sea cucumber ovum. *J. Agric. Food Chem.* **2019**, *67*, 12283–12292. [CrossRef] [PubMed]
63. Amalraj, A.; Pius, A. Bioavailability of calcium and its absorption inhibitors in raw and cooked green leafy vegetables commonly consumed in India—An in vitro study. *Food Chem.* **2015**, *170*, 430–436. [CrossRef]
64. Chi, C.F.; Wang, B.; Deng, Y.Y.; Wang, Y.M.; Deng, S.G.; Ma, J.Y. Isolation and characterization of three antioxidant pentapeptides from protein hydrolysate of monkfish (*Lophius litulon*) muscle. *Food Res. Int.* **2014**, *55*, 222–228. [CrossRef]
65. Chen, Y.; Jin, H.; Yang, F.; Jin, S.; Liu, C.; Zhang, L.; Huang, J.; Wang, S.; Yan, Z.; Cai, X.; et al. Physicochemical, antioxidant properties of giant croaker (*Nibea japonica*) swim bladders collagen and wound healing evaluation. *Int. J. Biol. Macromol.* **2019**, *138*, 483–491. [CrossRef] [PubMed]
66. Liao, W.; Chen, H.; Jin, W.; Yang, Z.; Cao, Y.; Miao, J. Three newly isolated calcium-chelating peptides from tilapia bone collagen hydrolysate enhance calcium absorption activity in intestinal caco-2 cells. *J. Agric. Food Chem.* **2020**, *68*, 2091–2098. [CrossRef] [PubMed]

Disclaimer/Publisher's Note: The statements, opinions and data contained in all publications are solely those of the individual author(s) and contributor(s) and not of MDPI and/or the editor(s). MDPI and/or the editor(s) disclaim responsibility for any injury to people or property resulting from any ideas, methods, instructions or products referred to in the content.

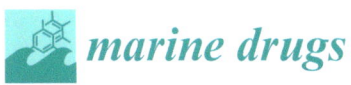

Article

Glucoregulatory Properties of a Protein Hydrolysate from Atlantic Salmon (*Salmo salar*): Preliminary Characterization and Evaluation of DPP-IV Inhibition and Direct Glucose Uptake In Vitro

Christian Bjerknes [1,*], Sileshi Gizachew Wubshet [2], Sissel Beate Rønning [2], Nils Kristian Afseth [2], Crawford Currie [1], Bomi Framroze [1] and Erland Hermansen [1,3]

[1] Hofseth Biocare ASA, Keiser Wilhelms Gate 24, 6003 Ålesund, Norway; cc@hofsethbiocare.no (C.C.); bf@hofsethbiocare.no (B.F.); ehe@hofsethbiocare.no (E.H.)
[2] Nofima AS, Osloveien 1, 1433 Ås, Norway; sileshi.wubshet@nofima.no (S.G.W.); sissel.beate.ronning@nofima.no (S.B.R.); nils.kristian.afseth@nofima.no (N.K.A.)
[3] Faculty of Medicine and Health Sciences, Norwegian University of Science and Technology (NTNU), Larsgårdsvegen 2, 6009 Ålesund, Norway
* Correspondence: chbj@hofsethbiocare.no

Abstract: Metabolic disorders are increasingly prevalent conditions that manifest pathophysiologically along a continuum. Among reported metabolic risk factors, elevated fasting serum glucose (FSG) levels have shown the most substantial increase in risk exposure. Ultimately leading to insulin resistance (IR), this condition is associated with notable deteriorations in the prognostic outlook for major diseases, including neurodegenerative diseases, cancer risk, and mortality related to cardiovascular disease. Tackling metabolic dysfunction, with a focus on prevention, is a critically important aspect for human health. In this study, an investigation into the potential antidiabetic properties of a salmon protein hydrolysate (SPH) was conducted, focusing on its potential dipeptidyl peptidase-IV (DPP-IV) inhibition and direct glucose uptake in vitro. Characterization of the SPH utilized a bioassay-guided fractionation approach to identify potent glucoregulatory peptide fractions. Low-molecular-weight (MW) fractions prepared by membrane filtration (MWCO = 3 kDa) showed significant DPP-IV inhibition (IC_{50} = 1.01 ± 0.12 mg/mL) and glucose uptake in vitro ($p \leq 0.0001$ at 1 mg/mL). Further fractionation of the lowest MW fractions (<3 kDa) derived from the permeate resulted in three peptide subfractions. The subfraction with the lowest molecular weight demonstrated the most significant glucose uptake activity ($p \leq 0.0001$), maintaining its potency even at a dilution of 1:500 ($p \leq 0.01$).

Keywords: marine protein hydrolysate; DPP-IV inhibition; glucose uptake; glucoregulatory peptides; bioactive peptides; salmon protein hydrolysate; metabolic disease

1. Introduction

Metabolic disorders entail a fundamental malfunction in the body's processing of nutrients, often stemming from an imbalance in nutrient intake, particularly in terms of excessive caloric consumption. In the 21st century, metabolic disease poses a substantial challenge to public health, fueled by a relentless rise in its incidence. An important downstream manifestation of metabolic disorders is related to glucose metabolism. Today, over 11% of the US adult population has clinical type 2 diabetes (DM2) according to a 2022 Center of Disease Control report [1]. Although the pathophysiology of type 2 diabetes (DM2) and metabolic syndrome differs, insulin resistance serves as a central metabolic derangement in both conditions.

A common early sign of metabolic disruption is elevated insulin levels. Continuous hyperinsulinemia can result in a cluster of metabolic abnormalities referred to as metabolic syndrome (MetS). This syndrome is defined somewhat arbitrarily by a collection of metabolic abnormalities including hypertension, elevated triglycerides, hyperglycemia, low HDL cholesterol, and central obesity [2]. Fulfilling three or more criteria establishes the presence of clinical MetS. While obesity is a criterion, it does not universally define metabolic unhealthiness, as not all metabolically unhealthy individuals are obese [3]. Addressing insulin resistance through therapeutic interventions is crucial, as research has identified it as a significant factor in developing chronic diseases. Several chronic diseases, such as cardiovascular disease, cancer, and neurodegenerative disease, are prognostically worsened by the presence of such metabolic abnormalities [4–9].

High fasting plasma glucose (HFPG) is the metabolic risk factor that has undergone the most substantial increase over time [10]. HFPG induces compensatory hyperinsulinemia, which, over the long term, can result in insulin signaling defects in tissues normally responsive to insulin [11]. Chronically elevated plasma glucose cause long-term negative effects on various tissues, in large part from glucose being irreversibly and non-enzymatically bound to proteins, lipids, or nucleic acids, leading to the formation of advanced glycation end products (AGEs) [12]. The presence of AGEs increases the likelihood of inappropriate activation of inflammatory and oxidative stress pathways, which contributes to negative health consequences [13]. A practical, easily accessible method involving the use of nutraceuticals or functional foods would be an appealing means to attempt to both delay and prevent the onset and progression of chronic metabolic diseases.

Natural marine bioactive compounds have become a focus of highly intensive research in recent years, with researchers having successfully discovered and isolated over 12,000 novel metabolites [14]. Indeed, marine bioactive compounds and their health effects rank among the most extensively researched compounds in the last two decades [15,16]. Marine organisms that were once regarded as a source of nutrition, like the sea cucumber, are now viewed as reservoirs of valuable bioactive compounds that hold the potential to serve as therapeutics and drug candidates relevant in addressing human diseases [17]. A compelling category of marine bioactive compounds comprises bioactive peptides. Typically spanning from 3 to 20 amino acids in length, these functional fragments may influence physiological processes upon consumption, serving as active biological regulators. Bioactive peptides, often natural constituents of food, are found encrypted and inactive within a specified parent protein, becoming bioactive upon release. Fish-derived marine bioactive peptides and their by-products are typically obtained through biotechnological techniques, commonly enzymatic hydrolysis. This method involves a gentle manufacturing process in which enzymes break down proteins to produce a mixture of peptides, known as a protein hydrolysate [18,19]. Hydrolysates are crude mixtures of low-molecular-weight (MW) bioactive and non-bioactive peptides [20]. Results from one clinical trial demonstrated meaningful antihypertensive effects from shrimp-derived hydrolysates for individuals with mild-to-moderate hypertension. The physiological effects of bioactive peptides contained within protein hydrolysates are remarkably diverse, with some exhibiting multifunctionality [21]. Marine organisms exhibit various bioactivities relevant to metabolic pathways, encompassing glucoregulatory, blood pressure-regulating, anti-inflammatory, and antioxidant effects [22,23]. Notably, however, research on their potential bioactivities is ongoing and includes several other areas of investigation, including the immune system and aging processes [23]. These diverse effects, along with inherent attributes such as target specificity and general safety, have intensified researchers' interest in their development. Sustainability concerns have shifted research towards the utilization of fish processing discards, now regarded as secondary raw materials, in the development of bioactive peptides and production of value-added protein hydrolysates that are suitable for human consumption [24]. A common occurrence with the enzymatic hydrolysis of various fish species and their processing discards is the generation of glucoregulatory bioactive peptides capable of interacting with enzymes involved in glucose homeostasis [25,26].

Bioactive peptides liberated from Atlantic salmon (*Salmo salar*) are commonly observed to inhibit dipeptidyl peptidase IV (DPP-IV), and to exert various antioxidant effects [27]. DPP-IV inhibition prevents the breakdown of glucagon-like peptide 1 (GLP-1) and glucose-dependent insulinotropic polypeptide (GIP) that are released post-prandially, prolonging their half-life and amplifying the insulin effect on glucose homeostasis (Figure 1) [28]. Prolonged systemic circulation of incretins enhances the transcription, synthesis, and exocytosis of insulin from pancreatic islet cells, which constitutes the mechanism of amplifying the insulin response. Indeed, gliptins, a category of medications inhibiting DPP-IV enzymes, are drugs that exploit this mechanism in the management of type 2 diabetes (DM 2). Bioactive peptides targeting DPP-IV are typically derived from proline-rich motifs of collagenous proteins, such as those found in the skin of salmon. As shown by Harnedy and colleagues, significant DPP-IV inhibitory potential was demonstrated for a salmon-derived hydrolysate manufactured from processing discards [29]. Today, various commercially available marine protein hydrolysates based on processing discards are available. Similarly, Li-Chan and colleagues reported considerable DPP-IV inhibitory effects of a specific peptide, GPAE, derived from salmon gelatin, a partially hydrolyzed protein source [30]. Other glucoregulatory effects were demonstrated by Roblet and colleagues, showing enhanced glucose uptake in muscle cells in vitro following exposure to a salmon-frame hydrolysate [31]. Hydrolysates from other fish species, such as sardine [25], silver carp [26], and shark liver [32], have also been shown to exhibit diverse glucoregulatory properties. Animal research has yielded encouraging findings, indicating that interventions lasting six weeks with the use of hydrolysates demonstrate promise in alleviating insulin resistance [33]. Early indications from clinical trials have indicated that marine hydrolysates can have clinically beneficial metabolic effects [34–36].

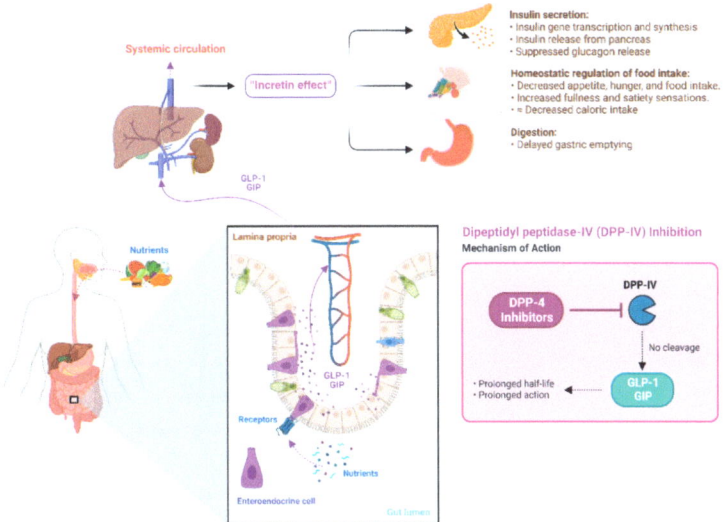

Figure 1. Illustration of the "incretin effect", which refers to the enhancement of insulin effectiveness due to the post-prandial secretion of incretins from intestinal enteroendocrine cells.

In prior investigations involving a salmon protein hydrolysate (SPH) derived from the processing discards of Norwegian Atlantic salmon (*Salmo salar*), some of the authors of the current paper demonstrated favorable changes in various metabolic biomarkers in small-scale clinical trials in response to daily SPH administration. These trials also uncovered favorable changes in body mass index (BMI). A noteworthy observation was the observation of significant improvements in hemoglobin and serum ferritin levels, in the absence of supplementary or additional dietary iron. A small, yet consistent reduction (ranging from 3% to 6%) in fasting plasma glucose has also been observed [37,38]. Further in vitro investigations into the SPH have revealed significant fold-change increases in gene expression, particularly genes that are recognized as central for antioxidant defense mechanisms, specifically HMOX, a change that was accompanied by the downregulation of proinflammatory genes, including ALOX12 [39]. Transcription and translation of ALOX12 yields a lipoxygenase involved in proinflammatory metabolite pathways, which may be one aspect contributing to pancreatic islet cell inflammation and injury, which is seen in the pathogenesis of DM [40–42].

The objective of this study was to assess whether the SPH housed bioactive peptides capable of exerting glucoregulatory properties. Glucoregulatory potential was assessed in terms of capacity for DPP-IV inhibition and glucose uptake in rat myocytes in vitro. Initial characterization of the SPH regarding its molecular weight and peptide composition was conducted to generate foundational knowledge about its composition. Bioassay-guided fractionation technology is employed in further developments in the presence of the specified bioactivity.

The overarching goal of this research is to advance the development of an SPH into a readily accessible and practical nutritional strategy that could potentially promote healthy metabolic function, properly substantiated by scientific publications.

This approach could represent a readily accessible, cost-effective, and easily implementable strategy, potentially offering broad benefits for human health in a sustainable manner.

2. Results

2.1. Characterization and Fractionation of SPH

Initially, peptides from the SPH were characterized by employing size-exclusion chromatography (SEC) and Fourier transform infra-red (FTIR) spectroscopy. SEC revealed the MW distribution of the crude SPH (Figure 2) to include peptides spanning a wide range of molecular weights. The average MW of the peptides for the crude SPH was calculated to be 3395 Daltons (Da).

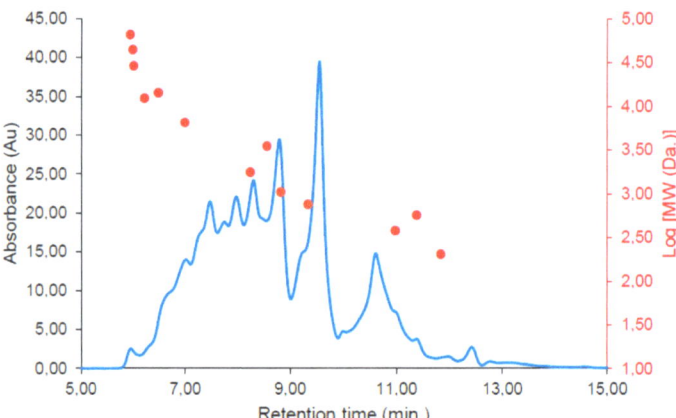

Figure 2. Size-exclusion chromatogram showing the molecular weight (MW) distribution of the SPH. The chromatogram was continuously monitored at 214 nanometers (nm). Correlations between the MW standards and retention time are presented as a dot plot overlayed in red.

As an initial fractionation protocol, filtration with a MW cut-off threshold of 3000 Da was employed. Both permeates (MW < 3 kDa) and retentates (MW > 3 kDa) were collected post-fractionation and analyzed further using SEC (Figure 3).

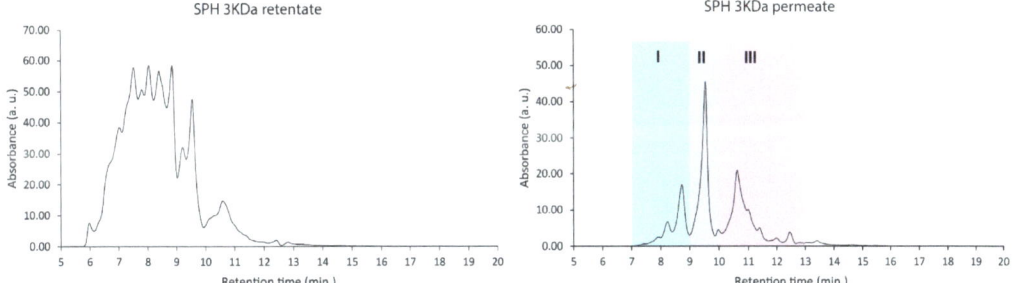

Figure 3. Molecular weight distributions (size-exclusion chromatogram) of the retentate (>3000 Da) and permeates (<3000 Da). Note that larger peptides and proteins elute earlier than smaller ones (see calibration data in Figure 2).

The retentate fraction, representing the portion of the SPH retained by the filtration membrane, exhibited an average MW of 4109 Da. Comparably, the permeate, which denotes the portion of the SPH solution passing through the filtration membrane, displayed a substantially lower average MW of 880 Da.

In addition to SEC, FTIR fingerprinting was used in order to benchmark the peptide composition of the SPH against a previously published database of laboratory- and industrial-scale hydrolysates [43]. The FTIR fingerprint of the SPH was projected onto a Principal Component Analysis (PCA) model based on a database containing 1300 registered hydrolysates. The FTIR fingerprint of the SPH shows that its peptide composition constitutes a relatively unique peptide profile, placing it relatively distant from most hydrolysate samples in the database (Figure 4). This can be attributed to both differences in the enzyme used (i.e., PC1) and raw material differences (i.e., PC3 and PC4) [43].

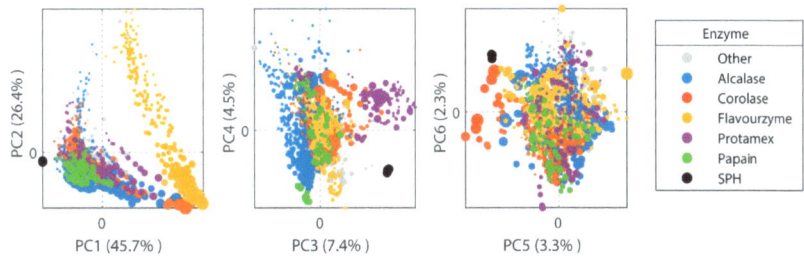

Figure 4. Scores of the first six FTIR-PCA components in a model based on 1300 protein hydrolysates. The dot size is proportional to hydrolysis time. Color represents employment of different enzymes in the manufacturing of a given hydrolysate (Alcalase represented by blue; Corolase represented by red; Flavourzyme represented by yellow; Protamex represented by purple; Papain represented by green). SPH samples (represented by black dots) were determined to be distant/unique from most of the database hydrolysates used for comparison.

2.2. Direct Glucose Uptake In Vitro

The effects of varying concentrations of crude SPH, permeate, and retentate are illustrated in Figure 5. L6 rat skeletal muscle cells treated with both crude SPH and 1.0 mg/mL permeate solution demonstrated significant increases in glucose uptake ($p \leq 0.001$ and $p \leq 0.0001$, respectively). Statistically significant effects were maintained at permeate concentrations of 0.1 mg/mL ($p \leq 0.05$). The permeate, consisting of smaller MW peptides, was the primary driver of this effect on glucose uptake. No significant effect in terms of glucose uptake was observed for cells treated with retentate solutions, composed of higher-MW peptides.

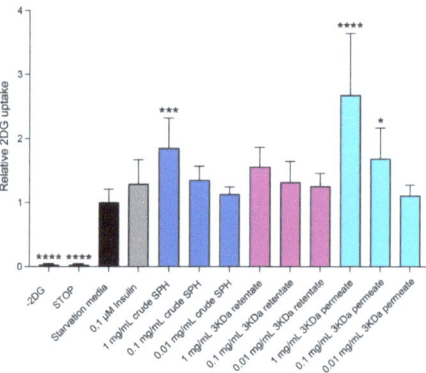

Figure 5. Effects of crude SPH, permeate, and retentate solutions on glucose uptake in L6 rat skeletal muscle cells in vitro. Bar plot of relative glucose uptake in cells treated with insulin or hydrolysates at indicated concentrations compared to control cells (i.e., untreated cells). The data are presented as the average of a cell culture experiment seeded out in triplicates ± SD. Asterisks denote significant differences (* $p < 0.05$, *** $p < 0.001$, **** $p < 0.0001$) compared to the control cells, calculated by one-way ANOVA using Dunnett's multiple comparison test.

To identify the most bioactive peptide fraction within the permeate, the permeate mixture was further fractionated using SEC (see Figure 3; colorized chromatogram). The resulting three subfractions, denoted as permeate I, permeate II, and permeate III, were composed of peptides in decreasing order of MW. The permeate III subfraction, comprising the smallest peptides, exhibited the highest activity in terms of directly facilitating glucose uptake into muscle cells ($p \leq 0.0001$; Figure 6). This subfraction exhibited a significant ($p \leq 0.01$) increase in glucose uptake even at the lowest tested concentration (fraction diluted 1:500), indicating a potent bioactive potential.

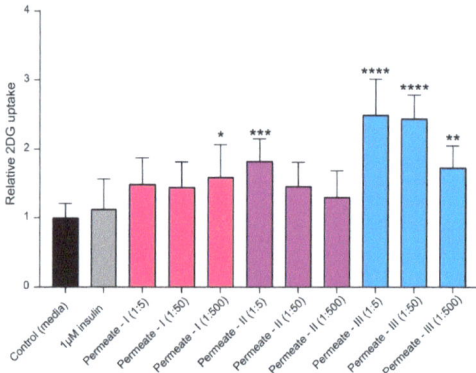

Figure 6. Effects of the subfractions permeate I, permeate II, and permeate III on insulin-independent glucose uptake in L6 rat skeletal muscle cells in vitro. Bar plot of relative glucose uptake in cells treated with insulin or hydrolysates at indicated concentrations compared to control cells (i.e., untreated cells). The data are presented as the average of a cell culture experiment seeded out in triplicates ± SD. Asterisks denote significant differences (* $p < 0.05$, ** $p < 0.01$, *** $p < 0.001$, **** $p < 0.0001$) compared to the control cells, calculated by one-way ANOVA using Dunnett's multiple comparison test.

2.3. DPP-IV Inhibition

Crude SPH, permeate, and retentates were screened for their glucoregulatory properties in terms of DPP-IV inhibition.

A capacity for DPP-IV inhibition was observed in all three types of samples, with the permeate specifically demonstrating the highest level of activity determined at an IC_{50} of 1.01 ± 0.12 mg/mL (Figure 7).

Table 1. IC_{50} values for crude SPH, permeate, and retentate along with their respective 95% confidence intervals (CIs).

	Crude SPH	Permeate	Retentate
Best-fit values			
Log IC_{50}	0.2613	0.004061	0.4062
Hill slope	0.8898	0.9853	0.9966
IC_{50}	1.825	1.009	2.548
95% CI (profile likelihood)			
Log IC_{50}	0.2350 to 0.2882	−0.04659 to 0.05563	0.3514 to 0.4647
Hill slope	0.84202 to 0.9421	0.8861 to 1.096	0.8746 to 1.137
IC_{50}	1.718 to 1.942	0.8983 to 1.137	2.246 to 2.915

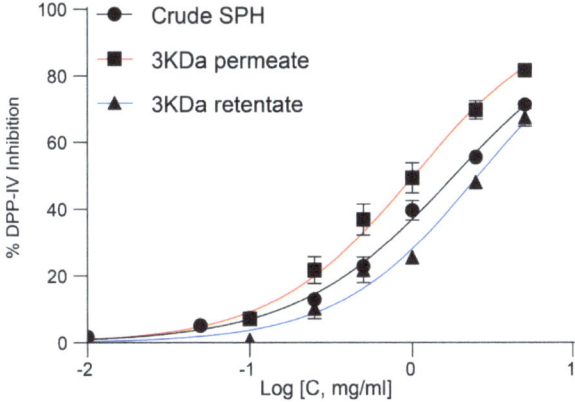

Figure 7. Dose–response curve illustrating DPP-IV inhibition activity of crude SPH, permeate, and retentate. Dose–response curves (left) and fitting results from IC_{50} value calculations (Table 1).

2.4. Liquid Chromatography–Mass Spectrometry (LC-MS) Peptide Identification

The fraction showing the most potential in terms of DPP-IV inhibition and glucose uptake effects underwent further analysis using MS-based peptidomics to enhance characterization and identify peptides. A total of 260 peptides were identified with a high "identification score". A complete list of the peptides with the details of the identification is available as supplementary data (See Supplementary Materials: 260 peptides). As an example, one of the proteins that several peptides were identified as deriving from was alpha fast skeletal muscle actin from *Salmo salar* (Figure 8).

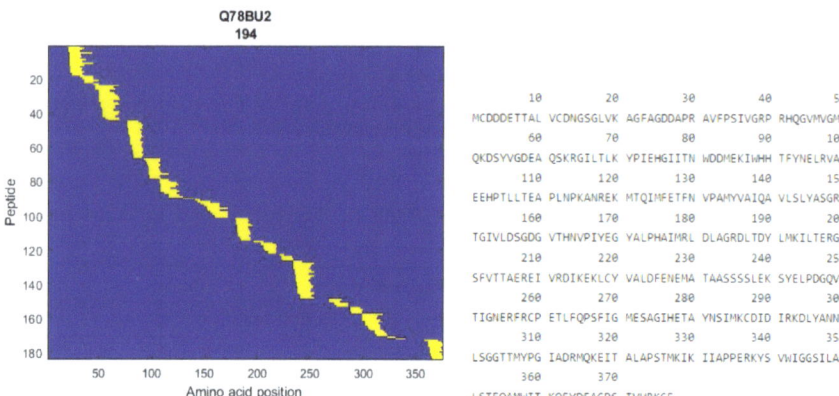

Figure 8. Heatmap of identified peptides in the permeate from alpha fast skeletal muscle actin from *Salmo salar* (**left**), and protein sequence of alpha fast skeletal muscle actin (**right**).

3. Discussion

In recent years, there has been a growing number of studies aiming to characterize and evaluate the feasibility and potential applicability of bioactivities in marine protein hydrolysates [44]. Marine hydrolysates are widely acknowledged as safe nutritional interventions, offering preventive and supportive approaches for managing metabolic disorders. Findings from clinical trials involving DPP-IV inhibitory hydrolysates have shown promising preliminary results, including improvements in fasting blood glucose (FBG) levels and glycosylated hemoglobin A1c (HbA1c) after three months of intervention [34]. Hence, the considerable health-promoting potential and feasibility of their utilization should warrant continued research efforts. On a population level, even modest improvements in a person's metabolic risk profile would likely lead to significant reductions in overall human disease burden and healthcare costs. As a component of a comprehensive strategy to address the rising prevalence of metabolic diseases, focusing research efforts on the development of nutraceutical interventions emerges as a valuable pursuit. This study aimed to collect initial insights into the potential metabolic advantages of an SPH, alongside conducting a characterization of this hydrolysate in terms of peptide composition.

Upon initial characterization, the SPH exhibited a peptide composition distinct from that of 1300 commercial and laboratory hydrolysates listed in a recently published database. This distinctiveness was apparent in the distribution of peptide sizes, a characteristic primarily influenced by predefined manufacturing parameters such as the enzymes, hydrolysis time, and composition of raw materials employed. The average MW was 3395 Da, comprising a broad spectrum of peptide sizes. The permeate, containing the smallest peptide fraction, demonstrated the highest DPP-IV inhibitory potency, with an IC_{50} of 0.8983 to 1.137 mg/mL, consistent with results from some published DPP-IV assay experiments on hydrolysates [45–47], with some studies reporting a comparably lower DPP-IV inhibitory capacity 20–30%) than the SPH [30,48]. We found that this activity was mediated by the peptide fraction composed of smaller-sized peptides with an average MW of 880 Da. Indeed, this aligns with results from Zhang et al., where the most potent inhibitors were seen for the peptide fractions lower than 3 kDa [49,50]. From the literature available over the last five years concerning purified DPP-IV inhibitory bioactive peptides, the majority were identified as di-, tri-, and oligopeptides, indicating peptides of smaller sizes [51]. Reportedly, inhibitors with smaller molecular weights exhibit superior performance as DPP-IV inhibitors compared to larger-sized peptides [52]. The permeate, comprising peptides with an average molecular weight of less than one kDa, aligns with the literature which suggests that smaller peptides exhibit superior DPP-IV inhibition activity compared to higher-molecular-weight fractions [53–55]. Moreover, the permeate surpassed both the retentate and crude SPH in terms of directly enhancing glucose uptake into rat myotubules. Glucose uptake was increased by approximately 2.5-fold compared to control conditions, and 2-fold compared to insulin at concentrations of 0.1 µM, a common in vitro dose for such assays. [56]. Through additional bioassay-guided fractionation of the permeate, the fraction containing the smallest peptides, designated as permeate-III, exhibited a significantly greater capacity for glucose uptake compared to the original permeate. This is in line with previously published reports, showing that glucose uptake was improved in muscle cells when stimulated with low MW peptides from soy and poultry by-products [31,57]. A mechanism mediating and facilitating glucose uptake seems to be a commonly occurrence for salmon-derived peptide fractions [58]. Even when diluted to a ratio of 1:500, the potency of permeate-III in achieving statistically significant effects was maintained for this low molecular weight fraction.

The findings presented here reveal the presence of glucoregulatory peptides within a potent subfraction derived from an SPH with a peptide composition unique from that of other industrial hydrolysates. The more potent permeate, consisting of smaller peptides with an average MW of 880 Da, suggests that shorter peptides are the main mediators of this bioactivity. Applying the average MW of the 20 common amino acids, this corresponds to a peptide chain of 8 amino acids, which is consistent with the characteristic chain length for DPP-IV inhibitory peptides [59]. Whether these are specific peptides demonstrating dual glucoregulatory properties or distinct peptides each performing a unique function is yet to be determined. Notably, one of the most intriguing aspects of bioactive peptides is their potential to be multifunctional, with a single peptide capable of exerting more than one effect. By targeting multiple pathways involved in glucose regulation, synergy may potentially offer enhanced efficacy in managing metabolic disruptions. Glucose can be transported into different tissues either by sodium-dependent glucose co-transporters, which do not depend on insulin, or by specialized glucose transporters known as GLUTs. The precise mechanism through which the presence of peptides facilitates glucose uptake remains to be understood. We can hypothesize whether GLUT-4 translocation to the plasma membrane might be responsible for some of the effect, occurring through the phosphoinositide 3-kinase pathway (PI3K-Akt) [46,60]. Bioactive peptides are reported to increase glucose uptake through both insulin-dependent and -independent pathways. Glucose uptake through insulin-independent pathways, specifically, frequently involves the activation of AMP-activated protein kinase (AMPK), presenting potential avenues for additional investigations for the SPH [61]. In a previous study, low-MW peptide fractions from soybean demonstrated enhanced glucose uptake in L6 muscle cells when insulin was present [31]. Although these peptides were found to activate AMPK, glucose uptake was not enhanced in the absence of insulin.

Potent glucoregulatory properties were also evident for the lower-MW peptide fraction in terms of DPP-IV inhibitory activities. The mechanism of enzyme inhibition, whether it involves competitive, uncompetitive, or non-competitive pathways, or even mixed modes by binding at either the active site and/or outside the catalytic site of the DPP-IV enzyme, awaits further clarification in future studies. Further investigations of the glucoregulatory properties described herein should consider fractionation as an initial measure to concentrate sufficient quantities of the potent low-molecular-weight constituents. In an initial peptide screening using LC-MS peptidomics, 260 peptides with unique sequences ranging from 8 to 25 amino acids in length were identified as highly likely to be bioactive and to exert relevant glucoregulatory effects. From the peptides derived from alpha fast skeletal muscle actin, we notice structural repeats in certain peptides, such as GP and PG sequences, which are common structures for DPP-IV inhibitory peptides [62]. Additionally, we observe proline flanked by leucine or valine residues, LP and VP, in some of the peptides, as a frequently reported feature in DPP-IV inhibitory peptides [25,63]. We can gain some insights into this specific peptide composition using predictive peptide tools. The list of 260 peptides was evaluated with an online predictive tool, Peptide Ranker, which employs neural networks to evaluate bioactivity based on peptide primary structure.

A rank of 0.0 represents high likelihood of no bioactivity being present, while a rank of 1.0 indicates the very highest likelihood of bioactivity present [64]. The prediction tool does not make predictions in terms of the nature of any given peptide, merely whether it is likely to be bioactive or not bioactive. A compilation of ranked peptides can be found in the supplementary materials (see Supplementary Materials: Ten Ranked Peptides). A rank threshold of 0.8 was chosen to filter only the peptides most likely to be bioactive, which affords a false positive rate of 6% for small peptides as reported by Bioware [65]. A total of 10 peptides out of the 260 listed peptides were assigned a rank higher than 0.8, suggesting a high likelihood of bioactivity with a corresponding low false positive rate, with lengths from 13 to 20 amino acids long. The ten ranked candidate peptides are seen harboring an abundance of Gly-Pro-type peptides, which may have been liberated from various types of collagen derived from the skin, head, and trimmings of the Atlantic salmon (*Salmo salar*) raw materials. Collagen is notably abundant in proline triplets, where proline typically occupies position 2 of these triplets, typically denoted as Gly-X-Y. Here, X and Y can represent any amino acid, although proline or hydroxyproline residues are typical [66]. Proline residues in the second position from the N-terminus are indeed a common structural feature of DPP-IV inhibitory bioactive peptides, a characteristic shared by every ranked peptide [67]. The peptides listed can be expected to exhibit varying degrees of DPP-IV inhibition based on this, with their potency likely influenced by the remaining portions of their primary sequences. Enzymatic hydrolysis of Atlantic salmon (*Salmo salar*) skin has produced peptides akin to the nine ranked peptides identified by Peptide Ranker, albeit shorter in length. Specifically, sequences reported included GPAE and GPGA, which exhibited potent IC_{50} values in terms of DPP-IV inhibition [30]. A glycine–proline type of peptide cannot, however, be a mandatory feature of peptides with DPP-IV inhibitory capacities, as novel peptides liberated from Atlantic salmon gelatin have yielded the peptide LDKVFR, which was determined to be quite potent [68]. Hydrophobic interactions of the peptide backbone with its DPP-IV target enzyme, along with other forces such as Van der Waals interactions, are those that would dictate how the peptide interacts with and modulates its target. The specific features contributing to the very highest potency of marine-derived DPP-IV inhibitory peptides, including their length and primary sequence, have not been fully elucidated at present.

The current findings are promising. Atlantic salmon (*Salmo salar*) processing by-products, often considered secondary raw materials in the production of value-added human-consumable products, are frequently identified as potent sources of glucoregulatory peptides. In one pre-clinical study on knockout mice, a fish protein hydrolysate was deemed to exert a capacity for beneficial glucoregulatory effects, with a potency on par with Metformin, a drug used in the management of type 2 diabetes [69]. A crucial future consideration is the bioavailability of such interventions, should such interventions be employed to address metabolic abnormalities. Certainly, addressing bioavailability remains crucial for ensuring the acceptance and effectiveness of purified hydrolysate interventions. At the same time, smaller peptides tend to exhibit greater resistance to gastrointestinal proteolysis, which may allow them to be absorbed into the circulation in an intact form [70,71]. The ranked peptides cannot be classified strictly as short peptides, however, should they become the most promising peptide candidates.

Even if the metabolic benefits of regular consumption of bioactive hydrolysates are modest, in the case of bioavailability limitations, the overall effects would be highly favorable on a population-wide scale. Another consideration is determining the extent of purification employed for a hydrolysate to enhance its glucoregulatory potency, while ensuring that this level of purification is still cost-effective and feasible for industrial-scale manufacturing. Additional in silico and in vitro investigations are necessary next steps to pinpoint the most potent and promising peptide candidates. These peptide candidates will subsequently undergo further characterization, including molecular docking investigations. Utilizing salmon raw materials sustainably to manufacture products with potentially meaningful health benefits appears to be an appealing and straightforward developmental trajectory. Since these peptides originate from food sources, they tend to be inherently safe for human consumption. In terms of conducting a comprehensive exploration of potential antidiabetic mechanisms, it would be intriguing to examine the possible presence of incretin mimetics within the SPH, as has been demonstrated for some hydrolysates [72]. Purified peptides will be further employed in appropriate pre-clinical animal models to assess their efficacy in an in vivo environment.

4. Conclusions

The current study provided initial characterization and bioactivity screening of a protein hydrolysate derived from Atlantic salmon (*Salmo salar*) raw materials. The initial analysis indicated that the SPH comprises relatively large peptides, with an average size of 3395 Da. The FTIR spectrum expressed a distinct signature compared to a large library of industrial hydrolysates, suggesting a unique peptide composition.

Bioactivity assaying unveiled potent glucoregulatory properties, operating through two distinct mechanisms. The permeate exhibited the highest potency, indicating that the glucoregulatory activity is mediated primarily by short-chained bioactive peptides. LC-MS-driven peptidomics identified more than 260 relevant peptides in the permeate, with 10 predicted to possess the highest bioactivity. The primary structures of these ten peptides displayed features commonly found in DPP-IV inhibitory peptides.

Biotransformation of salmon processing discards offers high-quality nutrition and potent glucoregulatory peptides, which, if applied on a population scale, could meaningfully alleviate the growing health burden of metabolic disease. Bioactive peptides emerge as promising and versatile biological tools suited for use in future personalized medicine.

A feasible and safe peptide intervention for general use, whether as crude hydrolysates or permeates offering health benefits, or as highly purified bioactive fractions, will require distinct considerations. Randomized clinical trials and bioavailability assessments are essential prerequisites to guarantee their successful application.

5. Materials and Methods

5.1. Manufacturing Salmon Protein Hydrolysate

The head, skin, trimmings, frames, and bones (regarded as secondary raw materials) of Atlantic salmon (*Salmo salar*), arriving from supplier-audited fileting plants, are received at the hydrolysis plant on a daily basis. Secondary raw materials are then ground up and directed into a hydrolysis tank after which food-grade enzymes, Foam Control 30, and water are added to generate a mixture. The product is heated in two steps to a final temperature of 95 °C, held for a period of 5 min. The final mixture is transferred and split into respective fractions. Upon centrifugation, a final separation of the mixture into an SPH fraction, partially hydrolyzed protein (PHP) fraction, salmon oil fraction, and collagenous hydroxyapatite fraction is generated. Subsequently, the protein concentrate is sent through a heat exchanger, is homogenized, and finally, is spray dried. The product is sieved and packed.

5.2. Sample Materials and Chemicals

SPH consists of a broad array of peptides derived from the enzymatic hydrolysis of proteins from salmon raw materials employing non-GMO protease enzymes. The degree of hydrolysis is estimated at 10%. The SPH appears as a light-yellow powder. It has a water-soluble protein content of >95%, of which >25% is composed of type I/III collagen peptides, with a fat content of <0.5%, and an ash content of <2.5%.

The amino acid composition is glutamic acid (13.9 g/100 g), aspartic acid (9.4 g/100 g), glycine (14.9 g/100 g), proline (7.6 g/100 g), lysine (7.0 g/100 g), alanine (7.5 g/100 g), and arginine (6.9 g/100 g). Hydroxyproline content was quantified to 4.18 g/100 g (ISO 13903:2005) [73]. Moreover, it contains meaningful amounts of vitamin B12 (cyanocobalamin), 27.9 µg/100 g (batch: sph 23012), as well as selenium (Se), 0.77 mg/kg (batch: sph 23012). Regular safety checks are performed by Eurofins as the process pertains to heavy metals, aflatoxins, dioxins, furans, and polychlorinated biphenyls. The SPH is screened negative for pesticides. The molecular weight peptide distribution is 5.5% for peptides <200 Da, 10.0% for peptides 200–500 Da, 14.1% for peptides 500–1000 Da, 20.4% for peptides 1000–2000 Da, 21.2% for peptides 2000–4000 Da, and 13.2% for peptides 4000–6000 Da, and remaining amounts are accounted for by higher-molecular-weight peptides.

Analytical grade acetonitrile, trifluoracetic acid (TFA), and monosodium phosphate used for size-exclusion chromatography (SEC) were purchased from Sigma-Aldrich (Oslo, Norway). A DPP4 inhibitor screening assay kit was purchased from Abcam (Amsterdam, Netherlands). Water was prepared by deionization and membrane filtration (0.22 µm) using a Millipore Milli-Q purification system (Molsheim, France).

5.3. FTIR-Based Fingerprinting and Benchmarking

Dry-film FTIR analysis was performed according to Wubshet et al. [74]. SPH was dissolved in ultrapure water to a concentration of 20 mg/mL, and 10 µL of such a sample was deposited onto a 96-slot Si-microtiter plate (Bruker Optik Gmbh, Germany) and dried at room temperature to form dry films. The sample was made in five replicates and measured by a High Throughput Screening eXTension (HTS-XT) unit coupled to a Tensor 27 spectrometer (both Bruker Optik Gmbh, Ettlingen, Germany). The spectra were recorded in the region between 4000 and 400 cm^{-1} with a spectral resolution of 4 cm^{-1} and an aperture of 5.0 mm. A second derivative was applied to the spectra using the Savitzky–Golay algorithm with a polynomial degree of two and a smoothing window size of 13 points. Similar to the database spectra published by Måge et al. [43], the spectra were normalized using a standard normal variate (SNV). For benchmarking, the FTIR fingerprints of SPH were projected into an in-house (Nofima, Ås, Norway) PCA model based on an FTIR spectral database of 1300 industrial and laboratory-produced hydrolysates, as described in Måge et al. [43].

5.4. Size-Exclusion Chromatography

The MW distributions of crude SPH, permeate, and retentate were analyzed with a size-exclusion chromatograph (SEC) according Wubshet et al. [74]. Briefly, 10 µL of the peptide solution (20 mg/mL) was separated in a BioSep-SEC-s2000 column (Phenomenex, Værløse, Denmark, 300 × 7.8 mm) coupled with a Dionex UltiMate 3000 HPLC system (Thermo Scientific, Waltham, MA, USA). The mobile phase was acetonitrile (30% (v/v)) in ultrapure water (70% (v/v)) containing 0.05% TFA. The flow rate was 0.9 mL/min, and the UV absorption was monitored at 214 nm. Molecular weight distribution and weight-average molecular weight (MW) of the crude hydrolysate and fractions were calculated using PSS winGPC UniChrom V 8.00 software (Polymer Standards Service, Mainz, Germany). Standards for calibration and calculations of molecular weight distribution and average MW were made as described in Wubshet et al. [74].

5.5. Filtration and SEC Fractionation

A solution of 10 mg/mL of SPH was prepared in ultra-filtered water and filtered through a Millex-HV PVDF syringe filter with a pore size of 0.45 mm (Merck Millipore, Billerica, MA, USA). The resulting crude SPH solution was subsequently fractionated using Amicon centrifugal filters, MWCO 3 kDa. The filtration procedure was carried out in accordance with the instructions provided by the manufacturer. Briefly, 15 mL (per single filtration) was loaded to the filters and centrifugation was performed at 4400 rpm for 20 min at 25 °C. Permeates and retentates from the filtration were collected and were freeze dried before further analysis.

Molecular-weight-based fractionation of the ProGo-permeate was performed using the same column and same method explained in Section 2.1 with higher loading. A total of three fractions were collected in the elution periods of 7–9 min (permeate I), 9–10 min (permeate II), and 10–13 min (permeate III). These three subfractions were freeze dried before further bioactivity evaluation.

5.6. Skeletal Muscle Glucose Uptake

Cellular models are essential for studying biology in controlled settings. They offer detailed understanding of the molecular pathways and cellular reactions associated with both healthy and diseased states. In this context, L6 myotubes are particularly useful. Their pattern of GLUT (glucose transporter) expression closely resembles that of fully differentiated mammalian muscle. Specifically, they exhibit high levels of GLUT4 and relatively low levels of GLUT1 and GLUT3 [75]. L6 rat myoblasts (CRL-1458, ATCC) were maintained in high glucose containing DMEM with 10% FBS, 0.1% penicillin/streptomycin, and 0.1% Fungizone. Glucose uptake experiments were performed on differentiated L6 rat myotubes (CRL-1458, ATCC), initiated as follows: Amounts of 5000 cells per well were seeded out in a white 96-well plate with a flat bottom using a high-glucose DMEM (ATCC 30–2002) cell culture medium with 10% FBS, 0.1% penicillin/streptomycin, and 0.1% Fungizone. After 4 days of proliferation, differentiation was initiated using a differentiation medium with high-glucose DMEM (ATCC 30–2002) 2% FBS, 0.1% penicillin/streptomycin, and 0.1% Fungizone. The differentiation medium was changed every day for three days, before the myotubes were placed in a starvation medium, containing DMEM with no glucose, phenol red, and glutamine (A1443001, ThermoFisher), and 0.1% penicillin/streptomycin and 0.1% Fungizone. Differentiation was monitored in the microscope throughout the experiment. After 18 h in the starvation medium, myotubes were incubated in the presence or absence of insulin and hydrolysates for 1 h at the concentrations indicated in the figure legend. Control cells were left in the starvation medium.

Glucose uptake was performed using the Glucose Uptake-Glo™ Assay (J1342, Promega) according to the manufacturer's instructions. In brief, cells pre-treated with insulin or hydrolysates for 1 h were washed with PBS, followed by 30 min incubation with 2-deoxyglucose (2DG). 2DG is transported across the cell membrane and undergoes intracellular phosphorylation, in the same manner as the breakdown of glucose during glycolysis. This process results in the formation of 2DG6P, which traps the substrate within the cell, leading to intracellular accumulation. However, due to steric hindrances, 2DG6P cannot be further processed in the glycolysis pathway. This allows for the assessment of 2DG uptake only. One hour after incubation with a 2DG6P detection reagent containing NADP+, reductase, and proluciferin enzymes, the intracellular 2DG6P is measured. The presence of 2DG6P reduces NADP+ to NADPH. This NADPH is then used by a reductase to convert proluciferin to luciferin. Luciferin serves as a substrate for luciferase, producing a luminescent signal proportional to the concentration of 2DG6P (See Figure 9). This allows for the quantification of 2DG uptake.

Luminescence was then recorded by a plate reader. Omitting 2DG or adding STOP buffer prior to 2DG incubation was used as negative controls. An amount of 0.1 µM insulin was employed as a positive control.

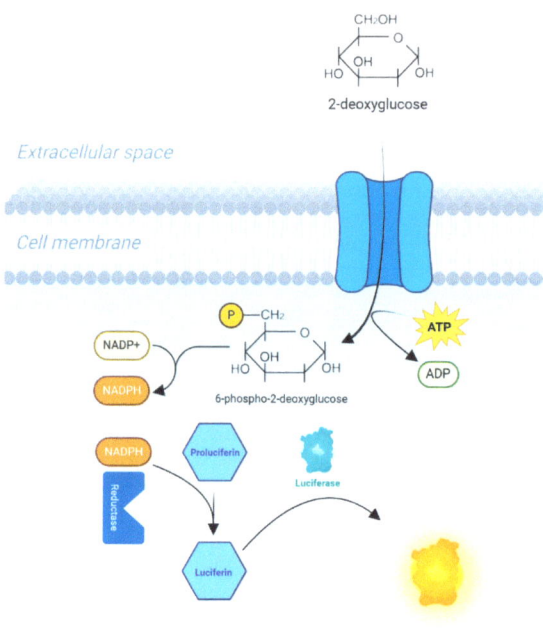

Figure 9. Illustration of the bioluminescence method for measuring glucose uptake in cells, based on the detection of 2-deoxyglucose-6-phosphate (2DG6P). First, 2DG is added to the cells, and is transported into the cell. Then stop and neutralization buffers are added to stop the reactions, lyse the cells, and eliminate the NADPH present inside the cells. The 2DG6P detection reagent is added; this will oxidize 2DG6P to 6-phosphodeoxygluconate and reduce NADP+ to NADPH. Proluciferin is then converted to luciferin, which acts as a substrate for a recombinant luciferase that produces a luminescence signal proportional to the concentration of 2DG6P.

5.7. DPP-IV Inhibition

DPP-IV inhibition of crude SPH, permeate, and retentate fractions was evaluated using a commercial fluorometric dipeptidyl peptidase-IV (DPP-IV) inhibitor screening assay kit (Ab133081) produced by Abcam (Berlin, Germany). The protocol for the assay followed the instructions provided by the manufacturer. All three samples were tested in 8 different concentrations (from 0.01 mg/mL to 5.0 mg/mL). Test solutions were prepared in the assay buffer and all concentrations were tested in triplicates.

Fluorescence intensity was measured with a Microplate Reader Synergy H1 (BioTek, Winooski, VT, USA) using an excitation wavelength of 355 nm and an emission wavelength of 455 nm. Inhibition of DPP-IV (I_{DPP-IV}) was calculated as follows:

$$I_{DPP-IV}(\%) = \left(\frac{initial\ activity - inhibitor}{intial\ activity} \right) \times 100$$

where *initial activity* is the activity of DPP-IV without the inhibitor present and *inhibitor* is the activity of DPP-IV with the sample present. In addition to the test samples, a positive control, sitagliptin, was tested in triplicate in the same plate. At a predetermined concentration provided with the assay kit, sitagliptin showed DPP-IV inhibition of 87.64% (± 0.07).

The data fitting and IC_{50} value calculation were performed using GraphPad Prism (La Jolla, CA, USA).

5.8. Liquid Chromatography–Mass Spectrometry de Novo Sequencing of Peptides

Peptides were resolved with loading buffer [2% (v/v) CAN and 0.05% (v/v) trifluoroacetic acid]. Peptides were loaded onto a trap column (Acclaim PepMap 100, C18, 5 μm, 100 Å, 300 μm i.d. × 5 mm, Thermo Fisher Scientific) and then backflushed with a loading buffer described below onto a 50 cm × 75 μm analytical column (Acclaim PepMap RSLC C18, 2 μm, 100 Å, 75 μm i.d. × 50 cm, nanoViper, Thermo Fisher Scientific, Bremen, Germany) for LC-MS/MS analysis. Conditions for ultra-high-performance LC were as follows: loading pump, flow rate 20 μL/min with loading buffer; 2% (v/v) ACN and 0.05% (v/v) formic acid (FA) and nano/cap pump, flow rate 0.3 μL/min with a gradient of two buffers, A [0.1% (v/v) FA] and B [80% (v/v) CAN, 0.08% (v/v) FA]. The LC gradient was run for 120 min, from 3.2 to 80% buffer B. Peptides from the 12 most intense peaks were fragmented, and the mass-to-charge values of these fragmented ions were measured (tandem mass spectrometry, MS/MS) with a Q-Exactive Quadrupole-Orbitrap mass spectrometer (Thermo Fisher Scientific, USA). The Q-Exactive mass spectrometer was set up as follows: a full scan (300–1500 m/z) at R = 140,000 was followed by (up to) 12 MS2 scans at R = 17,500 using an NCE setting of 28. Singly charged precursors were excluded for MS/MS, as were precursors with z > 5. Dynamic exclusion was set at 20 s. Finally, peptide identification was performed using MaxQuant, an integrated suite of algorithms specifically developed for high-resolution, quantitative MS data. Raw LC-HRMS/MS data were searched against a non-specific digest of *Salmo salar* (*Atlantic salmon*) proteins (UniProtKB database).

Supplementary Materials: The following supporting information can be downloaded at: https://www.mdpi.com/article/10.3390/md22040151/s1, 260 Peptides, IC50 results raw and Peptide Ranker.

Author Contributions: Conceptualization, S.G.W., C.B., E.H. and S.B.R.; methodology, S.G.W., S.B.R. and N.K.A.; software, S.G.W.; validation, C.B., E.H. and C.C.; formal analysis, S.G.W.; investigation, S.G.W. and S.B.R.; resources, S.G.W.; data curation, S.G.W.; writing—original draft preparation, C.B. and C.C.; writing—review and editing, C.B., E.H., C.C. and B.F.; visualization, C.B.; supervision, E.H.; project administration, E.H., S.G.W. and N.K.A.; funding acquisition, E.H. All authors have read and agreed to the published version of the manuscript.

Funding: This research was funded in its entirety by Hofseth Biocare ASA. No external financial support or funding was received in order to conduct the current research.

Institutional Review Board Statement: Not applicable.

Data Availability Statement: Data requests may be made to the authors of this paper.

Acknowledgments: The authors thank Nina Solberg, Ingrid Måge, and Katinka Dankel for their technical support. Each author has agreed to the acknowledgments mentioned above.

Conflicts of Interest: C.B., C.C., E.H., and B.F. are employees of and/or consultants for Hofseth Biocare ASA, who is the sponsor of the current study. The remaining authors declare that the research was conducted in the absence of any commercial or financial relationships that could be construed as potential conflicts of interest.

References

1. Centers for Disease Control and Prevention. National Diabetes Statistics Report: Estimates of Diabetes and Its Burden in the United States. Available online: https://www.cdc.gov/diabetes/data/statistics-report/index.html (accessed on 6 February 2024).
2. Huang, P.L. A comprehensive definition for metabolic syndrome. *Dis. Model. Mech.* **2009**, *2*, 231–237. [CrossRef] [PubMed]
3. De Geest, B.; Mishra, M. The metabolic syndrome in obese and non-obese subjects: A reappraisal of the syndrome X of Reaven. *Eur. J. Prev. Cardiol.* **2023**, *30*, 1193–1194. [CrossRef] [PubMed]
4. Laakso, M.; Kuusisto, J. Insulin resistance and hyperglycaemia in cardiovascular disease development. *Nat. Rev. Endocrinol.* **2014**, *10*, 293–302. [CrossRef]
5. Ormazabal, V.; Nair, S.; Elfeky, O.; Aguayo, C.; Salomon, C.; Zuñiga, F.A. Association between insulin resistance and the development of cardiovascular disease. *Cardiovasc. Diabetol.* **2018**, *17*, 122. [CrossRef] [PubMed]
6. Arcidiacono, B.; Iiritano, S.; Nocera, A.; Possidente, K.; Nevolo, M.T.; Ventura, V.; Foti, D.; Chiefari, E.; Brunetti, A. Insulin resistance and cancer risk: An overview of the pathogenetic mechanisms. *Exp. Diabetes Res.* **2012**, *2012*, 789174. [CrossRef] [PubMed]

7. Tsugane, S.; Inoue, M. Insulin resistance and cancer: Epidemiological evidence. *Cancer Sci.* **2010**, *101*, 1073–1079. [CrossRef] [PubMed]
8. Godsland, I.F. Insulin resistance and hyperinsulinaemia in the development and progression of cancer. *Clin. Sci.* **2009**, *118*, 315–332. [CrossRef] [PubMed]
9. Nguyen, T.T.; Ta, Q.T.H.; Nguyen, T.T.D.; Le, T.T.; Vo, V.G. Role of Insulin Resistance in the Alzheimer's Disease Progression. *Neurochem. Res.* **2020**, *45*, 1481–1491. [CrossRef] [PubMed]
10. Liang, R.; Feng, X.; Shi, D.; Yang, M.; Yu, L.; Liu, W.; Zhou, M.; Wang, X.; Qiu, W.; Fan, L.; et al. The global burden of disease attributable to high fasting plasma glucose in 204 countries and territories, 1990–2019: An updated analysis for the Global Burden of Disease Study 2019. *Diabetes Metab. Res. Rev.* **2022**, *38*, e3572. [CrossRef]
11. Khalid, M.; Alkaabi, J.; Khan, M.A.B.; Adem, A. Insulin Signal Transduction Perturbations in Insulin Resistance. *Int. J. Mol. Sci.* **2021**, *22*, 8590. [CrossRef]
12. Twarda-Clapa, A.; Olczak, A.; Białkowska, A.M.; Koziołkiewicz, M. Advanced Glycation End-Products (AGEs): Formation, Chemistry, Classification, Receptors, and Diseases Related to AGEs. *Cells* **2022**, *11*, 1312. [CrossRef]
13. Hurrle, S.; Hsu, W.H. The etiology of oxidative stress in insulin resistance. *Biomed. J.* **2017**, *40*, 257–262. [CrossRef]
14. Okechukwu, Q.N.; Adepoju, F.O.; Kanwugu, O.N.; Adadi, P.; Serrano-Aroca, Á.; Uversky, V.N.; Okpala, C.O.R. Marine-Derived Bioactive Metabolites as a Potential Therapeutic Intervention in Managing Viral Diseases: Insights from the SARS-CoV-2 In Silico and Pre-Clinical Studies. *Pharmaceuticals* **2024**, *17*, 328. [CrossRef]
15. Wang, R.; Zhao, H.; Pan, X.; Orfila, C.; Lu, W.; Ma, Y. Preparation of bioactive peptides with antidiabetic, antihypertensive, and antioxidant activities and identification of α-glucosidase inhibitory peptides from soy protein. *Food Sci. Nutr.* **2019**, *7*, 1848–1856. [CrossRef] [PubMed]
16. Lammi, C.; Aiello, G.; Boschin, G.; Arnoldi, A. Multifunctional peptides for the prevention of cardiovascular disease: A new concept in the area of bioactive food-derived peptides. *J. Funct. Foods* **2019**, *55*, 135–145. [CrossRef]
17. Hossain, A.; Dave, D.; Shahidi, F. Antioxidant Potential of Sea Cucumbers and Their Beneficial Effects on Human Health. *Mar. Drugs* **2022**, *20*, 521. [CrossRef] [PubMed]
18. Phetchthumrongchai, T.; Tachapuripunya, V.; Chintong, S.; Roytrakul, S.; E-kobon, T.; Klaypradit, W. Properties of Protein Hydrolysates and Bioinformatics Prediction of Peptides Derived from Thermal and Enzymatic Process of Skipjack Tuna (*Katsuwonus pelamis*) Roe. *Fishes* **2022**, *7*, 255. [CrossRef]
19. Admassu, H.; Gasmalla, M.A.A.; Yang, R.; Zhao, W. Bioactive Peptides Derived from Seaweed Protein and Their Health Benefits: Antihypertensive, Antioxidant, and Antidiabetic Properties. *J. Food Sci.* **2018**, *83*, 6–16. [CrossRef]
20. Lemes, A.C.; Sala, L.; Ores Jda, C.; Braga, A.R.; Egea, M.B.; Fernandes, K.F. A Review of the Latest Advances in Encrypted Bioactive Peptides from Protein-Rich Waste. *Int. J. Mol. Sci.* **2016**, *17*, 950. [CrossRef]
21. Jakubczyk, A.; Karaś, M.; Rybczyńska-Tkaczyk, K.; Zielińska, E.; Zieliński, D. Current Trends of Bioactive Peptides—New Sources and Therapeutic Effect. *Foods* **2020**, *9*, 846. [CrossRef]
22. Chi, C.-F.; Wang, B. Marine Bioactive Peptides—Structure, Function and Application. *Mar. Drugs* **2023**, *21*, 275. [CrossRef] [PubMed]
23. Yang, H.; Zhang, Q.; Zhang, B.; Zhao, Y.; Wang, N. Potential Active Marine Peptides as Anti-Aging Drugs or Drug Candidates. *Mar. Drugs* **2023**, *21*, 144. [CrossRef] [PubMed]
24. Phadke, G.G.; Rathod, N.B.; Ozogul, F.; Elavarasan, K.; Karthikeyan, M.; Shin, K.-H.; Kim, S.-K. Exploiting of Secondary Raw Materials from Fish Processing Industry as a Source of Bioactive Peptide-Rich Protein Hydrolysates. *Mar. Drugs* **2021**, *19*, 480. [CrossRef] [PubMed]
25. Rivero-Pino, F.; Espejo-Carpio, F.J.; Guadix, E.M. Production and identification of dipeptidyl peptidase IV (DPP-IV) inhibitory peptides from discarded *Sardine pilchardus* protein. *Food Chem.* **2020**, *328*, 127096. [CrossRef] [PubMed]
26. Zhang, Y.; Chen, R.; Chen, X.; Zeng, Z.; Ma, H.; Chen, S. Dipeptidyl Peptidase IV-Inhibitory Peptides Derived from Silver Carp (*Hypophthalmichthys molitrix* Val.) Proteins. *J. Agric. Food Chem.* **2016**, *64*, 831–839. [CrossRef] [PubMed]
27. Neves, A.C.; Harnedy, P.A.; O'Keeffe, M.B.; FitzGerald, R.J. Bioactive peptides from Atlantic salmon (*Salmo salar*) with angiotensin converting enzyme and dipeptidyl peptidase IV inhibitory, and antioxidant activities. *Food Chem.* **2017**, *218*, 396–405. [CrossRef] [PubMed]
28. Bodnaruc, A.M.; Prud'homme, D.; Blanchet, R.; Giroux, I. Nutritional modulation of endogenous glucagon-like peptide-1 secretion: A review. *Nutr. Metab.* **2016**, *13*, 92. [CrossRef] [PubMed]
29. Harnedy, P.A.; Parthsarathy, V.; McLaughlin, C.M.; O'Keeffe, M.B.; Allsopp, P.J.; McSorley, E.M.; O'Harte, F.P.M.; FitzGerald, R.J. Atlantic salmon (*Salmo salar*) co-product-derived protein hydrolysates: A source of antidiabetic peptides. *Food Res. Int.* **2018**, *106*, 598–606. [CrossRef] [PubMed]
30. Li-Chan, E.C.Y.; Hunag, S.-L.; Jao, C.-L.; Ho, K.-P.; Hsu, K.-C. Peptides Derived from Atlantic Salmon Skin Gelatin as Dipeptidyl-peptidase IV Inhibitors. *J. Agric. Food Chem.* **2012**, *60*, 973–978. [CrossRef]
31. Roblet, C.; Doyen, A.; Amiot, J.; Pilon, G.; Marette, A.; Bazinet, L. Enhancement of glucose uptake in muscular cell by soybean charged peptides isolated by electrodialysis with ultrafiltration membranes (EDUF): Activation of the AMPK pathway. *Food Chem.* **2014**, *147*, 124–130. [CrossRef]
32. Huang, F.; Wu, W. Antidiabetic effect of a new peptide from *Squalus mitsukurii* liver (S-8300) in streptozotocin-induced diabetic mice. *J. Pharm. Pharmacol.* **2005**, *57*, 1575–1580. [CrossRef]

33. Wang, J.; Du, K.; Fang, L.; Liu, C.; Min, W.; Liu, J. Evaluation of the antidiabetic activity of hydrolyzed peptides derived from *Juglans mandshurica* Maxim. fruits in insulin-resistant HepG2 cells and type 2 diabetic mice. *J. Food Biochem.* **2018**, *42*, e12518. [CrossRef]
34. Devasia, S.; Kumar, S.; Stephena, P.S.; Inoue, N.; Sugihara, F.; Suzuki, K. Double Blind, Randomized Clinical Study to Evaluate Efficacy of Collagen Peptide as Add on Nutritional Supplement in Type 2 Diabetes. *J. Clin. Nutr. Food Sci.* **2018**, *1*, 006–011.
35. Hovland, I.H.; Leikanger, I.S.; Stokkeland, O.; Waage, K.H.; Mjøs, S.A.; Brokstad, K.A.; McCann, A.; Ueland, P.M.; Slizyte, R.; Carvajal, A.; et al. Effects of low doses of fish and milk proteins on glucose regulation and markers of insulin sensitivity in overweight adults: A randomised, double blind study. *Eur. J. Nutr.* **2020**, *59*, 1013–1029. [CrossRef]
36. Musa-Veloso, K.; Paulionis, L.; Pelipyagina, T.; Evans, M. A Randomized, Double-Blind, Placebo-Controlled, Multicentre Trial of the Effects of a Shrimp Protein Hydrolysate on Blood Pressure. *Int. J. Hypertens.* **2019**, *2019*, 2345042. [CrossRef]
37. Framroze, B.; Vekariya, S.; Dhruv, S. A Placebo-Controlled Study of the Impact of Dietary Salmon Protein Hydrolysate Supplementation in Increasing Ferritin and Hemoglobin Levels in Iron-Deficient Anemic Subjects. *J. Nutr. Food Sci.* **2015**, *5*, 1.
38. Framroze, B.; Vekariya, S.; Swaroop, D. A Placebo-Controlled, Randomized Study on the Impact of Dietary Salmon Protein Hydrolysate Supplementation on Body Mass Index in Overweight Human Subjects. *J. Obes. Weight Loss Ther.* **2016**, *6*, 296. [CrossRef]
39. Framroze, B.; Havaldar, F.; Misal, S. An in vitro study on the regulation of oxidative protective genes in human gingival and intestinal epithelial cells after treatment with salmon protein hydrolysate peptides. *Funct. Foods Health Dis.* **2018**, *8*, 398–411. [CrossRef]
40. Imai, Y.; Dobrian, A.D.; Morris, M.A.; Taylor-Fishwick, D.A.; Nadler, J.L. Lipids and immunoinflammatory pathways of beta cell destruction. *Diabetologia* **2016**, *59*, 673–678. [CrossRef] [PubMed]
41. Burkart, V.; Kolb, H. Protection of islet cells from inflammatory cell death in vitro. *Clin. Exp. Immunol.* **1993**, *93*, 273–278. [CrossRef] [PubMed]
42. Lieb, D.C.; Brotman, J.J.; Hatcher, M.A.; Aye, M.S.; Cole, B.K.; Haynes, B.A.; Wohlgemuth, S.D.; Fontana, M.A.; Beydoun, H.; Nadler, J.L.; et al. Adipose tissue 12/15 lipoxygenase pathway in human obesity and diabetes. *J. Clin. Endocrinol. Metab.* **2014**, *99*, E1713–E1720. [CrossRef] [PubMed]
43. Måge, I.; Böcker, U.; Wubshet, S.G.; Lindberg, D.; Afseth, N.K. Fourier-transform infrared (FTIR) fingerprinting for quality assessment of protein hydrolysates. *LWT* **2021**, *152*, 112339. [CrossRef]
44. Jahandideh, F.; Bourque, S.L.; Wu, J. A comprehensive review on the glucoregulatory properties of food-derived bioactive peptides. *Food Chem. X* **2022**, *13*, 100222. [CrossRef] [PubMed]
45. Carrera-Alvarado, G.; Toldrá, F.; Mora, L. DPP-IV Inhibitory Peptides GPF, IGL, and GGGW Obtained from Chicken Blood Hydrolysates. *Int. J. Mol. Sci.* **2022**, *23*, 14140. [CrossRef]
46. Vilcacundo, R.; Martínez-Villaluenga, C.; Hernández-Ledesma, B. Release of dipeptidyl peptidase IV, α-amylase and α-glucosidase inhibitory peptides from quinoa (*Chenopodium quinoa* Willd.) during in vitro simulated gastrointestinal digestion. *J. Funct. Foods* **2017**, *35*, 531–539. [CrossRef]
47. Ketnawa, S.; Suwal, S.; Huang, J.-Y.; Liceaga, A.M. Selective separation and characterisation of dual ACE and DPP-IV inhibitory peptides from rainbow trout (*Oncorhynchus mykiss*) protein hydrolysates. *Int. J. Food Sci. Technol.* **2019**, *54*, 1062–1073. [CrossRef]
48. Chanon, S.; Durand, C.; Vieille-Marchiset, A.; Robert, M.; Dibner, C.; Simon, C.; Lefai, E. Glucose Uptake Measurement and Response to Insulin Stimulation in In Vitro Cultured Human Primary Myotubes. *J. Vis. Exp.* **2017**, *124*, e55743. [CrossRef]
49. Zhang, C.; Zhang, Y.; Wang, Z.; Chen, S.; Luo, Y. Production and identification of antioxidant and angiotensin-converting enzyme inhibition and dipeptidyl peptidase IV inhibitory peptides from bighead carp (*Hypophthalmichthys nobilis*) muscle hydrolysate. *J. Funct. Foods* **2017**, *35*, 224–235. [CrossRef]
50. Zhang, Y.; Liu, H.; Hong, H.; Luo, Y. Purification and identification of dipeptidyl peptidase IV and angiotensin-converting enzyme inhibitory peptides from silver carp (*Hypophthalmichthys molitrix*) muscle hydrolysate. *Eur. Food Res. Technol.* **2019**, *245*, 243–255. [CrossRef]
51. Farias, T.C.; de Souza, T.S.P.; Fai, A.E.C.; Koblitz, M.G.B. Critical Review for the Production of Antidiabetic Peptides by a Bibliometric Approach. *Nutrients* **2022**, *14*, 4275. [CrossRef]
52. Nong, N.T.P.; Hsu, J.L. Characteristics of Food Protein-Derived Antidiabetic Bioactive Peptides: A Literature Update. *Int. J. Mol. Sci.* **2021**, *22*, 9508. [CrossRef]
53. Xu, F.; Yao, Y.; Xu, X.; Wang, M.; Pan, M.; Ji, S.; Wu, J.; Jiang, D.; Ju, X.; Wang, L. Identification and Quantification of DPP-IV-Inhibitory Peptides from Hydrolyzed-Rapeseed-Protein-Derived Napin with Analysis of the Interactions between Key Residues and Protein Domains. *J. Agric. Food Chem.* **2019**, *67*, 3679–3690. [CrossRef]
54. Nongonierma, A.B.; Hennemann, M.; Paolella, S.; FitzGerald, R.J. Generation of wheat gluten hydrolysates with dipeptidyl peptidase IV (DPP-IV) inhibitory properties. *Food Funct.* **2017**, *8*, 2249–2257. [CrossRef]
55. Nongonierma, A.B.; Lamoureux, C.; FitzGerald, R.J. Generation of dipeptidyl peptidase IV (DPP-IV) inhibitory peptides during the enzymatic hydrolysis of tropical banded cricket (*Gryllodes sigillatus*) proteins. *Food Funct.* **2018**, *9*, 407–416. [CrossRef]
56. Morifuji, M.; Koga, J.; Kawanaka, K.; Higuchi, M. Branched-chain amino acid-containing dipeptides, identified from whey protein hydrolysates, stimulate glucose uptake rate in L6 myotubes and isolated skeletal muscles. *J. Nutr. Sci. Vitaminol.* **2009**, *55*, 81–86. [CrossRef]

57. Lima, R.d.C.L.; Berg, R.S.; Rønning, S.B.; Afseth, N.K.; Knutsen, S.H.; Staerk, D.; Wubshet, S.G. Peptides from chicken processing by-product inhibit DPP-IV and promote cellular glucose uptake: Potential ingredients for T2D management. *Food Funct.* **2019**, *10*, 1619–1628. [CrossRef]
58. Henaux, L.; Pereira, K.D.; Thibodeau, J.; Pilon, G.; Gill, T.; Marette, A.; Bazinet, L. Glucoregulatory and Anti-Inflammatory Activities of Peptide Fractions Separated by Electrodialysis with Ultrafiltration Membranes from Salmon Protein Hydrolysate and Identification of Four Novel Glucoregulatory Peptides. *Membranes* **2021**, *11*, 528. [CrossRef]
59. Doi, M.; Yamaoka, I.; Nakayama, M.; Mochizuki, S.; Sugahara, K.; Yoshizawa, F. Isoleucine, a blood glucose-lowering amino acid, increases glucose uptake in rat skeletal muscle in the absence of increases in AMP-activated protein kinase activity. *J. Nutr.* **2005**, *135*, 2103–2108. [CrossRef]
60. Morato, P.N.; Lollo, P.C.B.; Moura, C.S.; Batista, T.M.; Camargo, R.L.; Carneiro, E.M.; Amaya-Farfan, J. Whey Protein Hydrolysate Increases Translocation of GLUT-4 to the Plasma Membrane Independent of Insulin in Wistar Rats. *PLoS ONE* **2013**, *8*, e71134. [CrossRef]
61. Jahandideh, F.; Wu, J. A review on mechanisms of action of bioactive peptides against glucose intolerance and insulin resistance. *Food Sci. Hum. Wellness* **2022**, *11*, 1441–1454. [CrossRef]
62. Lacroix, I.M.E.; Li-Chan, E.C.Y. Evaluation of the potential of dietary proteins as precursors of dipeptidyl peptidase (DPP)-IV inhibitors by an in silico approach. *J. Funct. Foods* **2012**, *4*, 403–422. [CrossRef]
63. Harnedy-Rothwell, P.A.; McLaughlin, C.M.; O'Keeffe, M.B.; Le Gouic, A.V.; Allsopp, P.J.; McSorley, E.M.; Sharkey, S.; Whooley, J.; McGovern, B.; O'Harte, F.P.M.; et al. Identification and characterisation of peptides from a boarfish (*Capros aper*) protein hydrolysate displaying in vitro dipeptidyl peptidase-IV (DPP-IV) inhibitory and insulinotropic activity. *Food Res. Int.* **2020**, *131*, 108989. [CrossRef]
64. Mooney, C.; Haslam, N.J.; Pollastri, G.; Shields, D.C. Towards the improved discovery and design of functional peptides: Common features of diverse classes permit generalized prediction of bioactivity. *PLoS ONE* **2012**, *7*, e45012. [CrossRef]
65. Ucd, B. Peptide Ranker. Available online: http://bioware.ucd.ie/~compass/biowareweb/Server_pages/help/peptideranker/help.php (accessed on 19 March 2024).
66. Berg, R.A.; Prockop, D.J. The thermal transition of a non-hydroxylated form of collagen. Evidence for a role for hydroxyproline in stabilizing the triple-helix of collagen. *Biochem. Biophys. Res. Commun.* **1973**, *52*, 115–120. [CrossRef]
67. Xu, Q.; Zheng, L.; Huang, M.; Zhao, M. Exploring structural features of potent dipeptidyl peptidase IV (DPP-IV) inhibitory peptides derived from tilapia (*Oreochromis niloticus*) skin gelatin by an integrated approach of multivariate analysis and Gly-Pro-based peptide library. *Food Chem.* **2022**, *397*, 133821. [CrossRef]
68. Jin, R.; Teng, X.; Shang, J.; Wang, D.; Liu, N. Identification of novel DPP-IV inhibitory peptides from Atlantic salmon (*Salmo salar*) skin. *Food Res. Int.* **2020**, *133*, 109161. [CrossRef]
69. Parthsarathy, V.; McLaughlin, C.; Sharkey, S.; Harnedy-Rothwell, P.; Lafferty, R.; Allsopp, P.; Emeir, M.; FitzGerald, R.; O'Harte, F. Protein hydrolysates from boarfish (*Capros aper*) and Atlantic salmon (*Salmo salar*) skin gelatin improve metabolic control in genetically obese diabetic (ob/ob) mice. *J. Food Bioact.* **2021**, *16*, 48–57. [CrossRef]
70. Han, R.; Hernández Álvarez, A.J.; Maycock, J.; Murray, B.S.; Boesch, C. Comparison of alcalase- and pepsin-treated oilseed protein hydrolysates—Experimental validation of predicted antioxidant, antihypertensive and antidiabetic properties. *Curr. Res. Food Sci.* **2021**, *4*, 141–149. [CrossRef]
71. Gomez, H.L.R.; Peralta, J.P.; Tejano, L.A.; Chang, Y.-W. In Silico and In Vitro Assessment of Portuguese Oyster (*Crassostrea angulata*) Proteins as Precursor of Bioactive Peptides. *Int. J. Mol. Sci.* **2019**, *20*, 5191. [CrossRef]
72. Reimer, R.A. Meat hydrolysate and essential amino acid-induced glucagon-like peptide-1 secretion, in the human NCI-H716 enteroendocrine cell line, is regulated by extracellular signal-regulated kinase1/2 and p38 mitogen-activated protein kinases. *J. Endocrinol.* **2006**, *191*, 159–170. [CrossRef]
73. *ISO 13903:2005*; Animal Feeding Stuffs-Determination of Amino Acids Content. International Organization for Standardization: Geneva, Switzerland, 2005.
74. Wubshet, S.G.; Måge, I.; Böcker, U.; Lindberg, D.; Knutsen, S.H.; Rieder, A.; Rodriguez, D.A.; Afseth, N.K. FTIR as a rapid tool for monitoring molecular weight distribution during enzymatic protein hydrolysis of food processing by-products. *Anal. Methods* **2017**, *9*, 4247–4254. [CrossRef]
75. Abdelmoez, A.M.; Sardón Puig, L.; Smith, J.A.B.; Gabriel, B.M.; Savikj, M.; Dollet, L.; Chibalin, A.V.; Krook, A.; Zierath, J.R.; Pillon, N.J. Comparative profiling of skeletal muscle models reveals heterogeneity of transcriptome and metabolism. *Am. J. Physiol.-Cell Physiol.* **2020**, *318*, C615–C626. [CrossRef] [PubMed]

Disclaimer/Publisher's Note: The statements, opinions and data contained in all publications are solely those of the individual author(s) and contributor(s) and not of MDPI and/or the editor(s). MDPI and/or the editor(s) disclaim responsibility for any injury to people or property resulting from any ideas, methods, instructions or products referred to in the content.

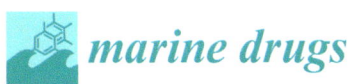

Article

Synthesis and Late-Stage Modification of (−)-Doliculide Derivatives Using Matteson's Homologation Approach

Markus Tost and Uli Kazmaier *

Organic Chemistry, Saarland University, Campus Building C4.2, D-66123 Saarbruecken, Germany; markus.tost@uni-saarland.de
* Correspondence: u.kazmaier@mx.uni-saarland.de; Tel.: +49-681-302-3409

Abstract: (−)-Doliculide, a marine cyclodepsipeptide derived from the Japanese sea hare, *Dolabella auricularia*, exhibits potent cytotoxic properties, sparking interest in the field of synthetic chemistry. It is comprised of a peptide segment and a polyketide moiety, rendering it amenable to Matteson's homologation methodology. This technique facilitates the diversification of the distinctive polyketide side chain, thereby permitting the introduction of functional groups in late stages for modifications of the derived compounds and studies on structure–activity relationships.

Keywords: actin binder; click chemistry; doliculide; Matteson homologation; SAR studies

1. Introduction

Isolation of (−)-doliculide (Figure 1) from the Japanese sea hare, *Dolabella auricularia*, was first reported almost 30 years ago by Yamada et al., along with its potent cytotoxicity against HeLa-S_3 cells (IC_{50} = 1 ng/mL) [1]. The mollusk itself may not necessarily be the producer of this cyclic depsipeptide, but metabolites isolated from *Dolabella auricularia* have been shown to originate from cyanobacteria and are therefore of dietary origin [2]. Due to their biological activities as anticancer agents, naturally derived cyclopeptides are interesting candidates for drug development, and so is doliculide [3–5].

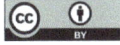

Figure 1. (−)-Doliculide.

Doliculide was found to act as a potent actin binder with a higher cell-membrane permeability than phalloidin and, thus, initiates actin aggregation, leading to inhibition of proliferation and apoptosis [6–10]. Subtoxic doses of doliculide lead to a transient change in reversible cytoskeleton dynamics and induction of premature senescence in p53 wild-type cells [11]. In a proof-of-concept study, doliculide was revealed to be a subtype-selective antagonist of the prostanoid E receptor 3 as a macromolecular target [12]. While the peptide and polyketide moieties of doliculide are both of some significance in actin binding, most synthetic derivatizations so far have focused on the peptide moiety, e. g., modifications in the (*R*)-Tyr-moiety, substitution of the iodo-(*R*)-Tyr part to Trp, or Gly to (*S*)-Ala [9,13,14].

Removal of the hydroxyl group within the polyketide moiety resulted in a notable sixfold reduction in cytotoxic activity against HeLa-S3 cells. Conversely, complete removal of the polyketide or all associated functionalities yielded derivatives that were inactive [13].

It was shown that doliculide stabilizes F-actin in a similar way to structurally related natural products such as jaspamide [15], geodiamolide [16], seragamide [17], or miuraenamide [18–20] (Figure 2) [21]. Even the double-bound geometry in the miuraenamides has no significant effect on cytotoxicity [22]. All these cyclodepsipeptides are hybrids of a small peptide fragment and a variably substituted polyketide unit. Here, an α- or β-amino acid can be incorporated, which might be substituted or unsaturated. In the case of doliculide, this third amino acid is even missing, while the polyketide fragment is longer compared to most of the other natural products (except for the miuraenamides). This prompted our assumption that the isopropyl group at the terminus of the polyketide may be a replacement for the third amino acid, and that this may also be variable.

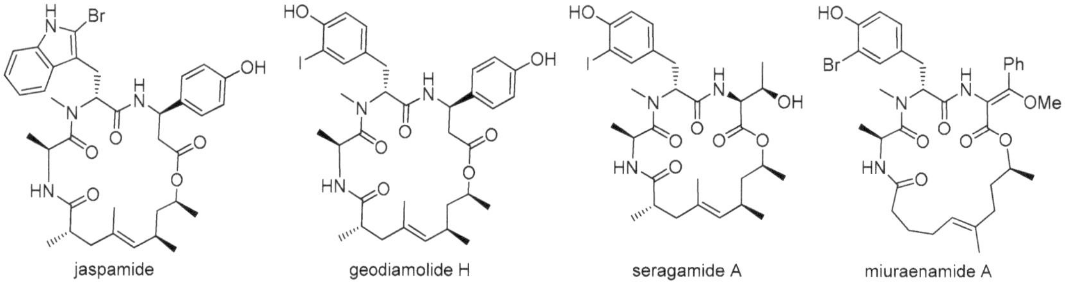

Figure 2. Structurally related F-Actin-stabilizing natural products.

2. Results and Discussion

As our group is experienced in the syntheses of such peptide–polyketide conjugates [23–26], this assumption led us to develop a straightforward synthesis of doliculide, and associated derivatives, based on Matteson homologation [27–29], allowing late-stage variation at exactly this position [30]. In an initial modification, it was demonstrated that replacing the isopropyl group by the smaller methyl group led to almost no change in its cytotoxic activity. In principle, Matteson homologation should allow for the synthesis of a variety of derivatives simply by varying the nucleophiles in the homologation steps [30–33]. Therefore, we decided to also incorporate allyl and propargyl moieties via Matteson homologation, which could then be further used for late-stage modification—generating a variety of doliculide derivatives for structure–activity relationship (SAR) studies.

2.1. Preparation of Modified Polyketide Fragments

Synthesis of the polyketide fragments started from the previously described boronic ester **1** [30], which was subjected to Matteson homologation with Cl$_2$CHLi to obtain homologated α-chloroboronic ester, **1a-Cl** (Scheme 1). To facilitate preparation of **2a**, compound **1a-Cl** was quickly worked up before it was reacted with a Knochel-type propargylic zinc reagent [34,35], which gave better yields than the corresponding Grignard reagent. Furthermore, **1a-Cl** was reacted with AllylMgBr in a one-pot fashion to deliver **2b**. Both boronic esters, **2a** and **2b**, were subsequently oxidized to the corresponding polyketide fragments, **3a** and **3b**.

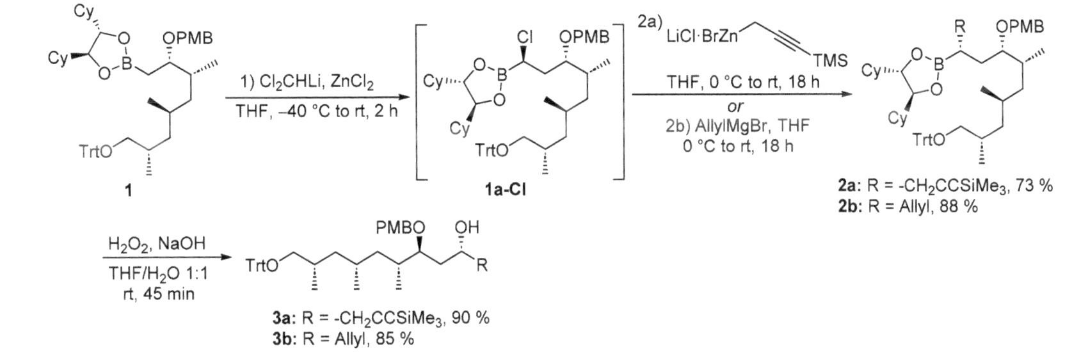

Scheme 1. Syntheses of the polyketide fragments **3**.

2.2. Syntheses of the Doliculide Core Structure

Steglich esterification of the alcohols, **3**, with modified (*R*)-Tyr, **4**, delivered the esters, **5**. Subsequent trityl deprotection and Jones oxidation generated acids, **6**, in acceptable yield even in the presence of the acid-labile Boc- and PMB-protecting groups (Scheme 2). The acids were then coupled with glycine *tert*-butyl ester to produce the peptides, **7**. After acidic cleavage of the Boc-, PMB- and *tert*-butyl-protection groups, cyclization using BOPCl (bis(2-oxo-3-oxazolidinyl)phosphinic chloride) as activator provided the corresponding cyclic peptides [36]. Unexpectedly, acidic treatment did not result in cleavage of the TMS-alkyne. Finally, CpRu(MeCN)$_3$PF$_6$-mediated removal of the allyl protecting group gave rise to both the TMS-protected alkyne, **8a**, and the allyl derivative, **8b** [22,37,38]. TMS deprotection of **8a** was achieved by treatment with TBAF and **8c** was obtained quantitatively.

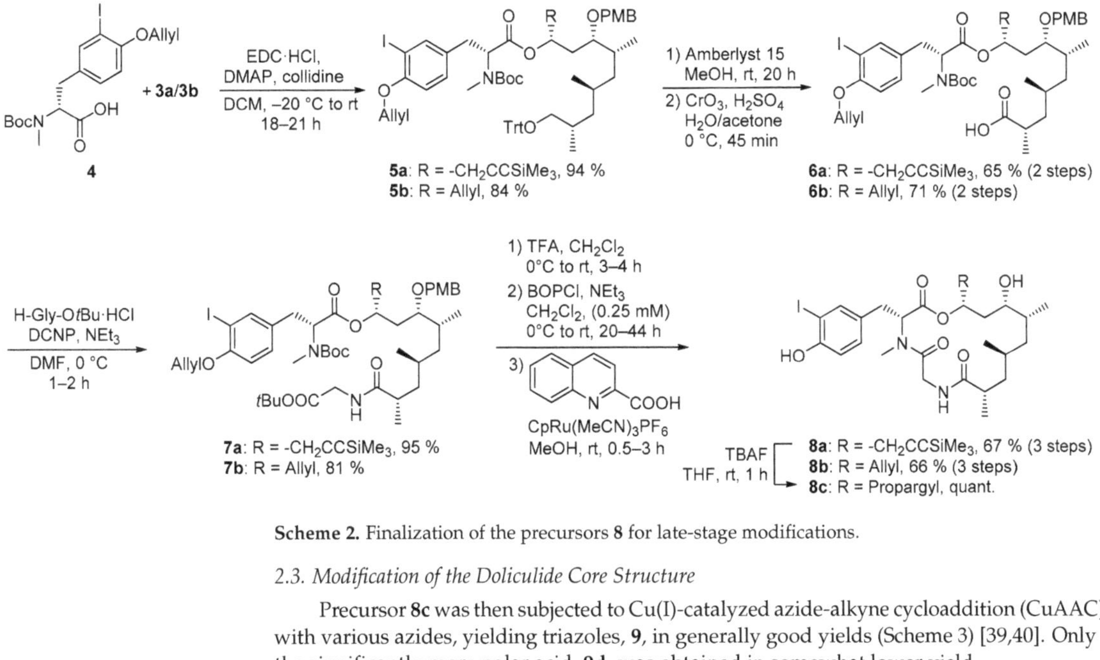

Scheme 2. Finalization of the precursors **8** for late-stage modifications.

2.3. Modification of the Doliculide Core Structure

Precursor **8c** was then subjected to Cu(I)-catalyzed azide-alkyne cycloaddition (CuAAC) with various azides, yielding triazoles, **9**, in generally good yields (Scheme 3) [39,40]. Only the significantly more polar acid, **9d**, was obtained in somewhat lower yield.

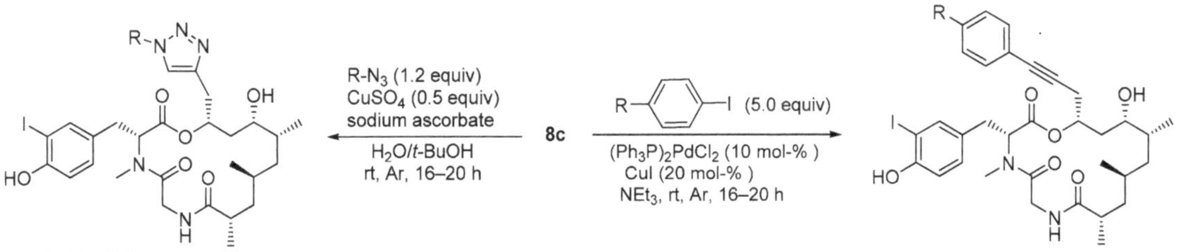

9a: R = Bn, 86 %
9b: R = *n*-Pentyl, 95 %
9c: R = BnOOCCH$_2$-, 94 %
9d: R = HO$_2$CCH$_2$(OC$_2$H$_4$)$_2$-, 66 %
9e: R = H(OC$_2$H$_4$)$_3$-, 80 %
9f: R = *t*-BuOOCNH(C$_2$H$_4$O)$_2$C$_2$H$_4$-, 92 %
9g: R = *t*-BuOOCNH(C$_2$H$_4$O)$_3$C$_2$H$_4$-, 80 %

10a: R = H, 58 %
10b: R = OMe, 75 %
10c: R = NO$_2$, 76 %

Scheme 3. Modifications of doliculide derivative **8c**.

In addition, alkyne **8c** was also used for Sonogashira couplings with several aryl iodides [41]. An excess of aryl iodide was used to prevent side-reactions which could occur with the electron-rich aryl iodide of the tyrosine moiety of **8c**. Good yields of **10** were obtained with both electron-rich and electron-poor iodoarenes.

Allyl derivative **8b** was subjected to a series of BEt$_3$/O$_2$-mediated radical thiol-ene reactions, giving rise to several functionalized thioethers, **11** (Scheme 4) [42,43]. Thioacetic acid could also be implemented, leading to the thioester **11f** in high yield. Only with ester and acid functionalities in the thiol component, the conversion was observed to be incomplete and, therefore, another 0.3 equiv. BEt$_3$ were subsequently added, leading to full conversion.

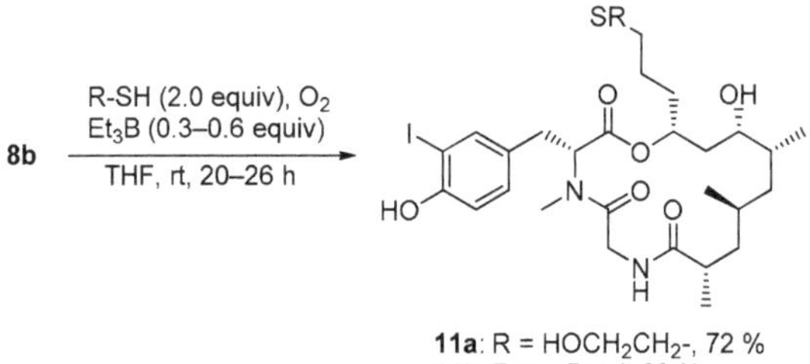

11a: R = HOCH$_2$CH$_2$-, 72 %
11b: R = *n*-Butyl, 83 %
11c: R = Bn, 55 %
11d: R = H$_3$CCH$_2$COOCH$_2$CH$_2$-, 79 %
11e: R = HO$_2$CCH$_2$-, 66 %
11f: R = H$_3$CCO-, 94 %

Scheme 4. Thiol-ene click reactions with precursor **8b**.

3. Cytotoxicity Evaluation of New Doliculide Derivatives

Finally, with the doliculide derivates now available, we undertook SAR studies to determine the impact of the modifications at the end of the polyketide chain. The cytotoxicity of the derivatives **8–11** was investigated towards five different cancer cell lines. The IC$_{50}$ values are given in Table 1 and compared to synthetic doliculide (**A**, entry 1).

Table 1. IC_{50} values of doliculide **A** and derivatives **8–11** towards different cancer cell lines [a].

Entry	Compound	IC_{50}				
		HepG2	CHO-K1	HCT-116	U-2 OS	KB3.1
1	A	16.4 ± 4.2 nM	110.8 ± 4.5 nM	8.8 ± 0.5 nM	25.2 ± 1.8 nM	38.0 ± 9.9 nM
2	8a	20.0 ± 4.5 μM	380 ± 44 nM	8.0 ± 7.3 nM	336 ± 146 nM	≤115 nM [b]
3	8b	>60.2 μM	264 ± 13 nM	16 ± 8 nM	521 ± 488 nM	103 ± 65 nM
4	8c	147 ± 65 nM	474 ± 147 nM	65 ± 16 nM	49 ± 33 nM	114 ± 49 nM
5	9a	>49.6 μM	24 ± 9 nM	309 ± 81 nM	≤ 80 nM [b]	47 ± 13 nM
6	9b	>50.1 μM	69 ± 12 nM	≤ 110 nM [b]	≤ 110 nM [b]	41 ± 14 nM
7	9c	>46.0 μM	23.8 ± 0.5 μM	3.81 ± 1.00 μM	14.4 ± 1.3 μM	21.9 ± 12.6 μM
8	9d	>46.2 μM	>46.2 μM	>46.2 μM	>46.2 μM	>46.2 μM
9	9e	>47.0 μM	>47.0 μM	8.55 ± 1.14 μM	23.0 ± 4.4 μM	10.5 ± 0.3 μM
10	9f	>41.7 μM	6.38 ± 2.81 μM	86 ± 79 nM	1.56 ± 0.67 μM	722 ± 180 nM
11	9g	>39.7 μM	12.9 ± 3.0 μM	432 ± 140 nM	2.94 ± 1.75 μM	3.29 ± 1.39 μM
12	10a	15.5 ± 0.3 μM	247 ± 145 nM	14.5 ± 0.6 nM	683 ± 87 nM	49 ± 29 nM
13	10b	>51.5 μM	1.46 ± 0.28 μM	153 ± 56 nM	1.88 ± 0.11 μM	459 ± 111 μM
14	10c	>50.4 μM	586 ± 205 nM	10 ± 3 nM	491 ± 95 nM	98 ± 41 nM
15	11a	>53.4 μM	765 ± 13 nM	22 ± 9 nM	129 ± 14 nM	196 ± 72 nM
16	11b	>52.5 μM	142 ± 85 nM	>52.5 μM	238 ± 10 nM	28 ± 3 nM
17	11c	>50.0 μM	391 ± 122 nM	10.8 ± 1.2 nM	582 ± 68 nM	37 ± 1 nM
18	11d	>49.4 μM	9.84 ± 3.87 μM	60 ± 13 nM	4.90 ± 3.87 μM	3.93 ± 1.14 μM
19	11e	>52.3 μM	39.8 ± 18.0 μM	6.21 ± 3.00 μM	>52.3 μM	>52.3 μM
20	11f	>53.6 μM	6.08 ± 2.32 μM	41 ± 23 nM	6.21 ± 1.74 μM	>53.6 μM
	Color code	<10.0 nM	10.0–100.0 nM	100.0 nM–1.0 μM	1.0–10.0 μM	>10.0 μM

[a] HepG2: human hepatocellular carcinoma; CHO-K1: mutagenized Chinese hamster ovary; HCT-116: human colon carcinoma; U-2 OS: human bone osteosarcoma; KB3.1: human epidermoid carcinoma cell line. [b] The individual results varied widely and were therefore given as a range.

Of all derivatives tested, only doliculide showed a high toxicity against most cancer cell lines. It was the only active compound against HepG2 (human hepatocellular carcinoma), and only propargyl-derivative **8c** showed any significant activity, although tenfold lower (entry 4). All other derivatives were almost inactive. Clearly, this cell line is extremely sensitive towards modification at this position. This derivative also showed good activity against U-2 OS (human bone osteosarcoma). Two triazole derivatives, **9a** and **9b**, were found to be the most active compounds against CHO-K1 (mutagenized Chinese hamster ovary carcinoma) (entries 5 and 6). Against KB3.1 (human epidermoid carcinoma cell line), they were comparably active with A or alkyne **10a**. The thioethers **11b** and **11c** were found to be the most active compounds in this series (entries 16 and 17). The human colon carcinoma cell line (HCT-116) was found to be by far the most sensitive cell line. IC_{50} values in the low nM range, and comparable to A, were obtained with several doliculide derivatives such as **8a**, **8b**, **10a**, **10c** or **11c** (entries 2, 3, 12, 14 and 17).

4. Materials and Methods

The General Synthetic Methods were as follows: All air- or moisture-sensitive reactions were carried out in dried glassware (>100 °C) under an atmosphere of nitrogen or argon. Anhydrous solvents were purchased from Acros Organics (now Thermo Fisher Scientific, Waltham, MA, USA) or dried before use (THF was distilled over Na/benzophenone, diisopropylamine over CaH_2, MeOH distilled with Magnesium and degassed via freeze–pump–thaw). $ZnCl_2$ was fused in vacuo at 0.1 mbar prior to use. Ethyl acetate (EtOAc), petroleum ether and n-pentane were additionally distilled before use. Reactions that required cooling were cooled using conventional methods (ice/water for 0 °C, dry ice/acetone for −40 °C or −78 °C). Reactions that required heating above rt were heated using an oil bath. Reactions were monitored by NMR or analytical TLC, which was performed on precoated silica gel on Macherey-Nagel (Dueren, NRW, Germany) TLC-PET foils (Polygram® SIL G/UV_{254}). Visualization was accomplished with UV-light (254 nm), $KMnO_4$ solution or Ce(IV)/ammonium molybdate solution. The products were purified by flash chromatography on Macherey-Nagel 60 silica gel columns (0.063–0.2 mm or 0.04–0.063 mm) or by automated flash chromatography on Büchi (Flawil, Switzerland) Pure C-815 Chromatography System and prepacked Teledyne Isco (Thousand Oaks, CA, USA) silica gel cartridges (RediSep Rf normal- Macherey-Nagelphase silica flash 30–70 µm columns). Reversed-phase flash chromatography was accomplished by automated flash chromatography on Büchi Reveleris Prep Chromatography System and Büchi FlashPure Select C18 30 µm spherical cartridges or Cole-Parmer Telos (Vernon Hills, IL, USA) C18 cartridges. Preparative HPLC was performed on a Büchi Reveleris Prep Chromatography System using a Phenomenex (Danaher Corporation, Washington, DC, USA) Luna C18(2) 100 Å column (250 × 21.1 mm, 5 µm). ^{1}H- and ^{13}C-NMR spectra were recorded with a Bruker (Billerica, MA, USA) AV II 400 [400 MHz (^{1}H), 100 MHz (13C)], a Bruker AV 500 [500 MHz, (^{1}H), 125 MHz (^{13}C)] or a Bruker Avance Neo 500 [500 MHz, (^{1}H), 125 MHz (^{13}C)] spectrometer in CDCl$_3$ or DMSO-D$_6$. NMR spectra were evaluated using NMR Processor Version 12.01 from Advanced Chemistry Development Inc. (ACD/Labs, Toronto, ON, Canada) or Bruker TopSpin Version 4.1.1. Chemical shifts are reported in ppm relative to Si(CH$_3$)$_4$ and the solvent residual peak was used as the internal standard. Selected signals for the minor diastereomers/rotamers are extracted from the spectra of the isomeric mixture. Multiplicities are reported as bs (broad signal), s (singlet), d (doublet), t (triplet), q (quartet) and m (multiplet). Signals marked with * in ^{13}C-NMR give broad signals. Structural assignments were made with additional information from gCOSY, gNOESY, gHSQC, or gHMBC experiments. Melting points were determined with a melting-point apparatus MEL-TEMP II by Laboratory Devices (Auburn, CA, USA) and are uncorrected. High-resolution mass spectra (HRMS) were recorded with a Finnigan (now Thermo Fisher Scientific) MAT95 spectrometer using the CI technique (CI) or a Bruker Daltonics 4G hr-ToF (ESI-ToF) or a Bruker solariX using the ESI technique (ESI-FTICR). Other HRMS were measured on a Thermo Fisher Scientific Orbitrap Q exactive mass spectrometer, equipped with a heated ESI source and a Thermo Finnigan (Thermo Fisher Scientific) Ultimate3000 HPLC (ESI-Q exactive). Optical rotations were measured in CHCl$_3$ with a Krüss (Hamburg, Germany) polarimeter P8000 T80 in thermostated (20 °C ± 1 °C) cuvettes and are given in 10^{-1}degcm^{2}g^{-1}. The radiation source used was a sodium vapor lamp (λ = 589 nm). The concentrations are given in g/100 mL.

The general procedure for Cu(I)-catalyzed azide alkyne cycloadditions (CuAAC) was as follows: The alkyne (1.0 equiv) and azide (1.2 equiv) were dissolved in a 1:1 mixture of *t*-BuOH and H$_2$O (0.05 M) in a 1.5 mL vial. Under a gentle stream of argon, sodium ascorbate (0.6 equiv, 1 M in H$_2$O), and copper(II) sulfate (0.5 equiv, 1 M in H$_2$O) were added, the vial sealed and the typically light-brownish suspension stirred overnight at rt (typically 16–20 h). The reaction mixture was concentrated and the residue purified by column chromatography.

The general procedure for Sonogashira cross-coupling of terminal alkyne was as follows: The alkyne (1.0 equiv), bis(triphenylphosphine)palladium(II) chloride (0.1 equiv), and copper(I) iodide (0.2 equiv) were added in a 1.5 mL vial and gently purged with argon for 5 min. Triethylamine (0.15 M) and the iodoarene (5.0 equiv) were added under a gentle stream of argon, the vial closed and the typically white suspension stirred overnight (typically 16–20 h) after which the reaction typically turned black. The suspension was diluted with MeCN, filtrated through a syringe filter (0.2 µm, PTFE), the solvent removed in vacuo, and the residue was subjected to chromatographic purification.

The general procedure for thiol-ene click reaction was as follows: The alkene (1.0 equiv) was gently purged with nitrogen and dissolved in THF abs. (0.1 M) in a 1.5 mL vial. Thiol (2.0 equiv) and Et$_3$B (0.3 equiv, 1 M in hexane) were subsequently added, and the vial closed. Initiation of the reaction was performed by addition of air (0.4 mL) via a syringe and the reaction mixture stirred overnight at rt (typically 20–26 h). The solvent was removed and the crude product was purified by chromatography.

4.1. Synthesis of the Polyketide Fragments

4.1.1. Synthesis of {(4R,6S,7R,9R,11S)-4-[(4S,5S)-4,5-Dicyclohexyl-1,3,2-dioxaborolan-2-yl]-6-[(4-methoxybenzyl)oxy]-7,9,11-trimethyl-12-(trityloxy)dodec-1-yn-1-yl}trimethylsilane (2a)

Nucleophile solution: Lithium chloride (746 mg, 17.6 mmol, 1.10 equiv) was fused under reduced pressure. Zinc (2.09 g, 32.0 mmol, 2.0 equiv, dust) was added and the mixture suspended in anhydrous THF (16.0 mL). 1,2-Dibromoethane (28.0 µL, 320 µmol, 0.02 equiv) was added and briefly heated to reflux. It was cooled to rt and trimethylsilyl chloride (102 µL, 800 µmol, 0.05 equiv) was added. The mixture was briefly heated to reflux again and cooled to rt. (3-bromoprop-1-yn-1-yl)trimethylsilane [34] (3.06 g, 16.0 mmol, 1.0 equiv) in anhydrous THF (16.0 mL) was added dropwise (exothermic) and stirred for 1 h dat rt. The stirrer was stopped, and the nucleophile solution decanted. Titration of the solution[1] gave a concentration of 0.36 M (approximately 73% of theory). LDA-solution: Diisopropylamine (1.37 mL, 9.63 mmol, 1.35 equiv) was dissolved in anhydrous THF (3.43 mL, 2.81 M) and cooled to −40 °C (acetone/dry ice). *n*-Butyllithium (3.57 mL, 8.91 mmol, 1.25 equiv, 2.5 M in hexane) was added dropwise, stirred for 10 min at −40 °C, warmed to rt and further stirred for 20 min. Homologation: Boronic ester **1** [30] (5.60 g, 7.13 mmol, 1.0 equiv) and DCM (1.38 mL, 21.4 mmol, 3.0 equiv) were dissolved in anhydrous THF (9.98 mL, 1.4 mL/mmol, 0.71 M) and cooled to −40 °C (acetone/dry ice). The previously prepared LDA solution was slowly added at this temperature and stirred for further 10 min after complete addition. A solution of zinc chloride (3.89 g, 28.5 mmol, 4.0 equiv) in anhydrous THF (17.1 mL, 0.6 mL/mmol, 1.67 M) was added, the reaction mixture warmed to rt and stirred for 2 h. Isolation and substitution: The reaction mixture was worked up with saturated NH_4Cl and *n*-pentane. The phases were separated, and the aqueous phase extracted twice with *n*-pentane. The combined organic extracts were dried over Na_2SO_4 and the solvent removed under reduced pressure. The resulting residue was taken up in anhydrous THF (28.5 mL, 0.25 M), cooled to 0 °C and the previously (freshly) prepared nucleophile solution (21.8 mL, 7.84 mmol, 1.1 equiv) was added dropwise. It was slowly warmed to rt and stirred for 18 h. The reaction mixture was worked up with saturated NH_4Cl and *n*-pentane. The phases were separated, the aqueous phase extracted twice with *n*-pentane and dried over Na_2SO_4. The solvent removed under reduced pressure and the resulting residue was subjected to chromatographic purification (SiO_2, petroleum ether:EtOAc 98:2–95:5). Boronic ester **2a** (4.67 g, 7.13 mmol, 73%) was obtained as colorless resin. R_f (**2a**) = 0.22 (silica, petroleum ether:EtOAc 95:5). $[\alpha]_D^{20}$ = −33.0 (c = 1.0, $CHCl_3$). ^{1}H-NMR (400 MHz, $CDCl_3$): δ = 0.13 (s, 9 H), 0.81 (d, *J* = 6.9 Hz, 3 H), 0.83 (d, *J* = 6.6 Hz, 1 H), 0.88–1.12 (m, 9 H), 1.13–1.21 (m, 6 H), 1.21–1.30 (m, 4 H), 1.35 (m, 1 H), 1.51 (m, 1 H), 1.54–1.61 (m, 4 H), 1.67 (m, 2 H), 1.71–1.81 (m, 6 H), 1.85 (m, 1 H), 1.95 (m, 1 H), 2.37 (m, 2 H), 2.83 (dd, *J* = 8.7, 6.9 Hz, 1 H), 2.99 (dd, *J* = 8.7, 5.1 Hz, 1 H), 3.40 (m, 1 H), 3.78–2-82 (m, 5 H), 4.34 (d, *J* = 11.1 Hz, 1 H), 4.47 (d, *J* = 11.1 Hz, 1 H), 6.84 (d, *J* = 8.7 Hz, 2 H), 7.20–7.26 (m, 5 H), 6.33 (m, 6 H), 7.46 (m, 6 H) ppm. ^{13}C-NMR (100 MHz, $CDCl_3$): δ = 0.00, 14.2, 18.4, 19.2*, 21.1, 22.2, 25.6, 25.8, 26.2, 27.3, 27.3, 28.4, 30.0, 31.1, 31.5, 40.5, 41.3, 42.8, 55.0, 68.2, 81.1, 83.3, 84.5, 85.9, 107.3, 113.4, 126.5, 127.4, 128.5, 128.9, 131.2, 144.3, 158.7 ppm. HRMS (ESI-FTICR) calcd. for $C_{59}H_{85}BNO_5Si^+$ $[M+NH_4]^+$: 925.63209 found 925.63421.

4.1.2. Synthesis of (4S,5S)-4,5-Dicyclohexyl-2-{(4R,6S,7R,9R,11S)-6-[(4-methoxybenzyl)oxy]-7,9,11-trimethyl-12-(trityloxy)dodec-1-en-4-yl}-1,3,2-dioxaborolane (2b)

LDA-solution: Diisopropylamine (800 µL, 5.61 mmol, 1.35 equiv) was dissolved in anhydrous THF (830 µL, 6.75 M) and cooled to −40 °C (acetone/dry ice). *n*-Butyllithium (3.24 mL, 5.19 mmol, 1.25 equiv, 1.6 M in hexane) was added dropwise, stirred for 10 min at −40 °C, warmed to rt and further stirred for 20 min. Homologation: Boronic ester **1** (3.26 g, 4.15 mmol, 1.0 equiv) and DCM (802 µL, 12.5 mmol, 3.0 equiv) were dissolved in anhydrous THF (5.81 mL, 1.4 mL/mmol, 0.71 M) and cooled to −40 °C (acetone/dry ice). The previously prepared LDA solution was slowly added at this temperature and stirred for further 10 min after complete addition. A solution of zinc chloride (2.26 g, 16.6 mmol,

4.0 equiv) in anhydrous THF (9.97 mL, 0.6 mL/mmol, 1.67 M) was added, the reaction mixture warmed to rt and stirred for 2 h. Substitution: The reaction mixture was cooled to 0 °C (ice/water) and allylmagnesium chloride (10.4 mL, 10.4 mmol, 2.5 equiv 1.0 M in diethyl ether) was slowly added. It was warmed to rt and stirred for 18 h. The reaction mixture was worked up with saturated NH$_4$Cl and n-pentane; the phases were separated and the aqueous phase extracted twice with n-pentane. The combined organic extracts were dried over Na$_2$SO$_4$ and the solvent removed under reduced pressure. The resulting residue was chromatographed (SiO$_2$, n-pentane:EtOAc 98:2–95:5) and boronic ester **2b** (3.09 g, 3.64 mmol, 88%) obtained as colorless resin. R$_f$ (**2b**) = 0.13 (silica, n-pentane:EtOAc = 97:3). $[\alpha]_D^{20}$ = −35.2 (c = 1.0, CHCl$_3$). ^{1}H-NMR (400 MHz, CDCl$_3$): δ = 0.74 (d, J = 6.7 Hz, 3 H), 0.76–0.81 (m, J = 6.5 Hz, 4 H), 0.83–1.04 (m, J = 6.6 Hz, 8 H), 1.06–1.23 (m, 9 H$_b$), 1.32 (ddd, J = 13.1, 7.5, 6.0 Hz, 1 H), 1.37–1.58 (m, 6 H), 1.64 (m, 2 H), 1.67–1.84 (m, 7 H), 1.90 (m, 1 H), 2.14 (ddddd, J = 13.8, 6.8, 6.8, 1.6, 1.6 Hz, 1 H), 2.19 (ddddd, J= 13.8, 6.8, 6.8, 1.6, 1.6 Hz, 1 H), 2.79 (dd, J = 8.6, 6.8 Hz, 1 H), 2.95 (dd, J = 8.7, 5.0 Hz, 1 H), 3.27 (m, 1 H), 3.74 (m, 2 H), 3.76 (s, 3 H), 4.29 (d, J = 11.2 Hz, 1 H), 4.43 (d, J = 11.1 Hz, 1 H), 4.90 (ddt, J = 10.1, 1.6, 1.6 Hz, 1 H), 4.97 (ddt, J = 17.0, 1.6, 1.6 Hz, 1 H), 5.78 (dddd, J = 17.0, 10.1, 6.9, 6.9 Hz, 1 H), 6.81 (d, J = 8.6 Hz, 2 H), 7.16–7.22 (m, 5 H), 7.26 (m, 6 H), 7.43 (m, 6 H) ppm. ^{13}C-NMR (100 MHz, CDCl$_3$): δ = 14.1, 18.8, 19.3*, 21.4, 25.9, 26.0, 26.5, 27.7, 27.7, 28.6, 30.7, 31.4, 31.7, 36.7, 41.1, 41.4, 43.1, 55.2, 68.3, 70.8, 81.8, 83.5, 86.1, 113.6, 114.9, 126.8, 127.6, 128.7, 129.4, 131.3, 138.7, 144.5, 158.9 ppm. HRMS (ESI-Q exactive) calcd. for C$_{56}$H$_{76}$BO$_5^+$ [M+H]$^+$: 838.5702 found 838.5651.

4.1.3. Synthesis of (4R,6S,7R,9R,11S)-6-[(4-Methoxybenzyl)oxy]-7,9,11-trimethyl-1-(trimethylsilyl)-12-(trityloxy)dodec-1-yn-4-ol (**3a**)

Boronic ester **2a** (4.70 g, 5.18 mmol, 1.0 equiv) was dissolved in THF (10.3 mL, 0.5 M) and cooled to 0 °C. Hydrogen peroxide (2.40 mL, 25.8 mmol, 5.0 equiv, 33% in H$_2$O) and sodium hydroxide (1.03 g, 25.8 mmol, 5.0 equiv) dissolved in H$_2$O (10.3 mL, 2.5 M) were added. The reaction mixture was warmed to rt and stirred for 60 min. Saturated NaCl solution was added, and the mixture extracted thrice with diethyl ether. The combined organic extracts were dried over Na$_2$SO$_4$ and the solvent removed under reduced pressure. The residue was chromatographed (SiO$_2$, petroleum ether:EtOAc 95:5–7:3) and **3a** (3.30 g, 4.63 mmol, 90%) obtained as colorless resin. In another fraction, (S,S)-Dicyclohexylethanediol (753 mg, 3.33 mmol, 64%) was obtained as colorless needles. R$_f$ (**3a**) = 0.59 (silica, n-pentane:EtOAc 8:2). $[\alpha]_D^{20}$ = −19.0 (c = 1.0, CHCl$_3$). ^{1}H-NMR (400 MHz, CDCl$_3$): δ = 0.15 (s, 9 H), 0.79 (d, J = 6.5 Hz, 1 H), 0.84 (d, J = 6.5 Hz, 3 H), 0.88–0.95 (m, 2 H), 1.00 (d, J = 6.5 Hz, 3 H), 1.23 (m, 1 H), 1.37 (m, 1 H), 1.45 (m, 1 H), 1.56 (m, 1 H), 1.67 (m, 1 H), 1.84 (m, 1 H), 1.99 (m, 1 H), 2.39 (m, 2 H), 2.66 (d, J = 4.2 Hz, 1 H), 2.82 (dd, J = 8.7, 6.6 Hz, 1 H), 2.99 (dd, J = 8.7, 5.0 Hz, 1 H), 3.55 (m, 1 H), 3.79 (s, 3 H), 3.95 (m, 1 H), 4.36 (d, J = 11.0 Hz, 1 H), 4.49 (d, J = 11.0 Hz, 1 H), 6.85 (d, J = 8.7 Hz, 2 H), 7.20–7.25 (m, 5 H), 7.29 (m, 6 H), 7.45 (m, 6 H) ppm. ^{13}C-NMR (100 MHz, CDCl$_3$): δ = 0.1, 14.4, 18.9, 21.2, 27.9, 28.8, 31.4, 31.5, 34.4, 41.3, 41.5, 55.3 (q, C-13), 67.4, 68.3, 70.8, 79.5, 86.2, 87.1, 103.6, 113.8, 126.8, 127.6, 128.8, 129.5, 130.6, 144.5, 159.2 ppm. HRMS (CI) calcd. for C$_{45}$H$_{59}$O$_4$Si$^+$ [M]$^+$: 691.4177 found 691.4205.

4.1.4. Synthesis of (4R,6S,7R,9R,11S)-6-[(4-Methoxybenzyl)oxy]-7,9,11-trimethyl-12-(trityloxy)dodec-1-en-4-ol (**3b**)

Boronic ester **2b** (3.00 g, 3.54 mmol, 1.0 equiv) was dissolved in THF (7.07 mL, 0.5 M) and cooled to 0 °C. Hydrogen peroxide (1.64 mL, 17.7 mmol, 5.0 equiv, 33% in H$_2$O) and sodium hydroxide (707 mg, 17.7 mmol, 5.0 equiv) dissolved in H$_2$O (7.07 mL, 2.5 M) were added. The reaction mixture was warmed to rt and stirred for 45 min. Saturated NaCl solution was added, and the mixture extracted thrice with diethyl ether. The combined organic extracts were dried over Na$_2$SO$_4$ and the solvent removed under reduced pressure. The residue was chromatographed (SiO$_2$, n-pentane:EtOAc 9:1–8:2) and **3b** (1.87 g, 43.0

mmol, 85%) obtained as colorless resin. R_f (**3b**) = 0.50 (silica, *n*-pentane:EtOAc 8:2). $[α]_D^{20}$ = −25.2 (c = 1.0, CHCl$_3$). ^{1}H-NMR (400 MHz, CDCl$_3$): δ = 0.79 (d, *J* = 6.7 Hz, 3 H), 0.81–0.91 (m, *J* = 6.5 Hz, 5 H), 0.99 (d, *J* = 6.7 Hz, 3 H), 1.20 (ddd, *J* = 13.5, 6.5, 6.5 Hz, 1 H), 1.32–1.47 (m, 3 H), 1.59 (ddd, *J* = 14.4, 9.5, 2.3 Hz, 1 H), 1.82 (m, 1 H), 2.00 (m, 1 H), 2.19 (m, 2 H), 2.29 (d, *J* = 4.5 Hz, 1 H), 2.82 (dd, *J* = 8.7, 6.7 Hz, 1 H), 2.98 (dd, *J* = 8.7, 5.1 Hz, 1 H), 3.55 (ddd, *J* = 9.4, 4.6, 2.3 Hz, 1 H), 3.79 (s, 3 H), 3.85 (m, 1 H), 4.36 (d, *J* = 11.1 Hz, 1 H), 4.51 (d, *J* = 11.1 Hz, 1 H), 5.05–5.13 (m, 2 H), 5.80 (ddt, *J* = 17.4, 9.8, 7.2 Hz, 1 H), 6.86 (d, *J* = 8.7 Hz, 2 H), 7.18–7.25 (m, 5 H), 7.29 (m, 6 H), 7.45 (m, 6 H) ppm. ^{13}C-NMR (100 MHz, CDCl$_3$): δ = 14.5, 18.8, 21.1, 27.8, 31.3, 31.4, 35.0, 41.1, 41.6, 42.2, 55.3 (q, C-12), 67.9, 68.3, 70.4, 78.9, 86.1, 113.8, 117.6, 126.8, 127.6, 128.7, 129.5, 130.6, 135.1, 144.5, 159.2 ppm. HRMS (ESI-Q exactive) calcd. for $C_{42}H_{52}O_4K^+$ [M+K]$^+$: 659.3497 found 659.3500.

4.2. Syntheses of the Doliculide Core Structure

4.2.1. Synthesis of (4R,6S,7R,9R,11S)-6-[(4-Methoxybenzyl)oxy]-7,9,11-trimethyl-1-(trimethylsilyl)-12-(trityloxy)dodec-1-yn-4-yl (R)-3-[4-(allyloxy)-3-iodophenyl]-2-[(tert-butoxycarbonyl)(methyl)amino]propanoate (**5a**)

Carboxylic acid **4**[30] (4.23 g, 9.18 mmol, 2.0 equiv) and alcohol **3a** (3.27 g, 4.59 mmol, 1.0 equiv) were dissolved in anhydrous DCM (92.0 mL, 0.05 M) and cooled to −20 °C. DMAP (196 mg, 1.61 mmol, 0.35 equiv), EDC·HCl (1.76 g, 9.18 mmol, 2.0 equiv) and collidine (1.22 mL, 9.18 mmol, 2.0 equiv) were added and the reaction mixture stirred at −20 °C (acetone/cryostat) for 21 h. The reaction mixture was worked up with EtOAc and 1 M KHSO$_4$. The organic phase was washed with saturated NaHCO$_3$ and brine. The organic extract was dried over Na$_2$SO$_4$ and the solvent removed under reduced pressure. The residue was chromatographed (SiO$_2$, petroleum ether:EtOAc 9:1–8:2) and ester **5a** (4.88 g, 4.30 mmol, 94%) obtained as colorless resin. R_f (**5a**) = 0.44 (silica, petroleum ether: EtOAc 8:2). $[α]_D^{20}$ = −13.1 (c = 1.0, CHCl$_3$). ^{1}H-NMR (500 MHz, 373 K, DMSO-D$_6$): δ = 0.13 (s, 9 H), 0.79 (d, *J* = 6.6 Hz, 3 H), 0.82 (d, *J* = 6.6 Hz, 3 H), 0.87–0.92 (m, 2 H), 1.18 (m, 1 H), 1.32 (s, 9 H), 1.37 (m, 1 H), 1.44 (m, 1 H), 1.70–1.78 (m, 3 H), 1.93 (m, 1 H), 2.56 (m, 2 H), 2.68 (s, 3 H), 2.85 (dd, *J* = 8.9, 6.6 Hz, 1 H), 2.91 (m, 1 H), 2.98 (dd, *J* = 8.9, 5.0 Hz, 1 H), 3.10 (dd, *J* = 14.4, 5.0 Hz, 1 H), 3.30 (m, 1 H), 3.75 (s, 3 H), 4.24 (d, *J* = 11.0 Hz, 1 H), 4.40 (d, *J* = 11.0 Hz, 1 H), 4.57 (m, 2 H), 4.69 (dd, *J* = 10.4, 5.0 Hz, 1 H), 5.08 (m, 1 H), 5.25 (dd, *J* = 1.6, 10.7 Hz, 1 H), 5.46 (dd, *J* = 1.6, 17.3 Hz, 1 H), 6.03 (ddt, *J* = 17.3, 10.7, 5.0 Hz, 1 H), 6.85–6.90 (m, 3 H), 7.14 (dd, *J* = 8.2, 2.2 Hz, 1 H), 7.17–7.26 (m, 5 H), 7.30 (m, 6 H), 7.39 (m, 6 H), 7.61 (d, *J* = 2.2 Hz, 1 H) ppm. ^{13}C-NMR (125 MHz, 373 K, DMSO-D$_6$): δ = −0.6, 13.8, 17.9, 20.5, 24.8, 27.5, 27.5, 30.7, 31.2, 31.2, 32.6, 32.7, 40.1, 40.8, 54.7, 59.6, 67.7, 69.1, 69.5, 69.8, 77.4, 78.7, 85.5, 86.0, 86.5, 102.4, 112.7, 113.3, 116.5, 126.3, 127.1, 127.8, 128.4, 129.5, 130.5, 131.7, 132.7, 138.7, 143.7, 154.0, 155.2, 158.4, 169.2 ppm. HRMS (ESI-ToF) calcd. for $C_{44}H_{67}INO_8Si^+$ [M−Trt+H]$^+$: 892.3675 found 892.3674.

4.2.2. Synthesis of (4R,6S,7R,9R,11S)-6-[(4-Methoxybenzyl)oxy]-7,9,11-trimethyl-12-(trityloxy)dodec-1-en-4-yl (R)-3-[4-(allyloxy)-3-iodophenyl]-2-[(tert-butoxycarbonyl)(methyl)amino]propanoate (**5b**)

Carboxylic acid **4** (2.49 g, 5.39 mmol, 2.0 equiv) and alcohol **3b** (1.67 g, 2.69 mmol, 1.0 equiv) were dissolved in anhydrous DCM (53.9 mL, 0.05 M) and cooled to -20 °C. DMAP (115 mg, 943 μmol, 0.35 equiv), EDC·HCl (1.03 g, 5.39 mmol, 2.0 equiv) and collidine (718 μL, 5.39 mmol, 2.0 equiv) were added and the reaction mixture stirred at -20 °C (acetone/cryostat) for 18 h. The reaction mixture was worked up with EtOAc and 1 M KHSO$_4$. The organic phase was washed with saturated NaHCO$_3$ and brine. The organic extract was dried over Na$_2$SO$_4$ and the solvent removed under reduced pressure. The residue was chromatographed (SiO$_2$, petroleum ether:EtOAc 9:1–8:2) and ester **5b** (2.41 g, 2.27 mmol, 84%) obtained as colorless resin. R_f (**5b**) = 0.35 (silica, *n*-pentane:EtOAc 8:2). $[α]_D^{20}$ = −8.0 (c = 1.0, CHCl$_3$). ^{1}H-NMR (500 MHz, 373 K, DMSO-D$_6$): δ = 0.77 (d, *J* = 6.7 Hz, 3 H), 0.82 (d, *J* = 6.4 Hz, 3 H), 0.83–0.91 (m, 2 H), 0.93 (d, 3 H), 1.16 (m, 1 H), 1.30–1.36 (m, 10 H), 1.42 (m, 1 H), 1.58 (m, 2 H), 1.73 (m, 1 H), 1.91 (m, 1 H), 2.33 (m, 2 H), 2.65 (s, 3 H), 2.85 (dd, *J* = 9.0, 6.4 Hz, 1 H), 2.90 (dd, *J* = 14.3, 10.0 Hz, 1 H), 2.97 (dd, *J* = 9.0, 5.3 Hz,

1 H), 3.08 (dd, J = 14.3, 5.3 Hz, 1 H), 3.27 (ddd, J = 8.1, 8.1, 3.8 Hz, 1 H), 3.75 (s, 3 H), 4.24 (d, J = 11.1 Hz, 1H), 4.38 (d, J = 11.1 Hz, 1 H), 4.57 (ddd, J = 5.0, 1.6, 1.8 Hz, 2 H), 4.65 (dd, J = 10.0, 5.3 Hz, 1 H), 5.02–5.13 (m, 3 H), 5.25 (ddt, J = 10.4, 1.6, 1.6 Hz, 1 H), 5.45 (ddt, J = 17.2, 1.8, 1.6 Hz, 1 H), 5.73 (ddt, J = 17.1, 10.2, 7.0 Hz, 1 H), 6.02 (ddt, J = 17.3, 10.4, 5.1 Hz, 1 H), 6.84–6.90 (m, 3 H), 7.14 (dd, J = 8.4, 2.1 Hz, 1 H), 7.19 (d, J = 8.5 Hz, 2 H), 7.23 (tt, J = 7.3, 1.2 Hz, 3 H), 7.30 (m, 6 H), 7.40 (m, 6 H), 7.80 (d, J = 2.0 Hz, 1 H) ppm. ^{13}C-NMR (125 MHz, 373 K, DMSO-D$_6$): δ = 13.8, 17.9, 20.5, 27.5, 27.5, 30.7, 31.1, 31.1, 32.6, 33.2, 38.1, 40.0, 40.8, 54.7, 59.6, 67.8, 69.1, 69.9, 71.2, 77.7, 78.7, 85.5, 86.0, 112.7, 113.3, 116.6, 117.0, 126.3, 127.1, 127.8, 128.4, 129.5, 130.5, 131.8, 132.7, 133.0, 138.6, 143.7, 154.0, 155.2, 158.4, 169.3 ppm. HRMS (ESI-Q exactive) calcd. for C$_{60}$H$_{74}$INO$_8$Na$^+$ [M+Na]$^+$: 1086.4351 found 1086.4358.

4.2.3. Synthesis of (4R,6S,7R,9R,11S)-12-Hydroxy-6-[(4-methoxybenzyl)oxy]-7,9,11-trimethyl-1-(trimethylsilyl)dodec-1-yn-4-yl (R)-3-[4-(allyloxy)-3-iodophenyl]-2-[(tert-butoxycarbonyl)(methyl)amino]propanoate (5a-1)

Trityl ether **5a** (2.52 g, 2.22 mmol, 1.0 equiv) was dissolved in MeOH (44.4 mL, 0.05 M). Amberlyst 15 (2.52 g, 100 m%) was added at rt and gently stirred for 20 h. EtOAc was added and the solid Amberlyst 15 was removed by filtration and stirred in ethyl acetate for 1 h. Amberlyst was again removed by filtration and both organic phases combined and washed with H$_2$O. The aqueous phase was extracted with ethyl acetate and the combined organic extracts were dried over Na$_2$SO$_4$. After removal of the solvent under reduced pressure, the residue was subjected to chromatographic purification (silica, n-pentane:EtOAc 7:3) and alcohol **5a-1** (1.69 g, 1.90 mmol, 85%) obtained as colorless resin. R$_f$ (**5a-1**) = 0.33 (silica, n-pentane:EtOAc 7:3). $[α]_D^{20}$ = −16.6 (c = 0.5, CHCl$_3$). ^{1}H-NMR (500 MHz, 373 K, DMSO-D$_6$): δ = 0.14 (s, 9 H), 0.83 (ddd, J = 13.8, 7.2, 7.2 Hz, 1 H), 0.85 (d, J = 6.6 Hz, 3 H), 0.86 (d, J = 6.9 Hz, 3 H), 0.89 (d, J = 6.6 Hz, 3 H), 0.94 (ddd, J = 13.8, 7.2, 7.2 Hz, 1 H), 1.23 (ddd, J = 13.8, 6.4, 6.4 Hz, 1 H), 1.30–1.37 (m, 10 H), 1.53–1.63 (m, 2 H), 1.71–1.77 (m, 2 H), 2.02 (m, 1 H), 2.54–2.60 (m, 2 H), 2.68 (s, 3 H), 2.91 (dd, J = 14.4, 10.4 Hz, 1 H), 3.11 (dd, J = 14.4, 5.0 Hz, 1 H), 3.16 (dd, J = 10.4, 6.6 Hz, 1 H), 3.30 (dd, J = 10.2, 5.2 Hz, 1 H), 3.33 (m, 1 H), 3.76 (s, 3 H), 4.27 (d, J = 11.3 Hz, 1 H), 4.44 (d, J = 11.3 Hz, 1 H), 4.58 (dt, J = 5.0, 1.6, 1.6 Hz, 2 H), 4.70 (dd, J = 10.4, 5.0 Hz, 1 H), 5.09 (m, 1 H), 5.26 (ddt, J = 10.6, 1.6, 1.6 Hz, 1 H), 5.46 (ddt, J = 17.3, 1.8, 1.8 Hz, 1 H), 6.03 (ddt, J = 17.3, 10.6, 4.9 Hz, 1 H), 6.87–6.92 (m, 3 H), 7.16 (dd, J = 8.5 Hz, J = 2.2 Hz, 1 H), 7.23 (m, 2 H), 7.61 (d, J = 2.2 Hz, 1 H) ppm. ^{13}C-NMR (125 MHz, 373 K, DMSO-D6): δ = −0.5, 13.9, 17.4, 20.6, 24.9, 27.3, 27.5, 31.0, 31.0, 32.6, 32.6, 32.6, 40.2, 40.7, 54.6, 59.6, 66.0, 69.1, 59.6, 69.8, 77.2, 78.8, 86.0, 86.5, 102.5, 112.7, 113.3, 116.6, 128.5, 129.6, 130.5, 131.7, 132.8, 138.7, 155.2, 155.2, 158.4, 169.3 ppm. HRMS (ESI-ToF) calcd. for C$_{44}$H$_{67}$INO$_8$Si$^+$ [M+H]$^+$: 892.3675 found 892.3660.

4.2.4. Synthesis of (4R,6S,7R,9R,11S)-12-Hydroxy-6-[(4-methoxybenzyl)oxy]-7,9,11-trimethyldodec-1-en-4-yl (R)-3-[4-(allyloxy)-3-iodophenyl]-2-[(tert-butoxycarbonyl)(methyl)amino]propanoate (5b-1)

Trityl ether **5b** (2.32 g, 2.18 mmol, 1.0 equiv) was dissolved in MeOH (43.7 mL, 0.05 M). Amberlyst 15 (2.32 g, 100 m%) was added at rt and gently stirred for 20 h. EtOAc was added and the solid Amberlyst 15 was removed by filtration and stirred in ethyl acetate for 1 h. Amberlyst was again removed by filtration and both organic phases combined and washed with H$_2$O. The aqueous phase was extracted with ethyl acetate and the combined organic extracts were dried over Na$_2$SO$_4$. After removal of the solvent under reduced pressure, the residue was subjected to chromatographic purification (silica, n-pentane:EtOAc 7:3) and alcohol **5b-1** (1.61 g, 1.94 mmol, 89%) obtained as colorless resin. R$_f$ (**5b-1**) = 0.33 (silica, n-pentane:EtOAc 7:3). $[α]_D^{20}$ = −11.6 (c = 1.0, CHCl$_3$). ^{1}H-NMR (500 MHz, 373 K, DMSO-D$_6$): δ = 0.80–0.85 (m, J = 7.0 Hz, 4 H), 0.86 (d, J = 6.7 Hz, 3 H), 0.89 (d, J = 6.6 Hz, 3 H), 0.94 (m, 1 H), 1.23 (m, 1 H), 1.31–1.38 (m, 10 H), 1.52–1.64 (m, 4 H), 1.99 (m, 1 H), 2.35 (m, 2 H), 2.66 (s, 3 H), 2.92 (dd, J = 14.3, 10.3 Hz, 1 H), 3.10 (dd, J = 14.3, 5.3 Hz, 1 H), 3.17 (dd, J = 10.2, 6.6 Hz, 1 H), 3.30 (m, J = 10.2, 5.2 Hz, 2 H), 3.77 (s, 3 H), 4.27 (d, J = 11.1 Hz, 1 H), 2.42 (d, J = 11.1 Hz, 1 H), 4.58 (ddd, J = 4.9, 1.7, 1.5 Hz, 2 H), 4.67 (dd, J = 10.3, 5.3 Hz, 1 H), 5.02–5.13 (m, 3 H), 5.26 (ddt, J = 10.7, 1.5, 1.5 Hz, 1 H), 5.45 (ddt, J = 17.3, 1.7, 1.5 Hz, 1

H), 5.75 (ddt, J = 17.1, 10.2, 7.0 Hz, 1 H), 6.03 (ddt, J = 17.2, 10.5, 5.1 Hz, 1 H), 6.87–6.93 (m, 3 H), 7.17 (dd, J = 8.4, 2.0 Hz, 1 H), 7.23 (d, J = 8.5 Hz, 2 H), 7.62 (d, J = 8.5 Hz, 1 H) ppm. ^{13}C-NMR (125 MHz, 373 K, DMSO-D$_6$): δ = 13.9, 17.2, 20.5, 27.3, 27.5, 31.0, 32.0, 32.5, 32.6, 33.0, 38.1, 40.1, 40.7, 54.7, 59.7, 66.0, 69.1, 69.9, 71.2, 77.4, 78.8, 86.0, 112.7, 113.3, 116.6, 117.0, 128.5, 129.5, 130.6, 131.8, 132.8, 133.0, 138.7, 154.1, 155.2, 158.4, 169.3 ppm. HRMS (ESI-ToF) calcd. for C$_{41}$H$_{61}$INO$_8{}^+$ [M+H]$^+$: 822.3436 found 822.3410.

4.2.5. Synthesis of (2S,4S,6R,7S,9R)-9-({(R)-3-[4-(Allyloxy)-3-iodophenyl]-2-[(tert-butoxycarbonyl)(methyl)amino]propanoyl}oxy)-7-[(4-methoxybenzyl)oxy]-2,4,6-trimethyl-12-(trimethylsilyl)dodec-11-ynoic Acid (**6a**)

Alcohol **5a-1** (3.18 g, 3.57 mmol, 1.0 equiv) was dissolved in acetone (35.7 mL, 0.1 M) and cooled to 0 °C. Jones reagent (2.97 mL, 8.91 mmol, 3 M in 16% H$_2$SO$_4$, 2.5 equiv) were added and the mixture stirred for 45 min at this temperature. The reaction mixture was quenched with *i*-PrOH and concentrated under reduced pressure. The residue was diluted with H$_2$O and EtOAc, the phases were separated and the aqueous phase extracted twice with EtOAc. The combined organic extracts were washed with brine, dried over Na$_2$SO$_4$. After removal of the solvent under reduced pressure, the residue chromatographically purified (silica, *n*-pentane:EtOAc 9:1–7:3) and acid **6a** (2.47 g, 2.72 mmol, 76%) obtained as colorless resin. R$_f$ (**6a**) = 0.33 (silica, *n*-pentane:EtOAc 7:3). $[α]_D^{20}$ = 0.6 (c = 0.5, CHCl$_3$). ^{1}H-NMR (500 MHz, 373 K, DMSO-D$_6$): δ = 0.14 (s, 9 H), 0.85 (d, J = 6.7 Hz, 3 H), 0.90 (d, J = 6.6 Hz, 3 H), 0.95–1.05 (m, 2 H), 1.08 (d, J = 7.0 Hz, 3 H), 1.20 (ddd, J = 13.4, 8.0, 5.0 Hz, 1 H), 1.33 (s, 9 H), 1.54 (m, 1 H), 1.70 (ddd, J = 13.5, 9.0, 4.7 Hz, 1 H), 1.75 (m, 2 H), 1.98 (m, 1 H), 2.41 (ddq, J = 9.0, 7.1, 4.8 Hz, 1 H), 2.57 (m, 2 H), 2.69 (s, 3 H), 2.92 (dd, J = 14.4, 10.8 Hz, 1 H), 3.12 (dd, J = 14.4, 5.2 Hz, 1 H), 3.30 (ddd, J = 8.0, 4.0, 4.0 Hz, 1 H), 3.77 (s, 3 H), 4.29 (d, J = 11.1 Hz, 1 H), 4.44 (d, J = 11.1 Hz, 1 H), 4.59 (ddd, J = 5.0, 1.7, 1.5 Hz, 2 H), 4.71 (dd, J = 10.5, 5.2 Hz, 1 H), 5.08 (m, 1 H), 5.26 (ddt, J = 10.7, 1.5, 1.5 Hz, 1 H), 5.45 (ddt, J = 17.3, 1.7, 1.5 Hz, 1 H), 6.03 (ddt, J = 17.2, 10.5, 5.0 Hz, 1 H), 6.86–6.93 (m, 3 H), 7.16 (dd, J = 8.4, 2.0 Hz, 1 H), 7.23 (d, J = 8.5 Hz, 2 H), 7.62 (d, J = 2.0 Hz, 1 H). ^{13}C-NMR (125 MHz, 373 K, DMSO-D6): δ = –0.46, 13.7, 17.6, 20.1, 25.0, 27.6, 28.1, 31.4, 31.4, 32.8, 33.0, 36.5, 40.2, 40.4, 54.9, 59.7, 69.3, 69.8, 70.0, 77.8, 79.0, 86.1, 86.7, 102.6, 112.9, 113.5, 116.8, 128.6, 129.7, 130.6, 131.9, 132.9, 138.8, 154.4, 155.4, 158.6, 169.5, 176.9. HRMS (ESI-ToF) calcd. for C$_{44}$H$_{65}$INO$_9$Si$^+$ [M+H]$^+$: 906.3468 found 906.3487.

4.2.6. Synthesis of (2S,4S,6R,7S,9R)-9-({(R)-3-[4-(Allyloxy)-3-iodophenyl]-2-[(tert-butoxycarbonyl)(methyl)amino]propanoyl}oxy)-7-[(4-methoxybenzyl)oxy]-2,4,6-trimethyldodec-11-enoic Acid (**6b**)

Alcohol **5b-1** (1.51 g, 1.82 mmol, 1.0 equiv) was dissolved in acetone (18.2 mL, 0.1 M) and cooled to 0 °C. Jones reagent (1.51 mL, 4.54 mmol, 3 M in 16% H$_2$SO$_4$, 2.5 equiv) were added and the mixture stirred for 45 min at this temperature. The reaction mixture was quenched with *i*-PrOH and concentrated under reduced pressure. The residue was diluted with H$_2$O and EtOAc, the phases were separated, and the aqueous phase was extracted twice with EtOAc. The combined organic extracts were washed with brine, dried over Na$_2$SO$_4$. After removal of the solvent under reduced pressure, the residue chromatographically purified (silica, *n*-pentane:EtOAc 9:1–7:3) and acid **6b** (1.23 g, 1.46 mmol, 80%) obtained as colorless resin. R$_f$ (**6b**) = 0.27 (silica, *n*-pentane:EtOAc 8:2). $[α]_D^{20}$ = –4.2 (c = 1.0, CHCl$_3$). ^{1}H-NMR (500 MHz, 373 K, DMSO-D$_6$): δ = 0.83 (d, J = 6.9 Hz, 3 H), 0.90 (d, J = 6.6 Hz, 3 H), 0.97 (ddd, J = 13.5, 8.4, 6.1 Hz, 1 H), 1.02 (ddd, J = 13.7, 8.4, 5.3 Hz, 1 H), 1.08 (d, J = 6.9 Hz, 3 H), 1.19 (ddd, J = 13.5, 7.7, 5.3 Hz, 1 H), 1.35 (s, 9 H), 1.52 (m, 1 H), 1.61 (m, 2 H), 1.68 (ddd, J = 13.7, 8.9, 4.8 Hz, 1 H), 1.97 (m, 1 H), 2.28–2.38 ((m, 2 H), 2.42 (ddq, J = 8.9, 6.9, 5.3 Hz, 1 H), 2.66 (s, 9 H), 2.92 (dd, J = 14.5, 10.1 Hz, 1 H), 3.11 (dd, J = 14.5, 5.5 Hz, 1 H), 3.28 (m, 1 H), 3.77 (s, 3 H), 4.27 (d, J = 11.1 Hz, 1 H), 4.42 (d, J = 11.1 Hz, 1 H), 4.59 (ddd, J = 4.9, 1.6, 1.6 Hz, 2 H), 4.68 (dd, J = 10.1, 5.4 Hz, 1 H), 5.03–5.13 (m, 3 H), 5.26 (ddt, J = 10.6, 1.6, 1.6 Hz, 1 H), 5.45 (ddt, J = 17.2, 1.6, 1.6 Hz, 1 H), 5.75 (ddt, J = 17.1, 10.2, 7.0 Hz,

1 H), 6.03 (ddt, J = 17.2, 10.5 Hz, J = 4.9 Hz, 1 H), 6.86–6.94 (m, 3 H), 7.17 (dd, J = 8.4, 2.0 Hz, 1 H), 7.23 (d, J = 8.5 Hz, 1 H), 7.63 (d, J = 2.0 Hz, 1 H) ppm. ^{13}C-NMR (125 MHz, 373 K, DMSO-D$_6$): δ = 13.7, 17.4, 20.0, 27.5, 27.9, 31.2, 31.2, 32.6, 33.4, 36.4, 38.1, 39.9, 40.3, 54.7, 59.6, 69.1, 70.0, 71.2, 77.9, 78.9, 86.0, 112.7, 113.3, 116.6, 117.0, 128.5, 129.5, 130.6, 131.8, 132.8, 133.1, 138.7, 154.1, 155.2, 158.4, 169.3, 176.7 ppm. HRMS (ESI-ToF) calcd. for C$_{41}$H$_{59}$INO$_9$$^+$ [M+H]$^+$: 836.3229 found 836.3228.

4.2.7. Synthesis of (4R,6S,7R,9S,11S)-12-{[2-(tert-Butoxy)-2-oxoethyl]amino}-6-[(4-methoxybenzyl)oxy]-7,9,11-trimethyl-12-oxo-1-(trimethylsilyl)dodec-1-yn-4-yl (R)-3-[4-(allyloxy)-3-iodophenyl]-2-[(tert-butoxycarbonyl)(methyl)amino]propanoate (**7a**)

Acid **6a** (2.42 g, 2.67 mmol, 1.0 equiv) and *tert*-butyl glycinate hydrochloride (595 mg, 3.55 mmol, 1.33 equiv) were dissolved in anhydrous DMF (13.3 mL, 0.2 M). NEt$_3$ (930 μL, 6.67 mmol, 0.726 gml^{-1}, 2.5 equiv) and diethyl cyanophosphonate (DCNP) (1.03 mL, 6.14 mmol, 1.075 gml^{-1}, 2.3 equiv) were added at 0 °C. After 1 h, brine and diethyl ether were added and the aqueous phase extracted twice with diethyl ether. The combined organic extracts were dried over Na$_2$SO$_4$ and the solvent removed under reduced pressure. After chromatographic purification (silica, *n*-pentane:EtOAc 8:2–7:3), amide **7a** (2.57 g, 2.52 mmol, 95%) was obtained as colorless resin. R$_f$ (**7a**) = 0.33 (silica, *n*-pentane:EtOAc 7:3). $[α]_D^{20}$ = −9.9 (c = 1.0, CHCl$_3$). Major rotamer: ^{1}H-NMR (500 MHz, CDCl$_3$): δ = 0.14 (s, 9 H), 0.84 (m, 3 H), 0.90 (d, J = 6.3 Hz, 3 H), 0.99 (m, 2 H), 1.10 (m, 1 H), 1.38 (s, 9 H), 1.43–1.52 (m, 10 H), 1.65–1.85 (m, 3 H), 2.03 (m, 1 H), 2.38 (m, 1 H), 2.55 (m, 2 H), 2.68 (s, 3 H), 2.87 (dd, J = 14.2, 10.5 Hz, 1 H), 3.08–3.28 (m, 2 H), 3.79 (s, 3 H), 3.91 (m, 2 H), 4.23 (m, 1 H), 4.41–4.55 (m, 3 H), 4.73 (dd, J = 10.5, 5.4 Hz, 1 H), 5.19 (m, 1 H), 5.28 (m, 1 H), 5.47 (m, 1 H), 5.95–5.92 (m, 2 H), 6.78 (d, J = 8.5 Hz, 1 H), 6.87 (m, 2 H), 7.12 (d, J = 7.9 Hz, 1 H), 7.26 (m, 2 H), 7.60 (s, 1 H) ppm. ^{13}C-NMR (125 MHz, CDCl$_3$): δ = 0.0, 14.0, 19.0, 21.1, 25.9, 28.0, 28.3, 41.7, 32.3, 33.5, 33.5, 33.9, 39.0, 41.0, 41.0, 41.9, 55.3, 59.9, 69.9, 70.7, 71.0, 78.6, 79.9, 82.0, 86.5, 87.2, 102.4, 112.5, 113.8, 117.5, 129.5, 129.9, 131.0, 132.0, 132.7, 139.8, 155.6, 156.0, 159.2, 169.2, 170.3, 176.4 (C-1) ppm. Minor rotamer: (selected signals) ^{1}H-NMR (500 MHz, CDCl$_3$): δ = 1.31 (s, 9 H), 2.74 (s, 3 H), 3.79 (s, 3 H), 7.03 (d, J = 7.9 Hz, 1 H), 7.61 (s, 1 H) ppm. ^{13}C-NMR (125 MHz, CDCl$_3$): δ = 13.8, 28.5, 31.2, 60.6, 70.4, 80.2, 86.5, 87.6, 130.8, 139.8, 154.9, 156.1, 170.2, 176.3 ppm. HRMS (ESI-ToF) calcd. for C$_{50}$H$_{75}$IN$_2$O$_{10}$Si$^+$ [M+H]$^+$: 1019.4308 found 1019.4310.

4.2.8. Synthesis of (4R,6S,7R,9S,11S)-12-{[2-(tert-Butoxy)-2-oxoethyl]amino}-6-[(4-methoxybenzyl)oxy]-7,9,11-trimethyl-12-oxododec-1-en-4-yl (R)-3-[4-(allyloxy)-3-iodophenyl]-2-[(tert-butoxycarbonyl)(methyl)amino]propanoate (**7b**)

Acid **6b** (1.19 g, 1.31 mmol, 1.0 equiv) and *tert*-butyl glycinate hydrochloride (293 mg, 1.75 mmol, 1.33 equiv) were dissolved in anhydrous DMF (6.56 mL, 0.2 M). NEt$_3$ (457 μL, 3.28 mmol, 0.726 gml^{-1}, 2.5 equiv) and diethyl cyanophosphonate (DCNP) (509 μL, 1.06 mmol, 1.075 gml^{-1}, 2.3 equiv) were added at 0 °C. After 2 h, brine and diethyl ether were added and the aqueous phase extracted twice with diethyl ether. The combined organic extracts were dried over Na$_2$SO$_4$ and the solvent removed under reduced pressure. After chromatographic purification (silica, *n*-pentane:EtOAc 8:2), amide **7b** (1.01 g, 1.06 mmol, 81%) was obtained as colorless resin. R$_f$ (**7b**) = 0.43 (silica, *n*-pentane:EtOAc 7:3). $[α]_D^{20}$ = −4.2 (c = 1.0, CHCl$_3$). ^{1}H-NMR (500 MHz, 373 K, DMSO-D$_6$): δ = 0.82 (d, J = 6.7 Hz, 3 H), 0.90 (d, J = 6.6 Hz, 3 H), 0.91–0.98 (m, 2 H), 1.04 (d, J = 6.9 Hz, 3 H), 1.16 (ddd, J = 13.4, 8.0, 5.0 Hz, 1 H), 1.35 (s, 9 H), 1.42 (s, 9 H), 1.48 (m, 1 H), 1.61 (m, 2 H), 1.71 (ddd, J = 13.5, 9.3, 4.3 Hz, 1 H), 1.97 (m, 1 H), 2.34 (m, 2 H), 2.43 (ddq, J = 9.3, 6.9, 5.0 Hz, 1 H), 2.67 (s, 3 H), 2.92 (dd, J = 14.3, 10.5 Hz, 1 H), 3.11 (dd, J = 14.3, 5.5 Hz, 1 H), 3.27 (m, 1 H), 3.67 (dd, J = 17.1, 6.0 Hz, 1 H), 3.72 (dd, J = 17.1, 6.0 Hz, 1 H), 3.77 (s, 3 H), 4.27 (d, J = 11.1 Hz, 1 H), 4.43 (d, = 11.1 Hz, 1 H), 4.58 (ddd, J = 4.9, 1.6, 1.6 Hz, 2 H), 4.69 (dd, J = 10.5, 5.5 Hz, 1 H), 5.02–5.13 (m, 3 H), 5.26 (ddt, J = 10.6, 1.6, 1.6 Hz, 1 H), 5.45 (dtt, J = 17.3, 1.8, 1.6 Hz, 1 H), 5.75 (ddt, J = 17.1, 10.2, 7.0 Hz, 1 H), 6.03 (ddt, J = 17.3, 10.5, 5.1 Hz, 1 H), 6.86–6.92 (m, 3 H), 7.17 (dd, J = 8.4, 2.1 Hz, 1 H), 7.23 (d, J = 8.7 Hz, 2 H), 7.63 (d, J = 2.0 Hz, 1 H), 7.71 (dd, J = 6.0, 6.0 Hz, 1 H) ppm. ^{13}C-NMR (125 MHz, 373 K, DMSO-D$_6$): δ = 13.6, 18.1, 20.2,

27.3, 27.5, 27.6, 31.2, 31.2, 32.6, 33.4, 37.0, 38.1, 40.2, 40.4, 41.0, 54.7, 59.6, 69.1, 70.0, 71.2, 78.1, 78.7, 79.8, 85.9, 112.7, 113.3, 116.5, 117.0, 128.5, 129.5, 130.6, 131.8, 132.7, 133.1, 138.7, 154.1, 155.2, 158.4, 168.4, 169.3, 175.4 ppm. HRMS (ESI-ToF) calcd. for $C_{47}H_{70}IN_2O_{10}^+$ [M+H]$^+$: 949.4070 found 949.4059.

4.2.9. Synthesis of (3R,9S,11S,13R,14S,16R)-3-[4-(Allyloxy)-3-iodobenzyl]-14-hydroxy-4,9,11,13-tetramethyl-16-[3-(trimethylsilyl)prop-2-yn-1-yl]-1-oxa-4,7-diazacyclohexadecane-2,5,8-trione (**7a-1**)

A solution of linear precursor **7a** (874 mg, 858 µmol, 1.0 equiv) in anhydrous DCM (3.86 mL, 4.5 mL/mmol, 0.22 M) was treated with TFA (2.57 mL, 3.0 mL/mmol, 0.33 M). It was warmed to rt and stirred for 90 min. The solvent was removed in N_2 stream and azeotropically distilled with benzene and dried in vacuo. Triethylamine (1.20 mL, 8.58 mmol, 10.0 equiv) and BOP-Cl (1.09 g, 4.29 mmol, 5.0 equiv) were dissolved in DCM (1.72 l, 0.5 mM) and cooled to 0 °C. The previously obtained residue was dissolved in DCM (172 mL, 200 mL/mmol) and added dropwise (overnight) to the solution at 0 °C. After complete addition, the mixture was warmed to rt and further stirred for 24 h. The reaction mixture was worked up with 0.1 M HCl and the organic phase washed with saturated NaHCO$_3$, saturated NH$_4$Cl and brine. The organic phase was dried over Na$_2$SO$_4$ and the solvent removed under reduced pressure. The residue was dissolved in MeOH (51.5 mL, 60 mL/mmol, 0.017 M) and ammonia (4.29 mL, 5 mL/mmol, 35% in H$_2$O) was added dropwise and stirred for 1 h. The solvent was removed under reduced pressure, the residue taken up on Isolute, reversed-phase chromatographed (Telos C18, H$_2$O:MeCN 80:20–MeCN) and **7a-1** (480 mg, 662 µmol, 77%) obtained as colorless powder after lyophilization. A sample was further purified by preparative HPLC (Luna C18, H$_2$O:MeCN 60:40–MeCN) for analytical purposes. R$_f$ (**7a-1**) = 0.33 (silica, *n*-pentane:EtOAc 1:1). $[\alpha]_D^{20}$ = −19.0 (c = 1.0, CHCl$_3$). ^{1}H-NMR (400 MHz, CDCl$_3$): δ = 0.18 (s, 9 H), 0.83 (d, *J* = 6.7 Hz, 3 H), 0.95 (d, *J* = 6.1 Hz, 3 H), 0.98–1.09 (m, 3 H), 1.11 (d, *J* = 6.6 Hz, 3 H), 1.19 (m, 1 H), 1.37 (ddd, *J* = 14.3, 11.2, 1.7 Hz, 1 H), 1.45–1.58 (m, 2 H), 1.98 (m, 1 H), 2.24 (bs, 1 H), 2.38 (ddq, *J* = 12.0, 6.6, 3.3 Hz, 1 H), 2.54 (d, = 6.1 H, 2 H), 2.89 (dd, *J* = 15.5, 12.0 Hz, 1 H), 2.93 (s, 3 H), 3.27 (dd, *J* = 17.0, 1.0 Hz, 1 H), 3.42 (dd, *J* = 15.4, 4.5 Hz, 1 H), 3.61 (ddd, *J* = 11.2, 3.8, 1.7 Hz, 1 H), 4.55 (ddd, *J* = 4.8, 1.6, 1.6 Hz, 2 H), 4.77 (dd, *J* = 17.0, 8.6 Hz, 1 H), 5.26 (ddt, *J* = 11.4, 6.1, 1.8 Hz, 1 H), 5.30 (ddt, *J* = 10.6, 1.6, 1.3 Hz, 1 H), 5.47 (dd, *J* = 12.0, 4.5 Hz, 1 H), 5.50 (ddt, *J* = 17.1, 1.6, 1.3 Hz, 1 H), 6.03 (ddt, *J* = 17.2, 10.4, 5.0 Hz, 1 H), 6.21 (d, *J* = 8.1 Hz, 1 H), 6.71 (d, *J* = 8.4 Hz, 1 H), 7.09 (dd, *J* = 8.4, 2.0 Hz, 1 H), 7.59 (d, *J* = 2.0 Hz, 1 H) ppm. ^{13}C-NMR (100 MHz, CDCl$_3$): δ = 0.0, 14.3, 17.6, 18.3, 26.4, 27.0, 30.5, 32.6, 33.1, 34.5, 39.0, 39.8, 42.7, 45.0, 57.8, 65.7, 69.7, 70.6, 86.8, 87.2, 102.0, 112.4, 117.7, 129.0, 130.7, 132.4, 139.1, 156.1, 171.0, 171.7, 177.4 ppm. HRMS (ESI-ToF) calcd. for $C_{33}H_{50}IN_2O_6Si^+$ [M+H]$^+$: 725.2477 found 725.2482.

4.2.10. Synthesis of (3R,9S,11S,13R,14S,16R)-16-allyl-3-[4-(allyloxy)-3-iodobenzyl]-14-hydroxy-4,9,11,13-tetramethyl-1-oxa-4,7-diazacyclohexadecane-2,5,8-trione (**7b-1**)

A solution of linear precursor **7b** (914 mg, 963 µmol, 1.0 equiv) in anhydrous DCM (4.33 mL, 4.5 mL/mmol, 0.22 M) was treated with TFA (2.89 mL, 3.0 mL/mmol, 0.33 M). It was warmed to rt and stirred for 90 min. The solvent was removed in N_2 stream and azeotropically distilled with benzene and dried in vacuo. Triethylamine (1.34 mL, 9.63 mmol, 10.0 equiv) and BOP-Cl (1.23 g, 4.82 mmol, 5.0 equiv) were dissolved in DCM (1.93 l, 0.5 mM) and cooled to 0 °C. The previously obtained residue was dissolved in DCM (193 mL, 200 mL/mmol) and added dropwise (overnight) to the solution at 0 °C. After complete addition, the mixture was warmed to rt and further stirred for 24 h. The reaction mixture was worked up with 0.1 M HCl and the organic phase washed with saturated NaHCO$_3$, saturated NH$_4$Cl and brine. The organic phase was dried over Na$_2$SO$_4$ and the solvent removed under reduced pressure. The residue was dissolved in MeOH (57.8 mL, 60 mL/mmol, 0.017 M) and ammonia (4.82 mL, 5 mL/mmol, 35% in H$_2$O) was added dropwise and stirred for 1 h. The solvent was removed under reduced pressure, the residue taken up on Isolute, reversed-phase chromatographed (FlashPure Select C18, H$_2$O:MeCN 90:10–MeCN), and **7b-1** (511 mg, 781 µmol, 81%) obtained as colorless powder after lyophilization. A sample was further purified by preparative HPLC (Luna C18, H$_2$O:MeCN 90:10–MeCN) for analytical purposes. $[\alpha]_D^{20}$ = −33.7 (c = 1.0, CHCl$_3$). ^{1}H-NMR (400 MHz, CDCl$_3$): δ = 0.82 (d, J = 6.7 Hz, 3 H), 0.95 (d, J = 6.1 Hz, 3 H), 0.98–1.08 (m, 3 H), 1.18 (m, 1 H), 1.31 (ddd, J = 13.9, 11.4, 2.0 Hz, 1 H), 1.42–1.55 (m, 2 H), 1.98 (m, 1 H), 2.07 (bs, 1 H), 2.35–2.43 (m, J = 6.7, 6.7 Hz, 3 H), 2.83 (dd, J = 15.3, 12.1 Hz, 1 H), 2.87 (s, 3 H), 3.24 (dd, J = 16.7, 1.0 Hz, 1 H), 3.38 (dd, J = 15.4, 4.5 Hz, 1 H), 3.60 (ddd, J = 11.4, 3.9, 1.8 Hz, 1 H), 4.54 (ddd, J = 4.9, 1.6, 1.6 Hz, 2 H), 4.78 (dd, J = 16.9, 8.7 Hz, 1 H), 5.04–5.14 (m, 2 H), 5.22–5.33 (m, J = 10.6, 1.5, 1.5 Hz, 2 H), 5.44 (dd, J = 12.2, 4.6 Hz, 1 H), 5.49 (dd, J = 17.3, 1.5, 1.5 Hz, 1 H), 5.74 (ddt, J = 17.0, 10.2, 6.9 Hz, 1 H), 6.03 (ddt, J = 17.2, 10.4, 5.0 Hz, 1 H), 6.24 (d, J = 8.3 Hz, 1 H), 6.70 (d, J = 8.4 Hz, 1 H), 7.08 (dd, J = 8.4, 2.0 Hz, 1 H), 7.58 (d, J = 2.0 Hz, 1 H) ppm. ^{13}C-NMR (100 MHz, CDCl$_3$): δ = 14.3, 17.6, 18.3, 27.0, 30.6, 32.6, 33.2, 34.4, 39.0, 39.7, 39.8, 42.7, 44.9, 57.7, 65.6, 69.7, 71.7, 86.7, 112.4, 117.7, 118.0, 128.9, 130.7, 132.4, 133.8, 139.4, 156.1, 171.3, 171.6, 177.5 ppm. HRMS (ESI-ToF) calcd. for C$_{30}$H$_{44}$IN$_2$O$_6$$^+$ [M+H]$^+$: 655.2239 found 655.2247.

4.2.11. Synthesis of (3R,9S,11S,13R,14S,16R)-14-Hydroxy-3-(4-hydroxy-3-iodobenzyl)-4,9,11,13-tetramethyl-16-[3-(trimethylsilyl)prop-2-yn-1-yl]-1-oxa-4,7-diazacyclohexadecane-2,5,8-trione (8a)

0.01 M catalyst solution: CpRu(II)(MeCN)$_3$PF$_6$ (16.4 mg, 37.8 µmol) was dissolved in anhydrous MeOH (3.42 mL) and stirred for 5 min (yellow solution). Quinoline-2-carboxylic acid (380 µL, 38 µmol, 0.1 M in anhydrous MeOH) was added and the mixture stirred for 30 min (dark red solution). Deprotection: Allyl ether **7a-1** (413 mg, 569 µmol, 1.0 equiv) was dissolved in anhydrous degassed MeOH (11.4 mL, 0.05 M) under an N$_2$-atmosphere. The previously prepared catalyst solution (2.85 mL, 28.5 µmol, 0.01 M) was added and the mixture stirred for 6 h at rt. The solvent was removed under reduced pressure, the residue taken up on Isolute and chromatographed (SiO$_2$, n-pentane:EtOAc 1:1–4:6) and alcohol **8a** (340 mg, 496 µmol, 87%) obtained as colorless powder after lyophilization. R$_f$ (**8a**) = 0.13 (silica, n-pentane: EtOAc 1:1). $[\alpha]_D^{20}$ = −20.1 (c = 1.0, CHCl$_3$). ^{1}H-NMR (400 MHz, CDCl$_3$): δ = 0.18 (s, 9 H), 0.84 (d, J = 6.7 Hz, 3 H), 0.94 (d, J = 6.0 Hz, 3 H), 1.01–1.10 (m, 3 H), 1.12 (d, J = 6.6 Hz, 3 H), 1.15–1.23 (m, 1 H), 1.42 (m, 1 H), 1.48–1.60 (m, 2 H), 1.98 (m, 1 H), 2.31 (bs, 1 H), 2.43 (m, 1 H), 2.55 (m, 2 H), 2.87 (dd, J = 15.2, 12.0 Hz, 1 H), 2.97 (s, 3 H), 3.21 (d, J = 16.6 Hz, 1 H), 3.42 (dd, J = 15.2, 4.3 Hz, 1 H), 3.63 (m, 1 H), 4.78 (dd, J = 16.7, 8.7 Hz, 1 H), 5.27 (dddd, J = 10.2, 6.6, 6.6, 1.6 Hz, 1 H), 5.52 (dd, J = 11.9, 4.4 Hz, 1 H), 6.36 (d, J = 6.8 Hz, 1 H), 6.83 (d, J = 8.3 Hz, 1 H), 6.95 (bs, 1 H), 7.05 (dd, J = 8.3, 1.1 Hz, 1 H), 7.47 (d, J = 1.1 Hz, 1 H) ppm. ^{13}C-NMR (100 MHz, CDCl$_3$): δ = 0.0, 14.3, 17.6, 18.4, 26.4, 27.1, 30.8, 32.6, 33.0, 34.6, 39.1, 39.6, 42.8, 44.9, 57.8, 65.9, 70.7, 85.2, 87.3, 102.0, 115.2, 129.5, 130.2, 138.2, 154.3, 170.6, 172.1, 177.6 ppm. HRMS (ESI-ToF) calcd. for C$_{30}$H$_{46}$IN$_2$O$_6$Si$^+$ [M+H]$^+$: 685.2164 found 685.2162.

4.2.12. Synthesis of (3R,9S,11S,13R,14S,16R)-16-Allyl-14-hydroxy-3-(4-hydroxy-3-iodobenzyl)-4,9,11,13-tetramethyl-1-oxa-4,7-diazacyclohexadecane-2,5,8-trione (8b)

0.01 M catalyst solution: CpRu(II)(MeCN)$_3$PF$_6$ (20.2 mg, 46.5 µmol) was dissolved in anhydrous MeOH (4.23 mL) and stirred for 5 min (yellow solution). Quinoline-2-carboxylic acid (470 µL, 470 µmol, 0.1 M in anhydrous MeOH) was added and the mixture stirred for 30 min (dark red solution). Deprotection: Allyl ether **7b-1** (463 mg, 707 µmol, 1.0 equiv) was dissolved in anhydrous degassed MeOH (14.1 mL, 0.05 M) under an N$_2$-atmosphere. The previously prepared catalyst solution (3.53 mL, 35.3 µmol, 0.01 M) was added and the mixture stirred for 90 min at rt. The solvent was removed under reduced pressure, the residue taken up on Isolute and chromatographed (SiO$_2$, n-pentane:EtOAc 1:1–2:8). The obtained residue was further purified by preparative HPLC (Luna C18, H$_2$O:MeCN

50:50–MeCN) and compound **8b** (354 mg, 576 µmol, 81%) obtained as colorless powder after lyophilization. R_f (**8b**) = 0.19 (silica, *n*-pentane:EtOAc 4:6). $[α]_D^{20}$ = −40.3 (c = 1.0, CHCl$_3$). ^{1}H-NMR (400 MHz, CDCl$_3$): δ = 0.83 (d, *J* = 6.9 Hz, 3 H), 0.96 (d, *J* = 6.1 Hz, 3 H), 1.00–1.10 (m, 3 H), 1.13 (d, *J* = 6.6 Hz, 3 H), 1.18 (m, 1 H), 1.25 (bs, 1 H), 1.34 (ddd, *J* = 14.0 Hz, *J* = 11.7, 2.0 Hz, 1 H), 1.48 (ddd, *J*= 14.0, 11.8, 2.0 Hz, 1 H), 1.52 (ddd, *J* = 12.1, 12.1, 1.5 Hz, 1 H), 1.99 (m, 1 H), 2.38 (dd, *J* = 7.0, 6.2 Hz, 2 H), 2.43 (ddd, *J* = 12.1, 6.6 Hz, 3.5 Hz, 1 H), 2.83 (dd, *J* = 15.4 Hz, 12.2 Hz, 1 H), 2.89 (s, 3 H), 3.23 (dd, *J* = 16.7, 1.6 Hz, 1 H), 3.40 (dd, *J* = 15.5, 4.5 Hz, 1 H), 3.62 (ddd, *J* = 11.6, 4.2, 2.1 Hz, 1 Hz), 4.80 (dd, *J* = 16.8, 8.7 Hz, 1 H), 5.06–5.15 (m, 2 H), 5.28 (ddt, *J* = 11.8, 6.2, 2.0 Hz, 1 H), 5.49 (dd, *J* = 12.1, 4.6 Hz, 1 H), 5.76 (ddt, *J* = 17.1, 10.2, 7.0 Hz, 1 H), 6.05 (bs, 1 H), 6.27 (d, *J* = 8.1 Hz, 1 H), 6.86 (d, *J* = 8.4 Hz, 1 H), 7.05 (dd, *J* = 8.3, 2.1 Hz, 1 H), 7.47 (d, *J* = 2.0 Hz, 1 H) ppm. ^{13}C-NMR (125 MHz, CDCl$_3$): δ = 14.3, 17.6, 18.4, 27.0, 30.7, 32.7, 33.2, 34.5, 39.1, 39.6, 39.8, 42.9, 44.9, 57.8, 65.8, 71.8, 85.5, 115.2, 118.0, 129.7, 130.4, 133.8, 138.0, 154.0, 171.1, 171.8, 177.6 ppm. HRMS (ESI-ToF) calcd. for C$_{27}$H$_{40}$IN$_2$O$_6$$^+$ [M+H]$^+$: 615.1926 found 615.1944.

4.2.13. Synthesis of (3R,9S,11S,13R,14S,16R)-14-Hydroxy-3-(4-hydroxy-3-iodobenzyl)-4,9,11,13-tetramethyl-16-(prop-2-yn-1-yl)-1-oxa-4,7-diazacyclohexadecane-2,5,8-trione (**8c**)

Compound **8a** (314 mg, 458 µmol, 1.0 equiv) was dissolved in anhydrous THF (9.17 mL, 0.05 M). TBAF (504 mL, 504 µmol, 1.1 equiv, 1 M solution in THF) was added at 0 °C and stirred for 15 min. The reaction was worked up with saturated NH$_4$Cl and the aqueous phase extracted twice with EtOAc. The combined organic phases were dried over Na$_2$SO$_4$, and the solvent removed under reduced pressure. The residue was chromatographed (FlashPure Select C18, H$_2$O:MeCN 90:10–MeCN) and alkyne **8c** (281 mg, 458 µmol, quant.) obtained as colorless powder after lyophilization. R_f (**8c**) = 0.22 (silica, *n*-pentane: EtOAc 1:1). $[α]_D^{20}$ = −35.1 (c = 0.5, CHCl$_3$). ^{1}H-NMR (500 MHz, CDCl$_3$): δ = 0.84 (d, *J* = 6.8 Hz, 3 H), 0.96 (d, *J* = 6.3 Hz, 3 H), 1.02–1.10 (m, 3 H), 1.12 (d, *J* = 6.7 Hz, 3 H), 1.20 (m, 1 H), 1.45–1.57 (m, 3 H), 1.98 (m, 1 H), 2.15 (t, *J* = 2.6 Hz, 1 H), 2.39–2.48 (m, 2 H), 2.61 (ddd, *J* = 17.1, 6.7, 2.6 Hz, 1 H), 2.88 (dd, *J* = 15.5, 11.9 Hz, 1 H), 2.94 (s, 3 H), 3.26 (d, *J* = 16.8 Hz, 1 H), 3.41 (dd, *J* = 15.5, 4.7 Hz, 1 H) 3.67 (m, 1 H), 4.81 (dd, *J* = 16.8, 8.7, 1 H), 5.26 (m, 1 H), 5.55 (dd, *J* = 11.9, 4.7 Hz, 1 H), 6.05 (bs, 1 H), 6.29 (m, 1 H), 6.86 (d, *J* = 8.2 Hz, 1 H), 7.06 (dd, *J* = 8.2, 2.0 Hz, 1 H), 7.49 (d, *J* = 2.0 Hz, 1 H) ppm. ^{13}C-NMR (125 MHz, CDCl$_3$): δ = 14.3, 17.6, 18.3, 24.9, 27.0, 30.5, 32.4, 34.7, 39.1, 39.8, 42.8, 45.0, 57.5, 65.9, 70.1, 71.4, 79.4, 85.5, 115.2, 129.8, 130.4, 138.1, 154.1, 170.6, 171.9, 177.5 ppm. HRMS (ESI-ToF) calcd. for C$_{27}$H$_{38}$IN$_2$O$_6$$^+$ [M+H]$^+$: 613.1769 found 613.1767.

4.3. Modification of the Doliculide Core Structure

4.3.1. Synthesis of (3R,9S,11S,13R,14S,16R)-16-[(1-Benzyl-1H-1,2,3-triazol-4-yl)methyl]-14-hydroxy-3-(4-hydroxy-3-iodobenzyl)-4,9,11,13-tetramethyl-1-oxa-4,7-diazacyclohexadecane-2,5,8-trione (**9a**)

According to the general procedure for CuAAC, alkyne **8c** (15.3 mg, 25.0 µmol, 1.0 equiv) was dissolved in a 1:1 mixture of *t*-BuOH:H$_2$O (500 µL, 0.05 M) and reacted with benzyl azide (4.0 mg, 30.0 µmol, 1.2 equiv), sodium ascorbate (15.0 µL, 15.0 µmol, 1 M in H$_2$O, 0.6 equiv), and copper(II) sulfate (12.5 µL, 12.5 µmol, 1 M in H$_2$O, 0.5 equiv). After stirring for 16 h, the mixture was concentrated and the obtained crude product was subjected to reversed-phase flash chromatography (FlashPure Select C18, H$_2$O:MeCN 90:10–MeCN). Triazole **9a** (17.5 mg, 23.5 µmol, 86%) was obtained as colorless powder after lyophilization. $[α]_D^{20}$ = −12.0 (c = 1.0, CHCl$_3$). ^{1}H-NMR (500 MHz, CDCl$_3$): δ = 0.81 (d, *J* = 6.9 Hz, 3 H), 0.94 (d, *J* = 6.1 Hz, 3 H), 1.01–1.09 (m, 3 H), 1.13 (d, *J* = 6.7 Hz, 3 H), 1.17 (m, 1 H), 1.43–1.55 (m, 3 H), 1.97 (m, 1 H), 2.44 (m, 1 H), 2.61 (dd, *J* = 15.3, 12.1 Hz, 1 H), 2.78 (s, 3 H), 2.98–3.08 (m, 2 H), 3.09–3.17 (m, 2 H), 3.63 (ddd, *J* = 9.0, 4.1, 4.1 Hz, 1 H), 4.71 (dd, *J* = 16.7, 8.9 Hz), 5.37 (dd, *J* = 12.1, 4.6 Hz, 1 H), 5.44 (m, 1 H), 5.55 (d, *J* = 14.8 Hz, 1 H), 5.59 (d, *J* = 14.8 Hz, 1 H), 6.34 (dd, *J* = 8.9, 2.4 Hz, 1 H), 6.80 (d, *J* = 8.3 Hz, 1 H), 6.95 (dd, *J* = 8.2, 1.4 Hz, 1 H), 7.28–7.37 (m, 5 H), 7.39 (d, *J* = 1.7 Hz, 1 H), 7.43 (s, 1 H) ppm. ^{13}C-NMR (125

MHz, CDCl$_3$): δ = 14.3, 17.6, 18.5, 27.0, 30.8, 31.5, 32.3, 33.1, 34.4, 39.1, 39.5, 42.9, 44.8, 54.0, 57.8, 65.8, 71.7, 85.1, 115.1, 121.9, 128.1, 128.7, 129.0, 129.4, 130.2, 135.0, 138.3, 143.9, 154.3, 171.1, 172.0, 177.7 ppm. HRMS (ESI-ToF) calcd. for C$_{34}$H$_{45}$IN$_5$O$_6$$^+$ [M]$^+$: 746.2409 found 746.2408.

4.3.2. Synthesis of (3R,9S,11S,13R,14S,16R)-14-hydroxy-3-(4-hydroxy-3-iodobenzyl)-4,9,11,13-tetramethyl-16-((1-pentyl-1H-1,2,3-triazol-4-yl)methyl)-1-oxa-4,7-diazacyclohexadecane-2,5,8-trione (**9b**)

According to the general procedure for CuAAC, alkyne **8c** (12.8 mg, 20.9 μmol, 1.0 equiv) was dissolved in a 1:1 mixture of *t*-BuOH:H$_2$O (418 μL, 0.05 M) and reacted with 1-azidopentane (2.8 mg, 25.1 μmol, 1.2 equiv), sodium ascorbate (12.5 μL, 12.5 μmol, 1 M in H$_2$O, 0.6 equiv) and copper(II) sulfate (10.5 μL, 10.5 μmol, 1 M in H$_2$O, 0.5 equiv). After stirring for 16 h, the mixture was concentrated and the obtained crude product was subjected to reversed-phase flash chromatography (FlashPure Select C18, H$_2$O:MeCN 90:10–MeCN). Triazole **9b** (14.4 mg, 19.8 μmol, 95%) was obtained as colorless powder after lyophilization. $[α]_D^{20}$ = −9.6 (c = 1.0, CHCl$_3$). ^{1}H-NMR (500 MHz, CDCl$_3$): δ = 0.81 (d, *J* = 6.6 Hz, 3 H), 0.88 (t, *J* = 7.1 Hz, 3 H), 0.94 (d, *J* = 6.0 Hz, 3 H), 0.99–1.08 (m, 3 H), 1.11 (d, *J* = 6.6 Hz, 3 H), 1.19 (m, 1 H), 1.24–1.39 (m, 4 H), 1.42–1.56 (m, 3 H), 1.89 (tt, *J* = 7.3, 7.3 Hz, 2 H), 1.97 (m, 1 H), 2.43 (m, 1 H), 2.70 (dd, *J* = 14.3, 11.2 Hz, 1 H), 2.94 (s, 3 H), 2.98 (dd, *J* = 15.3, 3.8 Hz, 1 H), 3.06 (dd, *J* = 15.3, 8.2 Hz, 1 H), 3.11–3.21 (m, 2 H), 3.53–3.74 (m, 2 H), 4.36 (t, *J* = 7.3 Hz, 2 H), 4.76 (dd, *J* = 16.6, 8.7 Hz, 1 H), 5.33 (dd, *J* = 11.1, 3.9 Hz, 1 H), 5.44 (m, 1 H), 6.44 (bs, 1 H), 6.77 (d, *J* = 7.8 Hz, 1 H), 6.92 (d, *J* = 7.8 Hz, 1 H), 7.40 (s, 1 H), 7.43 (s, 1 H) ppm. ^{13}C-NMR (125 MHz, CDCl$_3$): δ = 13.9, 14.4, 17.7, 18.4, 22.1, 27.0, 28.6, 30.1, 31.0, 31.6, 32.4, 33.2, 34.5, 39.0, 39.6, 42.8, 44.9, 50.3, 58.0, 65.8, 71.9, 86.0, 115.5, 121.7, 129.5, 129.5, 138.2, 143.5, 155.5, 171.3, 171.9, 177.6 ppm. HRMS (ESI-ToF) calcd. for C$_{32}$H$_{49}$IN$_5$O$_6$$^+$ [M+H]$^+$: 726.2722 found 726.2722.

4.3.3. Synthesis of Benzyl 2-(4-{[(3R,9S,11S,13R,14S,16R)-14-hydroxy-3-(4-hydroxy-3-iodobenzyl)-4,9,11,13-tetramethyl-2,5,8-trioxo-1-oxa-4,7-diazacyclohexadecan-16-yl]methyl}-1H-1,2,3-triazol-1-yl)acetate (**9c**)

According to the general procedure for CuAAC, alkyne **8c** (11.5 mg, 18.8 μmol, 1.0 equiv) was dissolved in a 1:1 mixture of *t*-BuOH:H$_2$O (374 μL, 0.05 M) and reacted with benzyl 2-azidoacetate (4.3 mg, 22.5 μmol, 1.2 equiv), sodium ascorbate (11.3 μL, 11.3 μmol, 1 M in H$_2$O, 0.6 equiv) and copper(II) sulfate (9.4 μL, 9.4 μmol, 1 M in H$_2$O, 0.5 equiv). After stirring for 16 h, the mixture was concentrated and the obtained crude product was subjected to reversed-phase flash chromatography (FlashPure Select C18, H$_2$O:MeCN 90:10–MeCN). Triazole **9c** (14.2 mg, 17.7 μmol, 94%) was obtained as colorless powder after lyophilization. $[α]_D^{20}$ = −13.0 (c = 1.0, CHCl$_3$). ^{1}H-NMR (500 MHz, CDCl$_3$): δ = 0.82 (d, *J* = 6.7 Hz, 3 H), 0.94 (d, *J* = 6.0 Hz, 3 H), 0.99–1.07 (m, 3 H), 1.10 (d, *J* = 6.6 Hz, 3 H), 1.16 (m, 1 H), 1.44–1.51 (m, 2 H), 1.58 (m, 1 H), 2.0 (m, 1 H), 2.42 (ddq, *J* = 12.1, 6.6 Hz, *J* = 3.4 Hz, 1 H), 2.78 (dd, *J* = 15.4, 12.4 Hz, 1 H), 2.80 (s, 3 H), 3.05 (dd, *J* = 16.6, 2.0 Hz, 1 H), 3.09 (dd, *J* = 16.3, 6.4 Hz, 1 H), 3.23 (dd, *J* = 16.3, 3.8 Hz, 1 H), 3.26 (dd, *J* = 15.4, 4.4 Hz, 1 H), 3.68 (m, 1 H), 4.70 (dd, *J* = 16.6, 9.2 Hz, 1 H), 5.19 (d, *J* = 12.2 Hz, 1 H), 5.25 (d, *J* = 12.2 Hz, 1 H), 5.33 (d, *J* = 17.5 Hz, 1 H), 5.37 (d, *J* = 17.5 Hz, 1 H), 5.47 (dd, *J* = 12.2, 4.4 Hz, 1 H), 5.58 (m, 1 H), 6.13 (dd, *J* = 9.2, 2.0 Hz, 1 H), 6.81 (d, *J* = 8.2 Hz, 1 H), 7.01 (dd, *J* = 8.2, 1.4 Hz, 1 H), 7.29–7.39 (m, 5 H), 7.46 (d, *J* = 1.7 Hz, 1 H), 7.68 (s, 1 H) ppm. ^{13}C-NMR (125 MHz, CDCl$_3$): δ = 14.2, 17.5, 18.5, 26.9, 30.7, 31.3, 32.2, 32.5, 34.2, 39.0 39.3, 43.1, 44.8, 50.8, 57.6, 65.8, 67.8, 71.1, 85.2, 115.1, 123.4, 128.4, 128.7, 128.7, 129.5, 130.4, 134.7, 138.3, 143.4, 154.2, 167.0, 171.2, 172.0, 177.9 ppm. HRMS (ESI-ToF) calcd. for C$_{29}$H$_{41}$IN$_5$O$_8$$^+$ [M−Bn+2H]$^+$: 714.1994 found 714.1991.

4.3.4. Synthesis of 2-{2-[2-(4-{[(3R,9S,11S,13R,14S,16R)-14-Hydroxy-3-(4-hydroxy-3-iodobenzyl)-4,9,11,13-tetramethyl-2,5,8-trioxo-1-oxa-4,7-diazacyclohexadecan-16-yl]methyl}-1H-1,2,3-triazol-1-yl)ethoxy]ethoxy}acetic Acid (9d)

According to the general procedure for CuAAC, alkyne **8c** (9.9 mg, 16.2 μmol, 1.0 equiv) was dissolved in a 1:1 mixture of t-BuOH:H_2O (324 μL, 0.05 M) and reacted with potassium 2-[2-(2-azidoethoxy)ethoxy)acetate (4.4 mg, 19.4 μmol, 1.2 equiv), sodium ascorbate (9.7 μL, 9.7 μmol, 1 M in H_2O, 0.6 equiv) and copper(II) sulfate (8.1 μL, 8.1 μmol, 1 M in H_2O, 0.5 equiv). After stirring for 18 h. DCM and brine were added to the reaction mixture, the phases separated and the aqueous phase extracted twice with DCM and once with $CHCl_3$/i-PrOH (3:1). The combined organic extracts were concentrated and the obtained crude product was subjected to reversed-phase flash chromatography (FlashPure Select C18, H_2O + 0.1% HCOOH:MeCN 90:10–MeCN). Triazole **9d** (8.5 mg, 10.6 μmol, 66%) was obtained as colorless powder after lyophilization. $[\alpha]_D^{20} = -4.1$ (c = 1.0, $CHCl_3$). ^{1}H-NMR (500 MHz, DMSO-D_6): δ = 0.68 (d, J = 6.9 Hz, 3 H), 0.84 (d, J = 6.3 Hz, 3 H), 0.87–0.92 (m, 3 H), 0.94 (d, J = 6.7 Hz, 3 H), 1.15 (m, 1 H), 1.22–1.38 (m, 3 H), 1.57 (bs, 1 H), 1.77 (m, 1 H), 2.47 (m, 1 H), 2.79 (dd, J = 15.0, 11.4 Hz, 1 H), 2.82 (s, 3 H), 2.92 (dd, J = 15.0, 4.6 Hz, 1 H), 2.98 (dd, J = 15.2, 6.0 Hz, 1 H), 3.01 (dd, J = 15.7, 3.1 Hz, 1 H), 3.09 (dd, J = 15.0, 4.6 Hz, 1 H), 3.34 (bs, 1 H), 3.51–3.58 (m, 5 H), 3.83 (t, J = 5.4 Hz, 2 H), 3.87 (s, 2 H), 4.49–4.60 (m, 3 H), 5.21 (dddd, J = 9.2, 6.0, 5.6, 4.6 Hz, 1 H), 5.38 (dd, J = 11.4, 4.6 Hz, 1 H), 6.78 (d, J = 8.2 Hz, 1 H), 6.97 (dd, J = 8.4, 2.0 Hz, 1 H), 7.47 (d, J = 2.0 Hz, 1 H), 7.93 (s, 1 H), 8.17 (dd, J = 8.6, 3.1 Hz, 1 H), 10.5 (bs, 1 H) ppm. ^{13}C-NMR (125 MHz, DMSO-D_6): δ = 14.4, 17.5, 18.6, 26.2, 30.5, 30.8, 31.0, 31.4, 34.5, 37.1, 38.6, 43.0, 44.7, 49.1, 56.6, 63.9, 68.3, 68.9, 69.5, 69.5, 70.8, 84.4, 114.7, 123.2, 129.6, 130.0, 138.4, 142.0, 155.2, 169.9, 170.7, 171.8, 176.2 ppm. HRMS (ESI-ToF) calcd. for $C_{33}H_{49}IN_5O_{10}^+$ [M+H]$^+$: 802.2519 found 802.2518.

4.3.5. Synthesis of (3R,9S,11S,13R,14S,16R)-14-Hydroxy-3-(4-hydroxy-3-iodobenzyl)-16-((1-(2-(2-(2-hydroxyethoxy)ethoxy)ethyl)-1H-1,2,3-triazol-4-yl)methyl)-4,9,11,13-tetramethyl-1-oxa-4,7-diazacyclohexadecane-2,5,8-trione (9e)

According to the general procedure for CuAAC, alkyne **8c** (14.8 mg, 24.2 μmol, 1.0 equiv) was dissolved in a 1:1 mixture of t-BuOH:H_2O (484 μL, 0.05 M) and reacted with 2-[2-(2-azidoethoxy]ethoxy)ethan-1-ol (5.1 mg, 29.1 μmol, 1.2 equiv), sodium ascorbate (14.5 μL, 14.5 μmol, 1 M in H_2O, 0.6 equiv) and copper(II) sulfate (12.1 μL, 12.1 μmol, 1 M in H_2O, 0.5 equiv). After stirring for 16 h, the mixture was concentrated and the obtained crude product was subjected to reversed-phase flash chromatography (FlashPure Select C18, H_2O + 0.1% HCOOH:MeCN 90:10–MeCN). Triazole **9e** (15.2 mg, 19.3 μmol, 80%) was obtained as colorless powder after lyophilization. $[\alpha]_D^{20} = -9.6$ (c = 1.0, $CHCl_3$). ^{1}H-NMR (500 MHz, $CDCl_3$): δ = 0.82 (d, J = 6.0 Hz, 3 H), 0.93 (d, J = 6.1 Hz, 3 H), 0.99–1.08 (m, 3 H), 1.12 (d, J = 6.6 Hz, 3 H), 1.17 (m, 1 H), 1.42–1.58 (m, 3 H), 1.88–2.07 (m, 3 H), 2.43 (ddq, J = 12.1, 6.6, 3.4 Hz, 1 H), 2.71 (dd, J = 15.3, 11.8 Hz, 1 H), 2.93 (s, 3 H), 2.99 (dd, J = 15.4, 4.1 Hz, 1 H), 3.07 (dd, J = 15.0, 7.9 Hz, 1 H), 3.13 (dd, J = 16.6, 1.5 Hz, 1 H), 3.17 (dd, J = 15.4, 4.6 Hz, 1 H), 3.58 (t, J = 4.4 Hz, 2 H), 3.60–3.65 (m, 5 H), 3.75 (dd, J = 4.1, 4.1 Hz, 2 H), 3.83–3.92 (m, 2 H), 4.57 (m, 2 H), 4.75 (dd, J = 16.6, 8.9 Hz, 1 H), 5.34 (dd, J = 11.8, 4.7 Hz, 1 H), 5.43 (m, 1 H), 6.41 (dd, J = 8.9, 1.5 Hz, 1 H), 6.82 (d, J = 8.1 Hz, 1 H), 6.97 (dd, J = 8.1, 1.7 Hz, 1 H), 7.44 (d, J = 1.7 Hz, 1 H), 7.73 (s, 1 H) ppm. ^{13}C-NMR (125 MHz, $CDCl_3$): δ = 14.3, 17.6, 18.5, 27.0, 31.0, 31.5, 32.4, 33.3, 34.4, 39.1, 39.6, 42.9, 44.9, 50.1, 58.0, 61.6, 65.9, 69.5, 70.2, 70.4, 72.2, 72.5, 85.0, 115.2, 123.4, 129.6, 130.2, 138.4, 143.6, 154.4, 171.2, 171.9, 177.8 ppm. HRMS (ESI-ToF) calcd. for $C_{33}H_{51}IN_5O_9^+$ [M+H]$^+$: 788.2726 found 788.2727.

4.3.6. Synthesis of tert-Butyl (2-{2-[2-(4-{[(3R,9S,11S,13R,14S,16R)-14-hydroxy-3-(4-hydroxy-3-iodobenzyl)-4,9,11,13-tetramethyl-2,5,8-trioxo-1-oxa-4,7-diazacyclohexadecan-16-yl]methyl}-1H-1,2,3-triazol-1-yl)ethoxy]ethoxy}ethyl)carbamate (**9f**)

According to the general procedure for CuAAC, alkyne **8c** (10.2 mg, 16.7 μmol, 1.0 equiv) was dissolved in a 1:1 mixture of *t*-BuOH:H$_2$O (334 μL, 0.05 M) and reacted with *tert*-butyl {2-[2-(2-aminoethoxy)ethoxy]ethyl}carbamate (5.5 mg, 20.0 μmol, 1.2 equiv), sodium ascorbate (10.0 μL, 10.0 μmol, 1 M in H$_2$O, 0.6 equiv) and copper(II) sulfate (8.3 μL, 8.3 μmol, 1 M in H$_2$O, 0.5 equiv). After stirring for 16 h, the mixture was concentrated and the obtained crude product was subjected to reversed-phase flash chromatography (FlashPure Select C18, H$_2$O + 0.1% HCOOH:MeCN 90:10–MeCN). Triazole **9f** (13.6 mg, 15.3 μmol, 92%) was obtained as colorless powder after lyophilization. $[\alpha]_D^{20}$ = −4.3 (c = 1.0, CHCl$_3$). ^{1}H-NMR (500 MHz, DMSO-D$_6$): δ = 0.68 (d, *J* = 6.7 Hz, 3 H), 0.84 (d, *J* = 6.1 Hz, 3 H), 0.86–0.93 (m, 3 H), 0.94 (d, *J* = 6.7 Hz, 3 H), 1.15 (m, 1 H), 1.22–1.35 (m, 3 H), 1.36 (s, 9 H), 1.77 (m, 1 H), 2.48 (m, 1 H), 2.80 (dd, *J* = 15.0, 11.7 Hz, 1 H), 2.81 (s, 3 H), 2.92 (dd, *J* = 15.1, 5.0 Hz, 1 H), 2.95–3.06 (m, 4 H), 3.09 (dd, *J* = 15.0, 4.3 Hz, 1 H), 3.34 (t, *J* = 6.0 Hz, 2 H), 3.45 (m, 2 H), 3.51 (m, 2 H), 3.57 (m, 1 H), 3.82 (ddd, *J* = 16.2, 10.8, 5.3 Hz, 1 H), 3.83 (ddd, *J* = 16.2, 11.1, 5.2 Hz, 1 H), 4.21 (d, *J* = 4.7 Hz, 1 H), 4.51–4.60 (m, 3 H), 5.21 (m, 1 H), 5.40 (dd, *J* = 11.5, 4.5 Hz, 1 H), 6.68–6.80 (m, 2 H), 6.98 (dd, *J* = 8.2, 1.8 Hz, 1 H), 7.47 (d, *J* = 1.8 Hz, 1 H), 7.91 (s, 1 H), 8.16 (dd, *J* = 8.6, 3.1 Hz, 1 H), 10.1 (bs, 1 H) ppm. ^{13}C-NMR (125 MHz, DMSO-D$_6$): δ = 14.4, 17.5, 18.6, 26.2, 28.2, 30.4, 30.8, 30.9, 31.3, 34.4, 37.1, 38.5, 39.7, 43.0, 44.7, 49.1, 56.5, 63.8, 68.0, 69.2, 69.4, 69.5, 70.7, 77.6, 84.3, 114.7, 123.2, 129.6, 130.1, 138.5, 141.9, 155.0, 155.6, 169.9, 170.7, 176.1 ppm. HRMS (ESI-ToF) calcd. for C$_{38}$H$_{60}$IN$_6$O$_{10}^+$ [M+H]$^+$: 887.3410 found 887.3397.

4.3.7. Synthesis of tert-Butyl [2-(2-{2-[2-(4-{[(3R,9S,11S,13R,14S,16R)-14-hydroxy-3-(4-hydroxy-3-iodobenzyl)-4,9,11,13-tetramethyl-2,5,8-trioxo-1-oxa-4,7-diazacyclohexadecan-16-yl]methyl}-1H-1,2,3-triazol-1-yl)ethoxy]ethoxy}ethoxy)ethyl]carbamate (**9g**)

According to the general procedure for CuAAC, alkyne **8c** (10.2 mg, 16.7 μmol, 1.0 equiv) was dissolved in a 1:1 mixture of *t*-BuOH:H$_2$O (334 μL, 0.05 M) and reacted with *tert*-butyl (2-{2-[2-(2-aminoethoxy)ethoxy]ethoxy}ethyl)carbamate (6.4 mg, 20.1 μmol, 1.2 equiv), sodium ascorbate (10.0 μL, 10.0 μmol, 1 M in H$_2$O, 0.6 equiv) and copper(II) sulfate (8.3 μL, 8.3 μmol, 1 M in H$_2$O, 0.5 equiv). After stirring for 16 h, the mixture was concentrated and the obtained crude product was subjected to reversed-phase flash chromatography (FlashPure Select C18, H$_2$O + 0.1% HCOOH:MeCN 90:10–MeCN) and further purified by preparative HPLC (Luna C18, H$_2$O + 0.1% HCOOH:MeCN 90:10–MeCN). Triazole **9g** (12.4 mg, 13.3 μmol, 80%) was obtained as colorless powder after lyophilization. $[\alpha]_D^{20}$ = −5.3 (c = 1.0, CHCl$_3$). ^{1}H-NMR (500 MHz, DMSO-D$_6$): δ = 0.68 (d, *J* = 6.7 Hz, 3 H), 0.84 (d, *J* = 6.3 Hz, 3 H), 0.86–0.92 (m, 3 H), 0.94 (d, *J* = 6.7 Hz, 3 H), 1.16 (m, 1 H), 1.22–1.34 (m, 3 H), 1.36 (s, 9 H), 1.77 (m, 1 H), 2.48 (m, 1 H), 2.75–2.82 (m, *J* = 15.3, 11.7 Hz, 4 H), 2.92 (dd, *J* = 15.1, 4.9 Hz, 1 H), 2.95–3.03 (m, 2 H), 3.04 (dt, *J* = 6.1, 6.1 Hz, 2 H), 3.09 (dd, *J* = 15.1, 4.6 Hz, 1 H), 3.36 (t, *J* = 6.1 Hz, 2 H), 3.45–3.47 (m, 4 H), 3.48 (m, 2 H), 3.51 (m, 2 H), 3.57 (m, 1 H), 3.83 (ddd, *J* = 16.3, 10.8, 5.2 Hz, 1 H), 3.83 (ddd, *J* = 16.3, 11.1, 5.2 Hz, 1 H), 4.21 (d, *J* = 4.0 Hz, 1 H), 4.49–4.61 (m, 3 H), 5.22 (m, 1 H), 5.40 (dd, *J* = 11.7, 4.5 Hz, 1 H), 6.68–6.77 (m, 2 H), 6.98 (dd, *J* = 8.3, 1.9 Hz, 1 H), 7.47 (d, *J* = 1.8 Hz, 1 H), 7.91 (s, 1 H), 8.16 (dd, *J* = 8.7, 3.2 Hz, 1 H), 10.2 (bs, 1 H) ppm. ^{13}C-NMR (125 MHz, DMSO-D$_6$): δ = 14.4, 17.5, 18.6, 26.2, 28.2, 30.4, 30.8, 30.9, 31.3, 34.4, 37.1, 38.5, 39.7, 43.0, 44.7, 49.1, 56.5, 63.8, 69.0, 69.2, 69.5, 69.5, 69.6, 69.7, 70.7, 77.6, 84.3, 114.7, 123.2, 129.6, 130.0, 138.5, 141.9, 155.1, 155.6, 169.9, 170.7, 176.1 ppm. HRMS (ESI-ToF) calcd. for C$_{40}$H$_{64}$IN$_6$O$_{11}^+$ [M+H]$^+$: 931.3672 found 931.3672.

4.3.8. Synthesis of (3R,9S,11S,13R,14S,16R)-14-Hydroxy-3-(4-hydroxy-3-iodobenzyl)-4,9,11,13-tetramethyl-16-(3-phenylprop-2-yn-1-yl)-1-oxa-4,7-diazacyclohexadecane-2,5,8-trione (**10a**)

According to the general procedure for Sonogashira couplings, alkyne **8c** (10.5 mg, 17.1 μmol) was reacted with $(PPh_3)_2PdCl_2$ (1.2 mg, 1.71 μmol, 0.1 equiv), iodobenzene (17.5 mg, 85.7 μmol, 5.0 equiv) and copper(I) iodide (0.7 mg, 3.4 μmol, 0.2 equiv) in NEt_3 (114 μL, 0.15 M) and stirred for 16 h. The obtained crude product was subjected to flash chromatography (RediSep Rf Silica, DCM–DCM:MeOH 90:10) and further purified by preparative HPLC (Luna C18, H_2O:MeCN 90:10–MeCN). Alkyne **10a** (6.8 mg, 9.9 μmol, 58%) was obtained as colorless powder after lyophilization. $[\alpha]_D^{20}$ = −0.3 (c = 1.0, $CHCl_3$). ^{1}H-NMR (500 MHz, $CDCl_3$): δ = 0.86 (d, J = 6.9 Hz, 3 H), 0.97 (d, J = 6.3 Hz, 3 H), 1.02–1.11 (m, 3 H), 1.13 (d, J = 6.7 Hz, 3 H), 1.20 (m, 1 H), 1.44 (ddd, J = 13.7, 11.4, 1.8 Hz, 1 H), 1.54 (m, 1 H), 1.60 (ddd, J = 13.7, 11.4 Hz, 1.8 Hz, 1 H), 2.02 (m, 1 H), 2.35 (bs, 1 H), 2.41 (ddq, J = 12.0, 6.6, 3.4 Hz, 1 H), 2.73 (d, J = 6.3 Hz, 1 H), 2.76 (dd, J = 15.6, 12.2 Hz, 1 H), 2.90 (s, 3 H), 3.25 (dd, J = 16.9, 1.7 Hz, 1 H), 3.35 (dd, J = 15.6, 4.6 Hz, 1 H), 3.66 (m, 1 H), 4.80 (dd, J = 16.8, 8.7 Hz, 1 H), 5.38 (ddt, J = 11.4, 6.4, 1.8 Hz, 1 H), 5.46 (dd, J = 12.1, 4.7 Hz, 1 H), 5.58 (bs, 1 H), 6.23 (dd, J = 8.7, 1.7 Hz, 1 H), 6.84 (d, J = 8.2 Hz, 1 H), 6.92 (dd, J = 8.3, 1.8 Hz, 1 H), 7.28 (d, J = 1.8 Hz, 1 H), 7.32–7.37 (m, 3 H), 7.43 (m, 2 H) ppm. ^{13}C-NMR (125 MHz, $CDCl_3$): δ = 14.3, 17.6, 18.4, 26.1, 27.1, 30.5, 32.6, 33.3, 34.5, 39.1, 39.7, 42.8, 45.0, 57.7, 65.9, 70.9, 82.8, 85.3, 85.7, 115.1, 123.1, 128.2, 128.5, 129.6, 130.4, 131.6, 137.8, 153.9, 171.2, 171.9, 177.5 ppm. HRMS (ESI-ToF) calcd. for $C_{33}H_{42}IN_2O_6^+$ [M+H]$^+$: 689.2062 found 689.2061.

4.3.9. Synthesis of (3R,9S,11S,13R,14S,16R)-14-Hydroxy-3-(4-hydroxy-3-iodobenzyl)-16-[3-(4-methoxyphenyl)prop-2-yn-1-yl]-4,9,11,13-tetramethyl-1-oxa-4,7-diazacyclohexadecane-2,5,8-trione (**10b**)

According to the general procedure for Sonogashira couplings, alkyne **8c** (11.3 mg, 18.4 μmol) was reacted with $(PPh_3)_2PdCl_2$ (1.3 mg, 1.85 μmol, 0.1 equiv), 1-iodo-4-methoxybenzene (21.6 mg, 92.3 μmol, 5.0 equiv) and copper(I) iodide (0.7 mg, 3.7 μmol, 0.2 equiv) in NEt_3 (123 μL, 0.15 M) and stirred for 16 h. The obtained crude product was subjected to flash chromatography (RediSep Rf Silica, DCM–DCM:MeOH 9:1). Alkyne **10b** (10.0 mg, 13.9 μmol, 75%) was obtained as colorless powder after lyophilization. $[\alpha]_D^{20}$ = +8.8 (c = 1.0, $CHCl_3$). ^{1}H-NMR (500 MHz, $CDCl_3$): δ = 0.85 (d, J = 6.9 Hz, 1 Hz, 3 H), 0.96 (d, J = 6.1 Hz, 3 H), 1.00–1.11 (m, 3 H), 1.13 (d, J = 6.6 Hz, 3 H), 1.19 (m, 1 H), 1.44 (m, 1 H), 1.54 (m, 1 H), 1.59 (m, 1 H), 2.01 (m, 1 H), 2.35–2.46 (m, J = 12.2, 6.6 Hz, 3.4 Hz, 1 H), 2.71 (d, J = 6.3 Hz, 2 H), 2.77 (dd, J = 15.6, 12.2 Hz, 1 H), 2.91 (s, 3 H), 3.23 (dd, J = 16.8, 1.8 Hz, 1 H), 3.35 (dd, J = 15.6, 4.6 Hz, 1 H), 3.66 (m, 1 H), 3.82 (s, 3 H), 4.80 (dd, J = 16.8, 8.7 Hz, 1 H), 5.36 (ddt, J = 11.4, 6.3, 2.0 Hz, 1 H), 5.47 (dd, J = 12.2, 4.6 Hz, 1 H), 6.12 (bs, 1 H), 6.29 (dd, J = 8.7, 1.8 Hz, 1 H), 6.83 (d, J = 8.4 Hz, 1 H), 6.87 (m, 2 H), 6.93 (dd, J = 8.4, 2.0 Hz, 1 H), 7.29 (d, J = 2.0 Hz, 1 H), 7.36 (m, 2 H) ppm. ^{13}C-NMR (125 MHz, $CDCl_3$): δ = 14.3, 17.6, 18.4, 26.1, 27.1, 30.5, 32.6, 33.2, 34.5, 39.1, 39.7, 42.8, 44.9, 55.3, 57.7, 65.9, 71.0, 82.6, 83.7, 85.4, 114.1, 115.1, 115.2, 129.5, 130.3, 133.0, 138.0, 154.1, 159.5, 171.1, 172.0, 177.5 ppm. HRMS (ESI-ToF) calcd. for $C_{34}H_{44}IN_2O_7^+$ [M+H]$^+$: 719.2188 found 719.2192.

4.3.10. Synthesis of (3R,9S,11S,13R,14S,16R)-14-Hydroxy-3-(4-hydroxy-3-iodobenzyl)-4,9,11,13-tetramethyl-16-[3-(4-nitrophenyl)prop-2-yn-1-yl]-1-oxa-4,7-diazacyclohexadecane-2,5,8-trione (**10c**)

According to the general procedure for Sonogashira couplings, alkyne **8c** (14.4 mg, 23.5 μmol) was reacted with $(PPh_3)_2PdCl_2$ (1.7 mg, 2.35 μmol, 0.1 equiv), 1-iodo-4-nitrobenzene (29.3 mg, 118 μmol, 5.0 equiv) and copper(I) iodide (0.9 mg, 4.7 μmol, 0.2 equiv) in NEt_3 (157 μL, 0.15 M) and stirred for 16 h. The obtained crude product was subjected to flash chromatography (RediSep Rf Silica, DCM–DCM:MeOH 9:1). Alkyne **10c** (13.1 mg, 17.9 μmol, 76%) was obtained as colorless powder after lyophilization. $[\alpha]_D^{20}$ = +11.7 (c = 1.0, $CHCl_3$). ^{1}H-NMR (500 MHz, $CDCl_3$): δ = 0.86 (d, J = 6.7 Hz, 3 H), 0.96 (d, J = 6.3 Hz, 3 H), 1.04–1.13 (m, 3 H), 1.14 (d, J = 6.6

Hz, 3 H), 1.21 (m, 1 H), 1.51–1.63 (m, 3 H), 1.99 (m, 1 H), 2.12 (bs, 1 H), 2.44 (ddq, J = 12.0, 6.6, 3.4 Hz, 1 H), 2.74–2.81 (m, 2 H), 2.87 (dd, J = 17.4, 5.3 Hz, 1 H), 2.92 (s, 3 H), 3.17 (dd, J = 16.6, 2.1 Hz, 1 H), 3.39 (dd, J = 15.3, 4.6 Hz, 1 H), 3.72 (m, 1 H), 4.78 (dd, J = 16.6, 8.8 Hz, 1 H), 5.38 (m, 1 H), 5.56 (dd, J = 11.9, 4.7 Hz, 1 H), 6.36 (dd, J = 8.8, 2.1 Hz, 1 H), 6.70–6.91 (m, J = 8.2 Hz, 2 H), 6.99 (dd, J = 8.3, 2.0 Hz, 1 H), 7.37 (d, J = 2.0 Hz, 1 H), 7.62 (m, 2 H), 8.20 (m, 2 H) ppm. ^{13}C-NMR (125 MHz, CDCl$_3$): δ = 14.3, 17.6, 18.5, 26.0, 27.1, 30.7, 32.5, 32.7, 34.8, 39.1, 39.5, 42.9, 44.9, 57.6, 66.0, 70.3, 81.6, 85.2, 90.9, 115.1, 123.7, 129.5, 130.0, 130.0, 132.5, 138.2, 147.0, 154.3, 170.5, 172.0, 177.6 ppm. HRMS (ESI-ToF) calcd. for C$_{33}$H$_{41}$IN$_3$O$_8^+$ [M+H]$^+$: 734.1933 found 734.1936.

4.3.11. Synthesis of (3R,9S,11S,13R,14S,16R)-14-Hydroxy-3-(4-hydroxy-3-iodobenzyl)-16-{3-[(2-hydroxyethyl)thio]propyl}-4,9,11,13-tetramethyl-1-oxa-4,7-diazacyclohexadecane-2,5,8-trione (**11a**)

According to the general procedure for thiol-ene click reactions, alkene **8b** (17.6 mg, 28.6 µmol) was dissolved in anhydrous THF (286 µL, 0.1 M) and reacted with 2-mercaptoethanol (5.00 µL, 57.3 µmol, 1.12 gml^{-1}, 2.0 equiv), triethylborane (34.4 µL, 8.59 µmol, 0.3 equiv, 0.25 M in hexane) and air (0.4 mL) and stirred for 20 h. The obtained crude product was subjected to reversed-phase chromatography (FlashPure Select C18, H$_2$O:MeCN 90:10–MeCN). Thioether **11a** (14.2 mg, 20.5 µmol, 72%) was obtained as colorless powder after lyophilization. $[α]_D^{20}$ = −14.9 (c = 1.0, CHCl$_3$). ^{1}H-NMR (500 MHz, CDCl$_3$): δ = 0.83 (d, J = 6.7 Hz, 3 H), 0.94 (d, J = 6.0 Hz, 3 H), 1.01–1.10 (m, 3 H), 1.12 (d, J = 6.6 Hz, 3 H), 1.17 (m, 1 H), 1.35 (ddd, J = 13.9, 11.5, 2.0 Hz, 1 H), 1.45 (ddd, J = 13.8, 11.6, 2.0 Hz, 1 H), 1.51 (m, 1 H), 1.62 (m, 2 H), 1.72 (m, 2 H), 1.97 (m, 1 H), 2.14–2.35 (m, 2 H), 2.43 (ddq, J = 11.7, 6.6, 3.4 Hz, 1 H), 2.55 (m, 2 H), 2.73 (m, 2 H), 2.86 (dd, J = 15.3, 12.1 Hz, 1 H), 2.93 (s, 3 H), 3.15 (dd, J = 16.7, 2.0 Hz, 1 H), 3.40 (dd, J = 15.3, 4.4 Hz, 1 H), 3.63 (ddd, J = 11.6, J = 4.0, 2.0 Hz, 1 H), 3.74 (t, J = 6.0 Hz, 2 H), 4.76 (dd, J = 16.7, 8.8 Hz, 1 H), 5.22 (m, 1 H), 5.49 (dd, J = 12.1, 4.4 Hz, 1 H), 6.40 (dd, J = 8.8, 2.0 Hz, 1 H), 6.83 (d, J = 8.2 Hz, 1 H), 7.04 (dd, J = 8.2, 1.8 Hz, 1 H), 7.48 (d, J = 1.8 Hz, 1 H) ppm. ^{13}C-NMR (125 MHz, CDCl$_3$): δ = 14.4, 17.6, 18.4, 25.6, 27.0, 30.9, 31.3, 32.6, 33.1, 34.0, 34.4 35.1, 39.1, 39.5, 43.0, 44.8, 58.0, 60.7, 66.0, 72.4 85.2, 115.2, 129.6, 130.2, 138.3, 154.3, 171.0, 171.9, 177.9 ppm. HRMS (ESI-ToF) calcd. for C$_{29}$H$_{46}$IN$_2$O$_7^+$ [M+H]$^+$: 693.2065 found 693.2076.

4.3.12. Synthesis of (3R,9S,11S,13R,14S,16R)-16-[3-(Butylthio)propyl]-14-hydroxy-3-(4-hydroxy-3-iodobenzyl)- 4,9,11,13-tetramethyl-1-oxa-4,7-diazacyclohexadecane-2,5,8-trione (**11b**)

According to the general procedure for thiol-ene click reactions, alkene **8b** (17.9 mg, 29.1 µmol) was dissolved in anhydrous THF (291 µL, 0.1 M) and reacted with 1-butanethiol (6.25 µL, 58.2 µmol, 0.84 gml^{-1}, 2.0 equiv), triethylborane (35.0 µL, 8.74 µmol, 0.3 equiv, 0.25 M in hexane) and air (0.4 mL) and stirred for 20 h. The obtained crude product was subjected to reversed-phase chromatography (FlashPure Select C18, H$_2$O:MeCN 90:10–MeCN). Thioether **11b** (17.0 mg, 24.1 µmol, 83%) was obtained as colorless powder after lyophilization. $[α]_D^{20}$ = −13.2 (c = 1.0, CHCl$_3$). ^{1}H-NMR (500 MHz, CDCl$_3$): δ = 0.83 (d, J = 6.9 Hz, 3 H), 0.90–0.97 (m, J = 6.7 Hz, 6 H), 1.01–1.10 (m, 3 H), 1.12 (d, J = 6.7 Hz, 3 H), 1.19 (m, 1 H), 1.32 (m, 1 H), 1.41 (m, 2 H), 1.45–1.53 (m, 2 H), 1.54–1.63 (m), 1.67 (m, 1 H), 1.76 (m, 1 H), 1.98 (m, 1 H), 2.44 (ddq, J = 11.6, 6.7, 3.2 Hz, 1 H), 2.46–2.58 (m, 4 H), 2.86 (dd, J = 15.3, 12.3 Hz, 1 H), 2.92 (s, 3 H), 3.22 (d, J = 16.7 Hz, 1 H), 3.41 (dd, J = 15.4, 4.4 Hz, 1 H), 3.62 (ddd, J = 11.4, 4.0, 2.0 Hz, 1 H), 4.77 (dd, J = 16.7, 8.6 Hz, 1 H), 5.20 (m, 1 H), 5.49 (dd, J = 12.3, 4.4 Hz, 1 H), 6.34 (m, 1 H), 6.83 (m, 1 H), 7.05 (dd, J = 8.3, 2.0 Hz, 1 H), 7.48 (d, J = 2.0 Hz, 1 H) ppm. ^{13}C-NMR (125 MHz, CDCl$_3$): δ = 13.7, 14.4, 17.6, 18.4, 22.0, 25.8, 27.0, 30.9, 31.7, 31.8, 32.0, 32.7, 33.5, 34.4, 34.4, 39.1, 39.6, 43.0, 44.9, 58.0, 65.9, 72.6, 85.3, 115.2, 129.5, 130.2, 138.2, 154.3, 171.1, 172.0, 177.7 ppm. HRMS (ESI-ToF) calcd. for C$_{31}$H$_{50}$IN$_2$O$_6$S$^+$ [M+H]$^+$: 705.2429 found 705.2426.

4.3.13. Synthesis of (3R,9S,11S,13R,14S,16R)-16-[3-(Benzylthio)propyl]-14-hydroxy-3-(4-hydroxy-3-iodobenzyl)-4,9,11,13-tetramethyl-1-oxa-4,7-diazacyclohexadecane-2,5,8-trione (11c)

According to the general procedure for thiol-ene click reactions, alkene **8b** (18.8 mg, 30.6 μmol) was dissolved in anhydrous THF (306 μL, 0.1 M) and reacted with benzyl mercaptan (7.17 μL, 61.2 μmol, 1.06 gml^{-1}, 2.0 equiv), triethylborane (36.7 μL, 9.18 μmol, 0.3 equiv, 0.25 M in hexane) and air (0.4 mL) and stirred for 20 h. The obtained crude product was subjected to reversed-phase chromatography (FlashPure Select C18, H$_2$O:MeCN 90:10–MeCN). Thioether **11c** (12.5 mg, 16.9 μmol, 55%) was obtained as colorless powder after lyophilization. $[\alpha]_D^{20}$ = −6.7 (c = 1.0, CHCl$_3$). ^{1}H-NMR (500 MHz, CDCl$_3$): δ = 0.83 (d, *J* = 6.7 Hz, 3 H), 0.95 (d, *J* = 6.1 Hz, 3 H), 1.02–1.09 (m, 3 H), 1.13 (d, *J* = 6.7 Hz, 3 H), 1.17 (m, 1 H), 1.29 (m, 1 H), 1.43 (m, 1 H), 1.48–1.59 (m, 3 H), 1.63 (m, 1 H), 1.71 (m, 1 H), 1.98 (m, 1 H), 2.39–2.47 (m, 3 H), 2.84 (dd, *J* = 15.4, 12.2 Hz, 1 H), 2.88 (s, 3 H), 3.22 (d, *J* = 16.6 Hz, 1 H), 3.38 (dd, *J* = 15.4, 4.4 Hz, 1 H), 3.60 (ddd, *J* = 11.4, 4.2, 2.0 Hz, 1 H), 3.71 (s, 2 H), 4.76 (dd, *J* = 16.6, 8.7 Hz, 1 H), 5.16 (m, 1 H), 5.46 (dd, *J* = 12.2, 4.4 Hz, 1 H), 6.29 (d, *J* = 8.7 Hz, 1 H), 6.85 (d, *J* = 8.2 Hz, 1 H), 7.04 (dd, *J* = 8.2, 2.0 Hz, 1 H), 7.24 (m, 1 H), 7.29–7.34 (m, 4 H), 7.47 (d, *J* = 2.0 Hz, 1 H) ppm. ^{13}C-NMR (125 MHz, CDCl$_3$): δ = 14.4, 17.6, 18.4, 25.4, 27.0, 30.8, 31.0, 32.6, 33.5, 34.4, 34.4, 36.5, 39.1, 39.6, 43.0, 44.9, 58.0, 65.8, 72.6, 85.4, 115.2, 127.0, 128.5, 128.8, 129.6, 130.3, 138.1, 138.4, 154.2, 171.2, 171.9, 177.7 ppm. HRMS (ESI-ToF) calcd. for C$_{34}$H$_{48}$IN$_2$O$_6$S$^+$ [M+H]$^+$: 739.2272 found 739.2298.

4.3.14. Synthesis of Ethyl 3-({3-[(3R,9S,11S,13R,14S,16R)-14-hydroxy-3-(4-hydroxy-3-iodobenzyl)-4,9,11,13-tetramethyl-2,5,8-trioxo-1-oxa-4,7-diazacyclohexadecan-16-yl]propyl}-thio)propanoate (11d)

According to the general procedure for thiol-ene click reactions, alkene **8b** (18.8 mg, 30.6 μmol) was dissolved in anhydrous THF (306 μL, 0.1 M) and reacted with ethyl 3-mercaptopropanoate (7.75 μL, 61.2 μmol, 1.06 gml^{-1}, 2.0 equiv), triethylborane (36.7 μL, 9.18 μmol, 0.3 equiv, 0.25 M in hexane) and air (0.4 mL). After stirring for 2 h, triethylborane (36.7 μL, 9.18 μmol, 0.3 equiv, 0.25 M in hexane) was added and stirred for another 24 h. The obtained crude product was subjected to reversed-phase chromatography (FlashPure Select C18, H$_2$O:MeCN 90:10–MeCN) and further purified by preparative HPLC (Luna C18, H$_2$O:MeCN 25:75–MeCN). Thioether **11d** (19.2 mg, 25.6 μmol, 79%) was obtained as colorless powder after lyophilization. $[\alpha]_D^{20}$ = −8.5 (c = 1.0, CHCl$_3$). ^{1}H-NMR (500 MHz, CDCl$_3$): δ = 0.83 (d, *J* = 6.7 Hz, 3 H), 0.95 (d, *J* = 6.0 Hz, 3 H), 1.00–1.09 (m, 3 H), 1.12 (d, *J* = 6.6 Hz, 3 H), 1.19 (m, 1 H), 1.27 (t, *J* = 7.2 Hz, 3 H), 1.33 (m, 1 H), 1.43–1.55 (m, 2 H), 1.56–1.71 (m, 3 H), 1.76 (m, 1 H), 1.85 (bs, 1 H), 1.98 (m, 1 H), 2.43 (m, 1 H), 2.55 (m, 2 H), 2.60 (t, *J* = 7.4 Hz, 2 H), 2.78 (t, *J* = 7.4 Hz, 2 H), 2.88 (dd, *J* = 15.3, 11.9 Hz, 1 H), 2.93 (s, 3 H), 3.22 (d, *J* = 16.5 Hz, 1 H), 3.41 (dd, *J* = 15.3, 4.0 Hz, 1 H), 3.62 (m, 1 H), 4.16 (q, *J* = 7.2 Hz, 2 H), 4.77 (dd, *J* = 16.5, 7.7 Hz, 1 H), 5.21 (m, 1 H), 5.48 (dd, *J* = 12.0, 4.2 Hz, 1 H), 6.33 (bs, 1 H), 6.84 (d, *J* = 8.2 Hz, 1 H), 7.06 (d, *J* = 7.9 Hz, 1 H), 7.50 (s, 1 H) ppm. ^{13}C-NMR (125 MHz, CDCl$_3$): δ = 14.2, 14.4, 17.6, 18.4, 25.6, 27.0, 27.0, 30.9, 31.7, 32.6, 33.5, 34.3, 34.4, 34.9, 39.1, 39.6, 43.0, 44.9, 58.1, 60.7, 65.9, 72.5, 85.2, 115.2, 129.6, 130.3, 138.2, 154.3, 171.2, 171.9, 172.0, 177.7 ppm. HRMS (ESI-ToF) calcd. for C$_{32}$H$_{50}$IN$_2$O$_8$S$^+$ [M+H]$^+$: 749.2327 found 749.2360.

4.3.15. Synthesis of 2-({3-[(3R,9S,11S,13R,14S,16R)-14-Hydroxy-3-(4-hydroxy-3-iodobenzyl)-4,9,11,13-tetramethyl-2,5,8-trioxo-1-oxa-4,7-diazacyclohexadecan-16-yl]propyl}-thio)acetic Acid (11e)

According to the general procedure for thiol-ene click reactions, alkene **8b** (19.1 mg, 31.1 μmol) was dissolved in anhydrous THF (296 μL, 0.1 M) and reacted with 2-mercaptoacetic acid (4.31 μL, 62.2 μmol, 1.33 gml^{-1}, 2.0 equiv), triethylborane (37.3 μL, 9.32 μmol, 0.3 equiv, 0.25 M in hexane) and air (0.4 mL). After stirring for 2 h, triethylborane (37.3 μL, 9.32 μmol, 0.3

equiv, 0.25 M in hexane) was added and stirred for another 18 h. The obtained crude product was subjected to reversed-phase chromatography (FlashPure Select C18, H$_2$O:MeCN 90:10–MeCN) and further purified by preparative HPLC (Luna C18, H$_2$O:MeCN 25:75–MeCN). Thioether **11e** (14.4 mg, 20.4 µmol, 66%) was obtained as colorless powder after lyophilization. $[\alpha]_D^{20} = -11.5$ (c = 1.0, CHCl$_3$). ^{1}H-NMR (500 MHz, CDCl$_3$): δ = 0.84 (d, J = 6.7 Hz, 3 H), 0.94 (d, J = 6.0 Hz, 3 H), 1.03–1.11 (m, 3 H), 1.11–1.18 (m, J = 6.6 Hz, 4 H), 1.36 (m, 1 H), 1.44 (m, 1 H), 1.56 (m, 1 H), 1.60–1.77 (m, 3 H), 1.82 (m, 1 H), 1.99 (m, 1 H), 2.46 (ddq, J = 12.1, 6.6, 3.4 Hz, 1 H), 2.62 (m, 2 H), 2.86 (dd, J = 15.5, 12.1 Hz, 1 H), 2.98 (s, 3 H), 3.16 (d, J = 16.8 Hz, 1 H), 3.23 (s, 2 H), 3.40 (dd, J = 15.4, 4.4 Hz, 1 H), 3.65 (ddd, J = 11.3, 4.1, 2.1 Hz, 1 H), 4.96 (dd, J = 16.8, 9.0 Hz, 1 H), 5.27 (m, 1 H), 5.55 (dd, J = 12.1, 4.4 Hz, 1 H), 6.72 (bs, 1 H), 6.84 (d, J = 8.2 Hz, 1 H), 7.04 (d, J = 8.4, 1.8 Hz, 1 H), 7.48 (d, J = 2.0 Hz, 1 H) ppm. ^{13}C-NMR (125 MHz, CDCl$_3$): δ = 14.2, 17.5, 18.3, 25.0, 26.9, 30.9, 31.9, 32.4, 33.4, 33.5, 34.3, 34.6, 39.2, 39.7, 42.9, 44.6, 57.7, 66.0, 72.1, 85.3, 115.2, 129.6, 130.3, 138.2, 154.3, 170.8, 171.8, 173.4, 178.5 ppm. HRMS (ESI-ToF) calcd. for C$_{29}$H$_{44}$IN$_2$O$_6$S$^+$ [M+H]$^+$: 707.1858 found 707.1884.

4.3.16. Synthesis of S-{3-[(3R,9S,11S,13R,14S,16R)-14-Hydroxy-3-(4-hydroxy-3-iodobenzyl)-4,9,11,13-tetramethyl-2,5,8-trioxo-1-oxa-4,7-diazacyclohexadecan-16-yl]propyl} ethanethioate (**11f**)

According to the general procedure for thiol-ene click reactions, alkene **8b** (18.0 mg, 29.3 µmol) was dissolved in anhydrous THF (293 µL, 0.1 M) and reacted with thioacetic acid (4.17 µL, 58.6 µmol, 1.07 gml^{-1}, 2.0 equiv), triethylborane (35.1 µL, 8.79 µmol, 0.3 equiv, 0.25 M in hexane) and air (0.4 mL) and stirred for 20 h. The obtained crude product was subjected to reversed-phase chromatography (FlashPure Select C18, H$_2$O:MeCN 90:10–MeCN). Thioether **11f** (19.0 mg, 27.5 µmol, 94%) was obtained as colorless powder after lyophilization. $[\alpha]_D^{20} = -11.6$ (c = 1.0, CHCl$_3$). ^{1}H-NMR (500 MHz, CDCl$_3$): δ = 0.83 (d, J = 6.7 Hz, 3 H), 0.95 (d, J = 6.1 Hz, 3 H), 1.00–1.09 (m, 3 H), 1.12 (d, J = 6.6 Hz, 3 H), 1.18 (m, 1 H), 1.32 (m, 1 H), 1.45 (m, 1 H), 1.52 (m, 1 H), 1.56–1.66 (m, 3 H), 1.72 (m, 1 H), 1.99 (m, 1 H), 2.34 (s, 3 H), 2.44 (m, 1 H), 2.85 (t, J = 6.8 Hz, 2 H), 2.89 (m, 1 H), 2.93 (s, 3 H), 3.22 (d, J = 16.6 Hz, 1 H), 3.40 (dd, J = 15.4, 4.4 Hz, 1 H), 3.61 (ddd, J = 11.3, 4.0, 1.9 Hz, 1 H), 4.77 (dd, J = 16.8, 8.7 Hz, 1 H), 5.20 (m, 1 H), 5.48 (dd, J = 12.1, 4.3 Hz, 1 H), 6.33 (bs, 1 H), 6.74 (bs, 1 H), 6.83 (d, J = 8.4 Hz, 1 H), 7.06 (dd, J = 8.4, 1.8 Hz, 1 H), 7.49 (d, J = 1.8 Hz, 1 H) ppm. ^{13}C-NMR (125 MHz, CDCl$_3$): δ = 14.4, 17.6, 18.4, 25.9, 27.0, 28.7, 30.7, 30.9, 32.6, 33.6, 34.3, 34.4, 39.1, 39.6, 43.0, 44.9, 58.1, 65.8, 72.4, 85.3, 115.2, 129.6, 130.3, 138.2, 154.2, 171.2, 171.9, 177.7, 195.9 ppm. HRMS (ESI-ToF) calcd. for C$_{29}$H$_{44}$IN$_2$O$_7$S$^+$ [M+H]$^+$: 691.1908 found 691.1909.

4.4. Cytotoxicity Evaluation

The cell cultures were cultivated at 37 °C under an atmosphere containing 5% CO$_2$. Before usage, Dulbecco's Modified Eagle Medium (DMEM) from Gibco (Thermo Fisher Scientific) was supplemented with 10% fetal bovine serum (FBS) from Gibco. Cells were used between passage 5 and 30 and were split separately for at least two passages to obtain biological repeats. Cells were washed with PBS and 0.5 mL trypsin was added before treatment. Cells were then incubated for 5 min before adding 10 mL medium containing 10% FBS. Per well, 120 µL cell suspension 5 × 10^4 cells/mL (CHO-K1, HCT-116. U-2 OS, KB3.1) or 1 × 10^5 cells/mL (HepG2) cells were seeded in transparent 96-well cell bind plate and incubated for 2 h at 37 °C and an atmosphere of 5% CO$_2$. Each compound was tested in a serial dilution so that the starting concentration is 111 µg/mL, which is diluted by 1:3 as well as the internal solvent control prepared in DMEM with 10% FBS. After 5 d incubation at 37 °C and an atmosphere of 5% CO$_2$, 20 µL of 5 mg/mL MTT (thiazolyl blue tetrazolium bromide) in PBS was added per well and cells were further incubated until coloration of the cells. The medium was then discarded and 100 µL 2-propanol/10 N HCl (250:1) added to the cells. The plates were analyzed by measuring the absorbance at 570 nm and 630 nm as reference using a microplate reader Infinite® 200 Pro from Tecan (Männedorf, Switzerland). Absorption is then converted to cell viability expressed as percentage relative to the respective solvent control. The calculated percentage of growth inhibition were determined by sigmoidal curve fitting using GraphPad (Boston, MA, USA) Prism software (version 10.0.2). Two independent measurements were generated for mean and standard deviation.

5. Conclusions

We have successfully synthesized a variety of doliculide derivates with focus on late-stage modification at the terminal position of the polyketide fragment. The incorporation of an alkene as well as an alkyne moiety during the last step of the Matteson homologation allowed us to accomplish modifications via cycloadditions, Sonogashira couplings, and thiol-ene click reactions. The more polar derivatives generally led to a decreased activity. Apart from one synthesized derivative, all modifications at the *i*-Pr moiety presented herein led to inactivity against HepG2.

Supplementary Materials: The following supporting information can be downloaded at: https://www.mdpi.com/article/10.3390/md22040165/s1, ^{1}H and ^{13}C NMR spectra of compounds **2–11**.

Author Contributions: M.T. was performing the synthesis of doliculide derivatives and was involved in writing the manuscript. U.K. coordinated the project and synthesis and was involved in writing the manuscript. All authors have read and agreed to the published version of the manuscript.

Funding: This research was funded by Saarland University and by a grant of the Deutsche Forschungsgemeinschaft (Ka880/13-1 and Bruker Neo 500–447298507) to U.K.

Institutional Review Board Statement: Not applicable.

Informed Consent Statement: Not applicable.

Data Availability Statement: The authors confirm that the data supporting the findings of this study are available within the article or the Supplementary Materials.

Acknowledgments: We are grateful to Jennifer Herrmann and Alexandra Amann from Helmholtz Institute for Pharmaceutical Research Saarland (HIPS) for investigation of cytotoxic activity and Alexander Voltz from HIPS for support on mass spectrometry. We also thank Stefan Boettcher from Pharmaceutical and Medicinal Chemistry department, Saarland University, for support on mass spectrometry.

Conflicts of Interest: The authors declare no conflicts of interest.

References

1. Ishiwata, H.; Nemoto, T.; Ojika, M.; Yamada, K. Isolation and Stereostructure of Doliculide, a Cytotoxic Cyclodepsipeptide from the Japanese Sea Hare *Dolabella auricularia*. *J. Org. Chem.* **1994**, *59*, 4710–4711. [CrossRef]
2. Harrigan, G.G.; Luesch, H.; Yoshida, W.Y.; Moore, R.E.; Nagle, D.G.; Paul, V.J.; Mooberry, S.L.; Corbett, T.H.; Valeriote, F.A. Symplostatin 1: A Dolastatin 10 Analogue from the Marine Cyanobacterium *Symploca hydnoides*. *J. Nat. Prod.* **1998**, *61*, 1075–1077. [CrossRef] [PubMed]
3. Butler, M.S. The Role of Natural Product Chemistry in Drug Discovery. *J. Nat. Prod.* **2004**, *67*, 2141–2153. [CrossRef] [PubMed]
4. Newman, D.J.; Cragg, G.M. Natural Products as Sources of New Drugs over the Nearly Four Decades from 01/1981 to 09/2019. *J. Nat. Prod.* **2020**, *83*, 770–803. [CrossRef] [PubMed]
5. Zhang, J.N.; Xia, Y.X.; Zhang, H.J. Natural Cyclopeptides as Anticancer Agents in the Last 20 Years. *Int. J. Mol. Sci.* **2021**, *22*, 3973. [CrossRef] [PubMed]
6. Bai, R.; Covell, D.G.; Liu, C.; Ghosh, A.K.; Hamel, E. (−)-Doliculide, a New Macrocyclic Depsipeptide Enhancer of Actin Assembly. *J. Biol. Chem.* **2002**, *277*, 32165–32171. [CrossRef] [PubMed]
7. Franklin-Tong, V.E.; Gourlay, C.W. A Role for Actin in Regulating Apoptosis/Programmed Cell Death: Evidence Spanning Yeast, Plants and Animals. *Biochem. J.* **2008**, *413*, 389–404. [CrossRef] [PubMed]
8. Pollard, T.D.; Cooper, J.A. Actin, a Central Player in Cell Shape and Movement. *Science* **2009**, *326*, 1208–1212. [CrossRef]
9. Matcha, K.; Madduri, A.V.R.; Roy, S.; Ziegler, S.; Waldmann, H.; Hirsch, A.K.H.; Minnaard, A.J. Total Synthesis of (−)-Doliculide, Structure–Activity Relationship Studies and Its Binding to F-Actin. *ChemBioChem* **2012**, *13*, 2537–2548. [CrossRef] [PubMed]
10. Foerster, F.; Braig, S.; Chen, T.; Altmann, K.-H.; Vollmar, A.M. Pharmacological Characterization of Actin-Binding (−)-Doliculide. *Bioorg. Med. Chem.* **2014**, *22*, 5117–5122. [CrossRef] [PubMed]
11. Foerster, F.; Chen, T.; Altmann, K.-H.; Vollmar, A.M. Actin-Binding Doliculide Causes Premature Senescence in P53 Wild Type Cells. *Bioorg. Med. Chem.* **2016**, *24*, 123–129. [CrossRef] [PubMed]

12. Schneider, G.; Reker, D.; Chen, T.; Hauenstein, K.; Schneider, P.; Altmann, K. Deorphaning the Macromolecular Targets of the Natural Anticancer Compound Doliculide. *Angew. Chemie Int. Ed.* **2016**, *5*, 12408–12411. [CrossRef] [PubMed]
13. Ishiwata, I.; Sone, H.; Kigoshi, H.; Yamada, K. Enantioselective Total Synthesis of Doliculide, a Potent Cytotoxic Cyclodepsipeptide of Marine Origin and Structure-Cytotoxicity Relationships of Synthetic Doliculide Congeners. *Tetrahedron* **1994**, *50*, 12853–12882. [CrossRef]
14. Chen, T. Total Synthesis of the Marine Macrolide (-)-Doliculide and SAR Studies. Doctoral Thesis, ETH-Zürich, Zürich, Switzerland, 2015. [CrossRef]
15. Bubb, M.R.; Spector, I.; Beyer, B.B.; Fosen, K.M. Effects of Jasplakinolide on the Kinetics of Actin Polymerization. *J. Biol. Chem.* **2000**, *275*, 5163–5170. [CrossRef] [PubMed]
16. Freitas, V.M.; Rangel, M.; Bisson, L.F.; Jaeger, R.G.; Machado-Santelli, G.M. The Geodiamolide H, Derived from Brazilian Sponge *Geodia corticostylifera*, Regulates Actin Cytoskeleton, Migration and Invasion of Breast Cancer Cells Cultured in Three-dimensional Environment. *J. Cell. Physiol.* **2008**, *216*, 583–594. [CrossRef] [PubMed]
17. Tanaka, C.; Tanaka, J.; Bolland, R.F.; Marriott, G.; Higa, T. Seragamides A–F, New Actin-Targeting Depsipeptides from the Sponge *Suberites japonicus* Thiele. *Tetrahedron* **2006**, *62*, 3536–3542. [CrossRef]
18. Sumiya, E.; Shimogawa, H.; Sasaki, H.; Tsutsumi, M.; Yoshita, K.; Ojika, M.; Suenaga, K.; Uesugi, M. Cell-Morphology Profiling of a Natural Product Library Identifies Bisebromoamide and Miuraenamide A as Actin Filament Stabilizers. *ACS Chem. Biol.* **2011**, *6*, 425–431. [CrossRef] [PubMed]
19. Moser, C.; Rüdiger, D.; Förster, F.; von Blume, J.; Yu, P.; Küster, B.; Kazmaier, U.; Vollmar, A.M.; Zahler, S. Persistent inhibition of pore-based cell migration by sub-toxic doses of miuraenamide, an actin filament stabilizer. *Sci. Rep.* **2017**, *7*, 16407. [CrossRef] [PubMed]
20. Wang, S.; Meixner, M.; Yu, L.; Karmann, L.; Kazmaier, U.; Vollmar, A.M.; Antes, I.; Zahler, S. Turning the Actin Nucleating Compound Miuraenamide into Nucleation Inhibitors. *ACS Omega* **2021**, *6*, 22165–22172. [CrossRef]
21. Desriac, F.; Jégou, C.; Balnois, E.; Brillet, B.; Le Chevalier, P.; Fleury, Y. Antimicrobial Peptides from Marine Proteobacteria. *Mar. Drugs* **2013**, *11*, 3632–3660. [CrossRef] [PubMed]
22. Karmann, L.; Schultz, K.; Herrmann, J.; Müller, R.; Kazmaier, U. Totalsynthese und biologische Evaluierung von Miuraenamiden. *Angew. Chemie* **2015**, *127*, 4585–4590. [CrossRef]
23. Becker, D.; Kazmaier, U. Synthesis of Simplified Halogenated Chondramide Derivatives as new Actin-binding Agents. *Eur. J. Org. Chem.* **2015**, *2015*, 2591–2602. [CrossRef]
24. Becker, D.; Kazmaier, U. Synthesis and Biological Evaluation of Dichlorinated Chondramide Derivatives. *Eur. J. Org. Chem.* **2015**, *2015*, 4198–4213. [CrossRef]
25. Gorges, J.; Kazmaier, U. Matteson Homologation-Based Total Synthesis of Lagunamide A. *Org. Lett.* **2018**, *20*, 2033–2036. [CrossRef] [PubMed]
26. Andler, O.; Kazmaier, U. Total synthesis of apratoxin A and B using Matteson's homologation approach. *Org. Biomol. Chem.* **2021**, *19*, 4866–4870. [CrossRef] [PubMed]
27. Matteson, D.S. Boronic Esters in Stereodirected Synthesis. *Tetrahedron* **1989**, *45*, 1859–1885. [CrossRef]
28. Matteson, D.S. Boronic Esters in Asymmetric Synthesis. *J. Org. Chem.* **2013**, *78*, 10009–10023. [CrossRef]
29. Matteson, D.S.; Collins, D.S.L.; Aggarwal, V.K.; Ciganek, E. The Matteson Reaction. *Org. React.* **2021**, *105*, 427–860. [CrossRef]
30. Tost, M.; Andler, O.; Kazmaier, U. A Matteson Homologation-Based Synthesis of Doliculide and Derivatives. *Eur. J. Org. Chem.* **2021**, *2021*, 6459–6471. [CrossRef]
31. Andler, O.; Kazmaier, U. A Straightforward Synthesis of Polyketides via Ester Dienolate Matteson Homologation. *Chem.-A Eur. J.* **2021**, *27*, 949–953. [CrossRef] [PubMed]
32. Andler, O.; Kazmaier, U. Application of Allylzinc Reagents as Nucleophiles in Matteson Homologations. *Org. Lett.* **2021**, *23*, 8439–8444. [CrossRef] [PubMed]
33. Kinsinger, T.; Kazmaier, U. Application of Vinyl Nucleophiles in Matteson Homologations. *Org. Lett.* **2022**, *24*, 3599–3603. [CrossRef] [PubMed]
34. Krasovskiy, A.; Knochel, P. A LiCl-Mediated Br/Mg Exchange Reaction for the Preparation of Functionalized Aryl- and Heteroarylmagnesium Compounds from Organic Bromides. *Angew. Chem. Int. Ed.* **2004**, *43*, 3333–3336. [CrossRef] [PubMed]
35. Sämann, C.; Knochel, P. A Convenient Synthesis of α-Substituted β,γ-Unsaturated Ketones and Esters via the Direct Addition of Substituted Allylic Zinc Reagents Prepared by Direct Insertion. *Synthesis* **2013**, *45*, 1870–1876. [CrossRef]
36. Che, W.; Wen, D.C.; Zhu, S.; Zhou, Q. Enantioselective Total Synthesis of (−)-Doliculide Using Catalytic Asymmetric Hydrogenations. *Helv. Chim. Acta* **2019**, *102*, e1900023. [CrossRef]
37. Tanaka, S.; Saburi, H.; Ishibashi, Y.; Kitamura, M. CpRuIIPF6/Quinaldic Acid-Catalyzed Chemoselective Allyl Ether Cleavage. A Simple and Practical Method for Hydroxyl Deprotection. *Org. Lett.* **2004**, *6*, 1873–1875. [CrossRef]
38. Kappler, S.; Karmann, L.; Prudel, C.; Herrmann, J.; Caddeu, G.; Müller, R.; Vollmar, A.M.; Zahler, S.; Kazmaier, U. Synthesis and Biological Evaluation of Modified Miuraenamides. *Eur. J. Org. Chem.* **2018**, *2018*, 6952–6965. [CrossRef]
39. Rostovtsev, V.V.; Green, L.G.; Fokin, V.V.; Sharpless, K.B. A Stepwise Huisgen Cycloaddition Process: Copper(I)-Catalyzed Regioselective "Ligation" of Azides and Terminal Alkynes. *Angew. Chem. Int. Ed.* **2002**, *41*, 2596–2599. [CrossRef]
40. Haldón, E.; Nicasio, M.C.; Pérez, P.J. Copper-Catalysed Azide–Alkyne Cycloadditions (CuAAC): An Update. *Org. Biomol. Chem.* **2015**, *13*, 9528–9550. [CrossRef] [PubMed]

41. Chinchilla, R.; Nájera, C. The Sonogashira Reaction: A Booming Methodology in Synthetic Organic Chemistry. *Chem. Rev.* **2007**, *107*, 874–922. [CrossRef]
42. Posner, T. Beiträge Zur Kenntniss Der Ungesättigten Verbindungen. II. Ueber Die Addition von Mercaptanen an Ungesättigte Kohlenwasserstoffe. *Berichte Dtsch. Chem. Ges.* **1905**, *38*, 646–657. [CrossRef]
43. Gorges, J.; Kazmaier, U. BEt 3-Initiated Thiol–Ene Click Reactions as a Versatile Tool To Modify Sensitive Substrates. *Eur. J. Org. Chem.* **2015**, *2015*, 8011–8017. [CrossRef]

Disclaimer/Publisher's Note: The statements, opinions and data contained in all publications are solely those of the individual author(s) and contributor(s) and not of MDPI and/or the editor(s). MDPI and/or the editor(s) disclaim responsibility for any injury to people or property resulting from any ideas, methods, instructions or products referred to in the content.

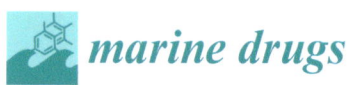

Article

Evaluation of the Biological Activities of Peptides from Epidermal Mucus of Marine Fish Species from Chilean Aquaculture

Claudio A. Álvarez [1,2,†], Teresa Toro-Araneda [2,†], Juan Pablo Cumillaf [3], Belinda Vega [2], María José Tapia [2], Tanya Roman [4], Constanza Cárdenas [4], Valentina Córdova-Alarcón [2,5], Carlos Jara-Gutiérrez [6,7], Paula A. Santana [8,*] and Fanny Guzmán [4,*]

1. Laboratorio de Cultivo de Peces Marinos, Facultad de Ciencias del Mar, Universidad Católica del Norte, Coquimbo 1781421, Chile; claudio.alvarez@ucn.cl
2. Laboratorio de Fisiología y Genética Marina (FIGEMA), Centro de Estudios Avanzados en Zonas Áridas (CEAZA), Coquimbo 1781421, Chile; teresa.toro@alumnos.ucn.cl (T.T.-A.); belinda.vega@ceaza.cl (B.V.); maria.tapia01@alumnos.ucn.cl (M.J.T.); valentina.cordova@ug.uchile.cl (V.C.-A.)
3. CRC Innovación, Puerto Montt 5507642, Chile; jpnenen@gmail.com
4. Núcleo Biotecnología Curauma, Pontificia Universidad Católica de Valparaíso, Valparaíso 2373223, Chile; tanya.roman.b@mail.pucv.cl (T.R.); constanza.cardenas@pucv.cl (C.C.)
5. Genomics on the Wave SpA, Viña del Mar 2520056, Chile
6. Centro Interdisciplinario de Investigación Biomédica e Ingeniería para la Salud—MEDING, Universidad de Valparaíso, Valparaíso 2362905, Chile; carlos.jara@uv.cl
7. Facultad de Medicina, Escuela de Kinesiología, Universidad de Valparaíso, Valparaíso 2362905, Chile
8. Instituto de Ciencias Aplicadas, Facultad de Ingeniería, Universidad Autónoma de Chile, Santiago 8910060, Chile
* Correspondence: paula.santana@uautonoma.cl (P.A.S.); fanny.guzman@pucv.cl (F.G.)
† The authors contributed equally to this work.

Abstract: The skin of fish is a physicochemical barrier that is characterized by being formed by cells that secrete molecules responsible for the first defense against pathogenic organisms. In this study, the biological activity of peptides from mucus of *Seriola lalandi* and *Seriolella violacea* were identified and characterized. To this purpose, peptide extraction was carried out from epidermal mucus samples of juveniles of both species, using chromatographic strategies for purification. Then, the peptide extracts were characterized to obtain the amino acid sequence by mass spectrometry. Using bioinformatics tools for predicting antimicrobial and antioxidant activity, 12 peptides were selected that were chemically produced by simultaneous synthesis using the Fmoc-Tbu strategy. The results revealed that the synthetic peptides presented a random coil or extended secondary structure. The analysis of antimicrobial activity allowed it to be discriminated that four peptides, named by their synthesis code 5065, 5069, 5070, and 5076, had the ability to inhibit the growth of *Vibrio anguillarum* and affected the copepodite stage of *C. rogercresseyi*. On the other hand, peptides 5066, 5067, 5070, and 5077 had the highest antioxidant capacity. Finally, peptides 5067, 5069, 5070, and 5076 were the most effective for inducing respiratory burst in fish leukocytes. The analysis of association between composition and biological function revealed that the antimicrobial activity depended on the presence of basic and aromatic amino acids, while the presence of cysteine residues increased the antioxidant activity of the peptides. Additionally, it was observed that those peptides that presented the highest antimicrobial capacity were those that also stimulated respiratory burst in leukocytes. This is the first work that demonstrates the presence of functional peptides in the epidermal mucus of Chilean marine fish, which provide different biological properties when the fish face opportunistic pathogens.

Keywords: mucus; peptide; *Seriola lalandi*; *Seriolella violacea*; antimicrobial; antioxidant; respiratory burst

Citation: Álvarez, C.A.; Toro-Araneda, T.; Cumillaf, J.P.; Vega, B.; Tapia, M.J.; Roman, T.; Cárdenas, C.; Córdova-Alarcón, V.; Jara-Gutiérrez, C.; Santana, P.A.; et al. Evaluation of the Biological Activities of Peptides from Epidermal Mucus of Marine Fish Species from Chilean Aquaculture. *Mar. Drugs* **2024**, *22*, 248. https://doi.org/10.3390/md22060248

Academic Editors: Bin Wang and Chang-Feng Chi

Received: 7 May 2024
Revised: 23 May 2024
Accepted: 25 May 2024
Published: 28 May 2024

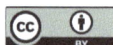

Copyright: © 2024 by the authors. Licensee MDPI, Basel, Switzerland. This article is an open access article distributed under the terms and conditions of the Creative Commons Attribution (CC BY) license (https://creativecommons.org/licenses/by/4.0/).

1. Introduction

In Chile, spearheading initiatives, such as the Chilean Aquaculture Diversification Programs (PDACH), have actively fostered the commercial farming of native species such as *Seriola lalandi* (yellowtail kingfish) and *Seriolella violacea* (palm ruff) because of their fast growth, adaptability to various growing conditions, and good commercial value [1–4]. Indeed, it becomes imperative to proactively address health concerns as these species undergo intensive cultivation and aquaculture practices intensify the inherent risks associated with disease proliferation.

While wild fish commonly bear a burden of parasites, the controlled environment of aquaculture tends to exacerbate this exponentially. This heightened parasite presence adversely affects the immune system, predisposing the fish to secondary infections caused by bacteria, viruses, and fungi [5]. Specifically focusing on *S. lalandi*, parasites such as *Caligus lalandei* and *Zeuxapta seriousolae* have been identified, residing in the gills and skin, respectively [6]. Moreover, the intensification of aquaculture practices creates a conducive environment for the proliferation of bacteria belonging to the genus Vibrio. These microorganisms, known for their ability to independently grow and reproduce in water, pose a significant threat to the health of cultivated species [7,8]. Indeed, in the cultivation of yellowtail kingfish in China, the emergence of shoots affected by vibriosis-related diseases has been documented [6].

The fish tegument, comprising layers like the cuticle, epidermis, basal membrane, dermis, and hypodermis, acts as a defensive barrier [9,10]. The cuticle, derived from secretions of epithelial and calciform cells, contains mucopolysaccharides, specific immunoglobulins, and fatty acids [11]. The epidermis, a non-keratinized stratified flat epithelium, is primarily cellular in structure [10]. Playing a crucial role in superficial wound repair, the skin and mucus collaborate in the healing process. Immediately following an injury, mucus laden with numerous lymphocytes covers the wound [9]. Subsequently, marginal wound cells proliferate, forming a protective layer that gradually completes the healing process [9]. Mucus secretions, encompassing proteins like mucin glycoproteins, agglutinins, reactive C protein, immunoglobulins (IgM), and enzymes, such as peroxidase, serve as physical protectors and immunological effectors [12]. Additionally, the mucus contains energetic molecules providing information on glucose metabolism and the internal metabolic state of the animals. It also contains molecules related to protein metabolism and defense against infections, including antimicrobial peptides [13]. Studies on marine species like juvenile gilthead sea bream, European sea bass, and meagre have demonstrated the antimicrobial activity of mucus [13]. However, a more in-depth knowledge of the specific molecules within epidermal mucus is essential to identify their role as a defense mechanism against pathogens and to assess the overall health of the fish. Peptides constitute a significant category of bioactive molecules [14].

Among the extensively studied peptides in diverse animal species are antimicrobial peptides (AMPs), also recognized as host defense peptides (HDPs) [15,16]. Characterized by their small size (less than 10 kDa), AMPs can either be encoded in the genome or generated through the proteolysis of larger polypeptides [17]. They are highly conserved and are produced across a spectrum of organisms, ranging from higher vertebrates to plants [16], with their expression identified in tissues of organs such as the kidney, skin, gills, and intestine. The amino acid sequence of each peptide imparts distinct biological properties, and some peptides exhibit multifunctionality [18]. HDPs may possess antioxidant, antihypertensive, immunomodulatory, antimicrobial, antifungal, and anticoagulant properties [18]. In teleost fish, 19 peptide families with antimicrobial, immunomodulatory, and/or antioxidant activities have been identified. These peptides demonstrate diverse secondary structures, contributing to their multifunctionality and versatility in biological activities [16].

This work focuses on the identification and characterization of peptides derived from the epidermal mucous secretions of aquaculture species, specifically *S. Lalandi* and *S. violacea*. After successful identification, these peptides were chemically synthesized and their antimicrobial and antioxidant properties and the ability to regulate respiratory burst in fish leukocytes were systematically assessed. The main objective of this comprehensive approach is to deepen the understanding of protective capacities inherent in these peptides sourced from fish mucus, with a vision towards their potential utilization as novel marine drugs, leveraging their multifunctional properties.

2. Results

2.1. Identification and Characterization of Peptides in Epidermal Mucus of S. lalandi and S. violacea

The peptidomic analysis identified a total of 237 peptides in the mucus of S. violacea and 52 peptides for S. lalandi. The obtained peptide sequences were input into online databases equipped with algorithms that evaluate net charge, amphipathicity, presence of basic amino acids like lysine and arginine, and the presence of amino acids such as tryptophan and cysteine. Following this theoretical comprehensive analysis, 12 peptides were selected to investigate in vitro activity, as detailed in Table 1.

Table 1. Characterization of chemically synthesized peptides identified from fish epidermal mucus.

Peptide ID	Residue	Fish Specie	MW * (Da)	Sequence	RT * (min)
5065	8	Seriolella violacea	977.29	FGVKWVKN	5.5
5066	9	Seriolella violacea	905.11	CTAGETAPR	4.0
5067	9	Seriolella violacea	1038.31	CTKGETFPR	5.0
5068	10	Seriola lalandi	1087.35	SRSALSLRTP	5.5
5069	10	Seriola lalandi	1186.49	SRSALWLRTP	5.8
5070	10	Seriola lalandi	1092.46	LGKFKGRSPC	5.8
5076	9	Seriola lalandi	974.28	LGLFKGRSP	5.5
5077	9	Seriola lalandi	1064.38	AERLTPCFK	5.6
5078	8	Seriola lalandi	904.12	AERLTPAF	5.8
5079	9	Seriolella violacea	1042.32	KWTGNLAPR	5.4
5080	9	Seriolella violacea	943.18	KSTGNLAPR	4.3
5081	8	Seriolella violacea	890.21	FGVKVVKN	5.0

* MW: molecular weight; RT: retention time.

The selected peptides underwent chemical synthesis to validate their biological activity. Each peptide was assigned a synthesis code, as outlined in Table 1. To ensure correct synthesis and purity, mass chromatograms and reverse-phase HPLC spectra were recorded (Supplementary Figures S1 and S2). During the analysis, the retention time (RT) was compared, revealing that peptides with numbers 5069, 5070, and 5078 exhibited the highest hydrophobicity with an RT of 5.8 min. Conversely, peptides 5066 and 5080, with retention times of 4.0 and 4.3 min, respectively, were identified as the most hydrophilic (Table 1).

In silico modeling indicated that none of the peptides exhibited a defined secondary structure, implying the absence of α-helix or β-sheets (Figure 1 and Supplementary Figure S3). This finding was corroborated by CD analysis for four of the peptides (Figure 1), which showed characteristic spectra with a minimum between 190 and 200 nm, indicative of peptides with a random coil structure.

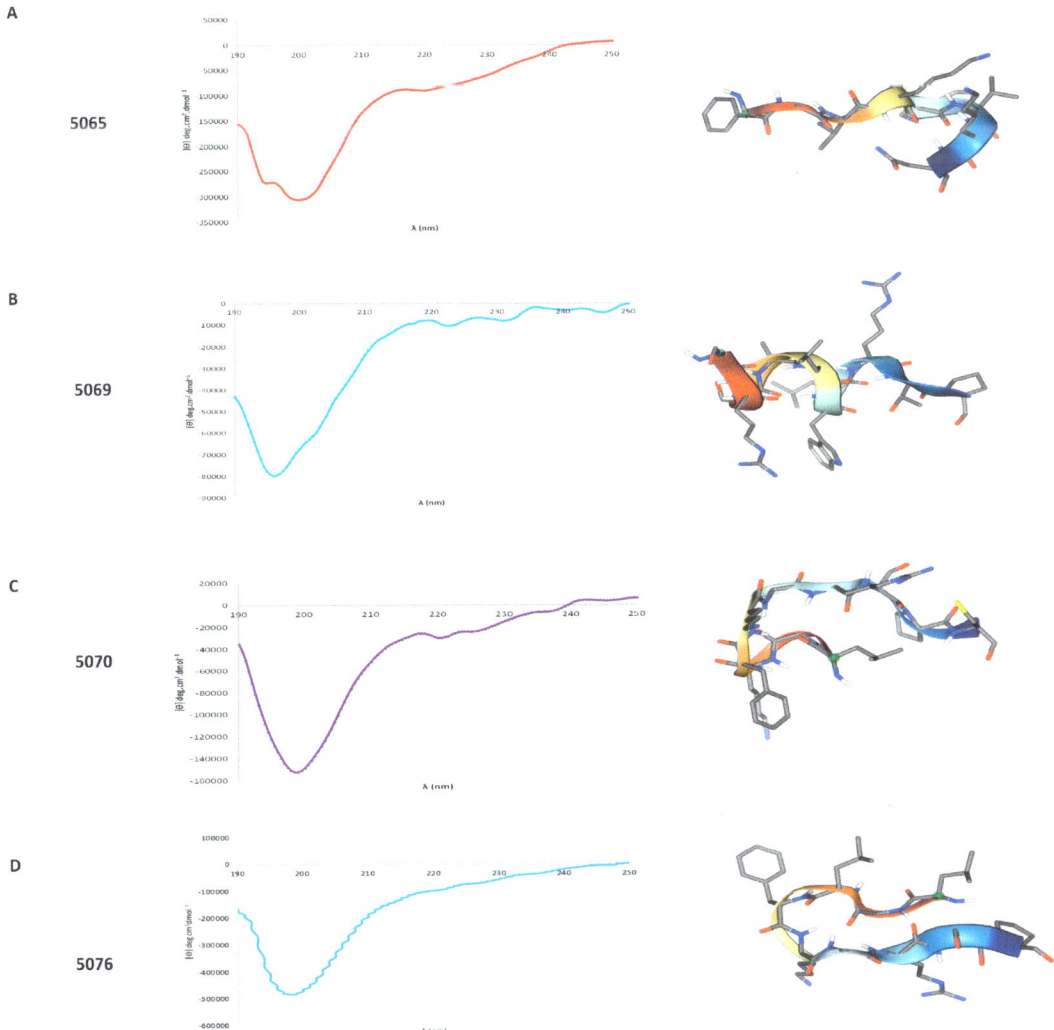

Figure 1. Characterization of secondary structure of peptides. Spectra of circular dichroism for peptides (**A**) 5065; (**B**) 5069; (**C**) 5070; and (**D**) 5076 in 30% v/v trifluoroethanol in water (left). On the right, 3D-structure model of peptides.

2.2. Antimicrobial Activity of Peptides Identified in the Mucus of S. lalandi and S. violacea

To conduct an initial screening of the antibacterial activity of the 12 synthesized peptides, their capacity to inhibit the growth of *Escherichia coli* at a concentration of 100 µM was assessed. The results indicated that peptides 5069, 5076, 5065, and 5070 were the greatest inhibitors of *E. coli* growth (Figure 2). Conversely, the remaining peptides exhibited similar or higher bacterial growth compared to the untreated control.

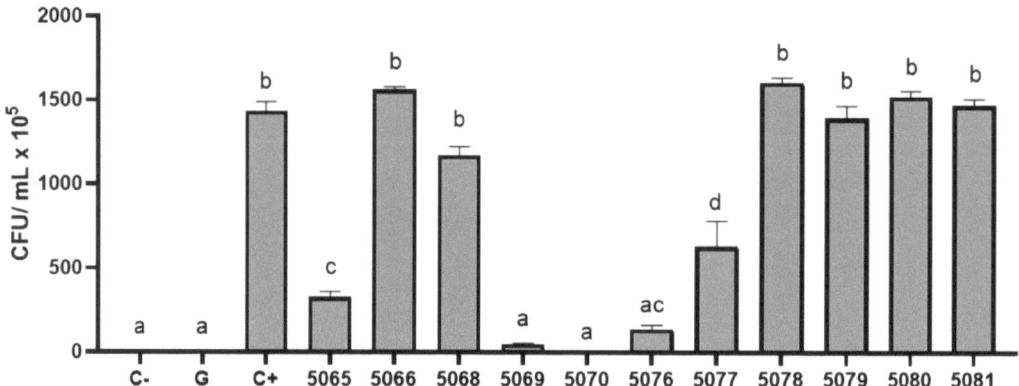

Figure 2. Antibacterial activity of synthetic peptides identified in the mucus of *S. lalandi* and *S. violacea* against *Escherichia coli*. The growth of *E. coli* is expressed in colony-forming units (CFU/mL) after application of 100 μM of synthetic peptides. As a negative control (C−) culture media without bacterial inoculum was used. Positive control (C+) was growth of *E. coli* without treatment. Treatment with gentamicin was used as positive antibacterial activity (G). Significant differences with respect to C+ are indicated with a different letter ($p > 0.05$).

For the four peptides that showed activity, MIC was determined for three bacterial strains (Table 2). Peptide 5065 exhibited an MIC of 6.25 μM against *V. ordalii*, 12.5 μM against *V. anguillarum*, and 25 μM against *E. coli*. Peptide 5069 had the same MIC of 12.5 μM for the two Vibrio strains and 25 μM against *E. coli*. Finally, peptides 5070 and 5076 shared the same MIC of 25 μM against all bacteria, with the exception that peptide 5076 exhibited no activity against *V. anguillarum* at the maximum peptide concentration tested here (100 μM).

Table 2. Minimum inhibitory concentration (MIC) of selected peptides against bacterial strains.

Peptide	MIC (μM)		
	Vibrio anguillarum	Vibrio ordalii	Escherichia coli
5065	12.5	6.25	25
5069	12.5	12.5	25
5070	25	25	25
5076	>100	25	25

For the peptides exhibiting antibacterial activity, their antiparasitic efficacy against the ectoparasite *C. rogercresseyi* was investigated. The activity was assessed after 48 h (Figure 3A) and 96 h (Figure 3B) of exposing *C. rogercresseyi* copepods to the synthetic peptides at concentrations of 50 μM and 150 μM. The results showed that, after 48 h, peptides 5069 and 5079 successfully reduced the survival percentage of *C. rogercresseyi* copepods but only at a concentration of 150 μM. Meanwhile, at 96 h post-exposure, peptides 5069, 5070, and 5079 exhibited antiparasitic activity at both concentrations evaluated. Notably, peptides 5069 and 5079 achieved almost 100% effectiveness at 50 μM. It was also observed that peptide 5065 only exhibited activity at 150 μM (Figure 3).

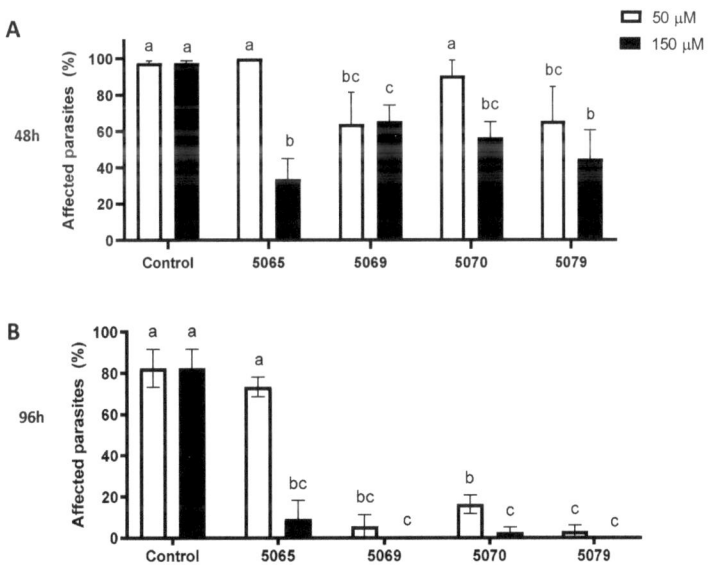

Figure 3. Antiparasitic activity of synthetic peptides against copepodite stage of *C. rogercresseyi*. Affected parasites was expressed as a percentage. The effect of the peptides at 50 and 150 µM on the copepodite stage was evaluated at (**A**) 48 h and (**B**) 96 h. Seawater-only conditions were employed as the control for copepodite survival. Statistically significant differences from the control are indicated by distinct letters ($p > 0.05$).

2.3. Antioxidant Activity of Peptides Identified in the Mucus of S. lalandi and S. violacea

Often, the term "antimicrobial" falls short in describing the diverse range of properties exhibited by peptides derived from natural sources, as novel functionalities continue to be unveiled. Hence, in our research, we extend our investigation to encompass the assessment of the antioxidant capabilities of these molecules as well. The antioxidant activity of the synthetic peptides was assessed using the DPPH and TRAP methods, with a comparison to the antioxidant capacity of a control peptide 4340 of marine origin [19] at the same concentration. The results from both assays are summarized in Table 3.

Table 3. Evaluation of antioxidant activity in synthetic peptides by DPPH and TRAP methods.

Peptide ID	DPPH (%RSC)				TRAP (TEAC µM)		
5065	6.883	±	1.204		7.078	±	0.914
5066	13.693	±	0.848	*	15.845	±	0.043
5067	31.031	±	1.233	***	53.164	±	3.251 **
5068	3.480	±	0.315		N.D.		
5069	4.564	±	0.695		6.428	±	0.998
5070	11.202	±	0.388	*	53.249	±	4.597 **
5076	2.048	±	0.102		0.813	±	0.358
5077	16.509	±	0.723	**	91.621	±	7.722 ***
5078	3.416	±	0.367		3.376	±	0.156
5079	3.526	±	1.060		5.544	±	0.355
5080	2.454	±	0.704		2.137	±	0.094
5081	5.084	±	1.051		2.287	±	0.536
4340	5.479	±	0.630		10.020	±	0.010

%RSC = radical scavenging capacity percentage values; TEAC = equivalent antioxidant capacity of TROLOX; N.D. = not determined. 4340 = reference antioxidant peptide (GPEPTGPTGAPQWLR). * $p < 0.05$; ** $p < 0.01$; *** $p < 0.001$.

For the DPPH method, peptides 5065 and 5081 exhibited similar activity to the control peptide. Conversely, peptides 5066, 5067, 5070, and 5077 demonstrated the highest antioxidant activity ($p > 0.001$). Among these four peptides, 5067 was the most effective, showing five times higher antioxidant activity than the control peptide, with a percentage radical scavenging value (%RSC) of 31.03%, compared to 5.48% for 4340 ($p > 0.001$). The remaining peptides did not display significant activity.

In the TRAP method, once again, peptides 5066, 5067, 5070, and 5077 showcased the highest antioxidant activity, with 5067 and 5077 exhibiting 10 times higher antioxidant activity than the control peptide 4340 ($p > 0.001$). The other peptides evaluated demonstrated very low activity, and even the activity of peptide 5068 was below the detection limit of the test.

2.4. The Respiratory Burst Stimulation Capacity of Leukocytes by Peptides from S. lalandi and S. violacea

The peptides demonstrating the highest antimicrobial and antioxidant activity were chosen to investigate their potential modulation of respiratory burst in fish leukocytes. Primary cultures of the anterior kidney were employed for this purpose.

The results are presented in terms of the stimulation index, representing the fold change compared to the unstimulated control. Peptide treatments were compared against the positive control (PMA-stimulated cells). The results indicate that peptides 5067 at a concentration of 100 µM, 5070 at 50 µM, and 5076 at 50 µM exhibited a respiratory burst stimulation similar to the positive control ($p > 0.05$). Additionally, peptides 5069 at 50 µM and 5076 at 100 and 200 µM demonstrated the most substantial stimulation of respiratory burst ($p > 0.05$) (Figure 4).

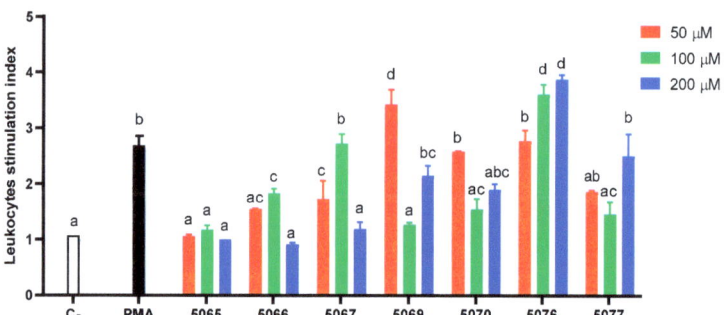

Figure 4. Effect of synthetic peptides on the activation of the respiratory burst process of anterior kidney leukocytes. Respiratory burst stimulation index of leukocytes treated with phosphate buffered saline (C−), Phorbol 12-myristate 13-acetate (PMA), and synthetic peptides (5065–5077) at three different concentrations (50, 100, and 200 µM) at 22 °C. Significant differences are indicated in different letters ($p > 0.05$).

3. Discussion

AMPs play a crucial role as innate immune system mediators in fish, particularly in protecting the mucosa of teleost [16]. This research conducted on the epidermal mucus of the marine fish species *Seriola lalandi* and *Seriolella violacea* identified and synthesized 12 peptides that were subsequently subjected to functional properties assessment.

Because fish mucus may contain compounds originating from the coexisting microbial community, directly attributing the identified sequences to the hosts is challenging. Regarding the observed homology in the blast search, it is crucial to consider that the sequences are relatively short, making matches easily identifiable. Very few peptides exhibit 100% identity in blast searches. Furthermore, when the blast excludes bacterial taxa, similar levels of homology are observed with other organisms such as plants, insects, fungi, parasites, and crustaceans. Similarly, restricting the search to teleost taxa (teleost fishes (taxid: 32443)) yields comparable results, with identity percentages falling within the same range as the previous searches. To conclusively determine whether the peptides correspond to the specific species we studied, data from the genomes, transcriptomes, or proteomes of these species are necessary.

Table 4 summarizes the proposed biological activities based on bioinformatics tools and the experimental outcomes for the 12 peptides identified in the epidermal mucus of *S. lalandi* and *S. violacea*. Among them, peptide 5070 was the one having the most robust functional properties, encompassing antibacterial, antiparasitic, antioxidant, and respiratory burst increasing. It was followed by peptides 5069 (antibacterial, antiparasitic, and respiratory burst increasing) and 5065 (antibacterial, antiparasitic, and antioxidant), while other peptides did not exhibit the analyzed activities.

Table 4. Summary and comparative analysis of simulated and experimentally determined biological activities for synthesized peptides.

Peptide ID	Fish Specie	Sequence	Theoretical Activity	Proven Biological Activity
5065	*Seriolella violacea*	FGVKWVKN	AM	AB/AOX/AP
5066	*Seriolella violacea*	CTAGETAPR	AM/AOX	AOX
5067	*Seriolella violacea*	CTKGETFPR	AM/AOX	AOX/IM
5068	*Seriola lalandi*	SRSALSLRTP	AM	N.D.
5069	*Seriola lalandi*	SRSALWLRTP	AM	AB/AP/IM
5070	*Seriola lalandi*	LGKFKGRSPC	AM	AB/AOX/AP/IM
5076	*Seriola lalandi*	LGLFKGRSP	AM	AB/IM
5077	*Seriola lalandi*	AERLTPCFK	AM	AOX
5078	*Seriola lalandi*	AERLTPAF	AM/AOX	N.D.
5079	*Seriolella violacea*	KWTGNLAPR	AM/AOX	AP
5080	*Seriolella violacea*	KSTGNLAPR	AM/AOX	N.D.
5081	*Seriolella violacea*	FGVKVVKN	AM/AOX	AOX

AM: antimicrobial activity; AOX: antioxidant activity; B: antibacterial activity; AP: antiparasitic activity; IM: immunomodulatory activity; N.D. = not determined.

The examination of results from antimicrobial, antioxidant, and respiratory burst tests in leukocytes provides insights into amino acid composition patterns associated with the functional roles these molecules play in the mucus secretions of teleost fish. This analysis aids in understanding the specific contributions of these peptides to the innate immune system and overall health status of the fish species under study.

The observed correlation between antibacterial activity and the abundance of lysine (K), arginine (R), or glycine (G) residues in the peptide sequences aligns with previous research findings. In fact, studies on peptides, particularly those belonging to the cathelicidin family, have highlighted that an increased presence of these amino acids enhances antimicrobial efficacy. For instance, the CATH-BRALE peptide from the fish Brachymystax lenok, rich in R and G residues, was a potent inhibitor of the Gram-negative bacteria *Aeromonas salmonicida* and *Aeromonas hydrophila*, with a low MIC value of 9.38 µM [20]. Similarly, peptides such as As-CATH4 and As-CATH5 from the cathelicidin family have shown enhanced survival against antibiotic-resistant pathogens in the Chinese crab *Eriocheir sinensis* [21].

The presence of basic amino acids in the sequences of AMPs is closely linked to antibacterial mechanisms, primarily involving electrostatic interactions between these cationic residues and the anionic surface of the bacterial membranes [22]. This relationship has been established for fish AMPs, exemplified by peptides like omIL-8α and ssIL-8α. These peptides, rich in basic amino acids, were studied by Santana et al. [23], demonstrating that their antibacterial action involves accumulation on bacterial surfaces followed by membrane permeabilization. While further investigation is required to unravel the exact mechanisms employed by the newly identified AMPs from the mucus of *S. lalandi* and *S. violacea*, the presence of basic amino acids in their composition suggests a potential involvement in membrane interactions as part of their antibacterial action. Therefore, the specific amino acid composition and secondary structure play a crucial role in determining the antimicrobial action of peptides.

The secondary structures, including alpha-helix or beta-sheet formations, are also important factors influencing how peptides interact with bacterial membranes or other targets, leading to their antimicrobial effects. Indeed, the presence of cysteine residues can contribute to antibacterial activity in certain peptides. Cysteine residues are unique among the amino acids because they contain a thiol group (-SH) that can form disulfide bonds with another cysteine residue. This capability to form disulfide bonds allows peptides to adopt specific structural conformations, such as stabilized beta-sheet structures [24]. For instance, a family of AMPs known as hepcidins, characterized by the presence of eight cysteine residues, includes peptides like HEP2p (GMKCKFCCNCCNLNGCGVCCRF) isolated from the flatfish turbot (*Scophthalmus maximus*). HEP2p has exhibited strong activity against Gram-negative bacteria such as *Edwardsiella tarda* (MIC = 1 μM) and *Vibrio anguillarum* (MIC = 2 μM). Administration of HEP2p in turbot increased its survival against *V. anguillarum* infections [25]. In the present study, none of the peptides exhibiting antibacterial activity against the tested strains, contain disulfide bridges. Additionally, the only peptide containing a single cysteine residue in its sequence (5070: LGKFKGRSPC) exhibits a random coil structure, as determined by both in silico analysis and circular dichroism spectroscopy. Therefore, the presence of certain amino acids, along with the arrangement of them in the peptide sequence, contribute to their antimicrobial properties [26,27]. Moreover, the presence of cysteine residues may promote dimerization, potentially enhancing its antimicrobial potency, as evidenced in previous investigations. Nevertheless, more studies are necessary to evaluate the influence of dimer formation on the antibacterial efficacy of the 5070 peptide.

In this investigation, we employed *Caligus rogerresseyi* as a model to assess activity against parasites due to the absence of established methods for the *S. lalandi* or *S. violacea* species. The ability of certain peptides to exhibit antiparasitic activity against *C. rogercresseyi* is an interesting finding. The presence of basic amino acids, such as lysine and arginine, can contribute to the antiparasitic action of peptides, similar to their role in antibacterial activities. However, the obtained results regarding the presence of aromatic amino acids, such as tryptophan in peptide 5079, highlight the diversity of factors that can influence the functional properties of these peptides. Aromatic amino acids, like tryptophan and phenylalanine, can contribute to the hydrophobicity and structural stability of peptides. This aspect gains relevance in the context of antiparasitic activity, exemplified by fish AMPs like piscidin, which contain tryptophan and histidine in its sequence [28,29]. Interestingly, the peptide 5079 lacks antibacterial activity but still exhibits antiparasitic activity, which suggests that it might have multiple modes of action or specific interactions with the parasite that are distinct from its antibacterial mechanisms. Understanding the mechanism of action of peptides against ectoparasites is crucial for developing targeted and effective treatments. Unraveling how these peptides interact with and affect ectoparasites could provide valuable insights into their potential as therapeutic agents. Future research efforts should involve detailed studies on the molecular and cellular interactions between these peptides and ectoparasites. Overall, this study provides valuable insights into the multifunctional roles of these peptides in the antimicrobial defense mechanisms of fish, encompassing antibacterial, antiparasitic, and potentially other pathogen-killing activities.

Beyond their antimicrobial activity, AMPs can also act as signaling and chemotactic molecules, serving as a link between immune and adaptive responses [30]. When phagocytes encounter a pathogen, membrane perturbation and phagocytosis can occur, triggering the respiratory burst and subsequent cellular activation. As described by Zughaier et al. [30], the formation of phagolysosomes and subsequent degranulation lead to the rapid release of these molecules into the phagocytic vacuole or the extracellular fluid. In such scenarios, AMPs can neutralize endotoxin-induced release of cellular cytokinins and nitric oxide. Therefore, inside phagocytes, AMPs enhance respiratory burst in leukocytes, promoting an increased release of reactive oxygen species (ROS). It is interesting to note that, in the present study, the peptides that stimulated respiratory burst, specifically peptides 5069, 5070, and 5079, were also the ones exhibiting potent antimicrobial activity. Similar findings have been reported for peptides derived from cathelicidins, such as HR-CATH identified in the tiger frog (*Hoplobatrachus rugulosus*). This peptide not only exhibited antibacterial activity against *Vibrio parahaemolyticus*, *Staphylococcus aureus*, and *Aeromonas hydrophila* but also induced increased chemotaxis and respiratory burst in RAW264.7 cells (a mouse leukemic monocyte/macrophage cell line) [31].

An additional example is the peptide NKHS27 derived from the seven-banded grouper (Hyporthodus septemfasciatus), which exhibited activity against both Gram-negative and Gram-positive bacteria. When applied in macrophage cultures, it not only demonstrated antimicrobial properties but also triggered respiratory burst in these cells. Moreover, NKHS27 positively influenced the expression of genes associated with the cellular immune response [32]. Similarly, the AMP LEAP-2A, identified in the liver of the cyprinid Hemibarbus labeo, demonstrated significant proinflammatory effects when combined with lipopolysaccharide (LPS) or phorbol 12-myristate 13-acetate (PMA). This combination induced a robust proinflammatory response in leukocytes, involving heightened activity of inducible nitric oxide synthase (iNOS), respiratory burst, and the proinflammatory cytokines IFN-γ, TNF-α, and IL-1β, as observed by Chen et al. [33]. This underscores that certain PAMs with antimicrobial activity can also modulate cellular responses in leukocytes, contributing to the elimination of pathogens, including the stimulation of respiratory burst, a mechanism observed in some peptides identified in the mucus of *S. lalandi* and *S. violacea* in the present study. This suggests a potential link between the ability to enhance the immune response (respiratory burst) and the peptides' effectiveness in combating microbial threats. The co-ordination of these two activities may contribute to a robust defense mechanism against pathogens. Further research should explore the specific mechanisms underlying this correlation and shed light on the multifaceted roles of these peptides in the immune response. Up to this point, AMPs that have been characterized as "immunomodulatory" have not revealed a straightforward correlation between their amino acid composition and the regulatory function of proinflammatory leukocyte responses. Consequently, this remains an area that requires further investigation to unravel the precise mechanisms by which these peptides stimulate and modulate immune cells, such as cytokines up-regulation.

Antioxidants play a crucial role in mitigating oxidative stress by neutralizing harmful free radicals within the fish body, including mucosal tissues. In the realm of immune enhancement, these antioxidant molecules function to safeguard immune cells from oxidative damage, thereby promoting their optimal functionality. Peptides, known for their diverse biological activities, particularly those rich in aromatic amino acid residues such as tyrosine (Y), histidine (H), tryptophan (W), and phenylalanine (F), have been implicated in contributing to antioxidant properties [34]. Amino acids featuring aromatic rings in their side chains act as hydrogen donors to electron-deficient radicals, enhancing the capacity to eliminate free radicals. For instance, histidine and tryptophan residues donate hydrogen atoms, effectively eliminating radicals and forming stabilized indole or phenoxy radicals, thereby establishing a conjugated electron system [35].

Peptides derived from marine fish, such as the peptides LHY and GAWA isolated from the Spanish sardine (*Sardinella aurita*), and those rich in phenylalanine and tryptophan obtained from whey protein hydrolysates have demonstrated antioxidant properties [34]. The present study aligns with this evidence, emphasizing the importance of aromatic amino acids for the antioxidant activity of peptides from the epidermal mucus of *S. lalandi* and *S. violacea*. Notably, the inclusion of cysteine in the sequences of antioxidant antimicrobial peptides further enhanced their efficacy. This is apparent in the case of peptides exhibiting high in vitro antioxidant capacity (5066, 5067, 5070, and 5077), as they not only contain aromatic amino acids but also feature a cysteine residue.

The antioxidant potential of cysteine residues in proteins and peptides stems from the sulfhydryl group in their side chain (–SH), possessing hydrogen-donating capacity against free radicals. Free radicals accept a hydrogen atom from the –SH group, transforming it into –S. This radical subsequently reacts with another -S or oxygen, converting into disulfide or alkylene sulfide (-SS-o SO_2), thereby concluding the free radical chain reaction [36]. Hence, cysteine is regarded as essential for antioxidant activity due to its remarkable capability to neutralize free radicals. For instance, research conducted with peptides isolated from horse mackerel (*Magalaspis cordyla*) identified the ACFL peptide sequence, which exhibited potent DPPH activity [36]. Other fish-derived peptides, such as TCSP from Pacific cod (*Gadus macrocehalus*), have demonstrated the ability to eliminate intracellular reactive oxygen species (ROS), protect DNA from oxidative damage, and significantly enhance cell viability under oxidative stress [37]. Additionally, two peptides identified in *Decapterus maruadsi*, a fish from the Carangidae family, displayed robust antioxidant activity, attributed to the presence of cysteines in their composition, functioning similarly to glutathione [38]. Therefore, the antioxidant peptides identified in the mucus of *S. lalandi* and *S. violacea* play a crucial role in managing free radicals within the mucus membranes of these fish.

4. Materials and Methods

4.1. Mucus Sampling from S. lalandi and S. violacea Juveniles

The mucus samples from juvenile *S. lalandi* and *S. violacea* were collected from 1-year-old individuals cultivated in the marine fish culture laboratory of the Universidad Católica del Norte. Initially, mucus was obtained from the fish cuticle by gently sliding and collecting it in a 50 mL tube, which was kept on ice throughout the process. The collected samples were then preserved at $-80\,^\circ$C until further use.

The mucus samples were thawed on ice and then homogenized using Mini-Beadbeater-24 Biospec equipment (Houston, TX, USA). The mucus was homogenized in a lysis buffer (50 mM TRIS-HCl 10 mM EDTA, pH 8.0) containing a commercial protease inhibitor (Sigma-Aldrich, Tokyo, Japan). Subsequently, the homogenized mixture was centrifuged at $3000\times g$ for 5 min at $4\,^\circ$C. The resulting supernatant was further centrifuged at $12,000\times g$ for 10 min at $4\,^\circ$C and stored at $-20\,^\circ$C until analysis.

For the isolation of peptide fractions, reverse-phase C-18 chromatographic columns (Themofisher, Tokyo, Japan) were utilized. The low-molecular-weight peptides (less than 10 kDa) were eluted with 10%, 20%, and 30% acetonitrile (ACN) in water [39]. Following elution, the samples were processed in SPEED-VAC equipment to remove organic solvents and subsequently lyophilized for further analysis.

4.2. Peptidomics Analysis

The peptide-enriched extracts from two mucus pools (100 µg lyophilized) for each fish species were subjected to analysis. The samples were suspended in 8 M urea in 50 mM NH_4HCO_3 and sonicated in an ultrasonic bath. Peptide quantification was carried out using the PierceTM Protein test. Subsequently, 10 µg of the peptide extracts underwent reduction (20 mM DTT in NH_4HCO_3 50 mM; 60 min, $32\,^\circ$C) and alkylation (55 mM iodoacetamide in NH_4HCO_3 50 mM; $25\,^\circ$C, 30 min, in the dark).

The resulting peptide mixtures were purified using a C18 tip (Polylcinc.) following the manufacturer's protocol. Finally, the peptide solution was dried and stored at $-20\,^\circ$C for subsequent LC-MS/MS analysis. The elution gradient for peptides involved a progression from 1% to 40% acetonitrile (ACN) over 60 min, followed by an increase from 40% to 60% ACN in water by 10 min, with a flow rate of 250 mL/min. The masses and sequences of the peptides were determined using an LTQ-Orbitrap Velos mass spectrometer (Thermo Scientific, Markham, ON, Canada).

4.3. Bioinformatics Analysis

The peptide sequences were submitted to online databases utilizing predictive algorithms to theoretically categorize the biological activities of the peptides identified from fish mucus. The antimicrobial activity was assessed at https://aps.unmc.edu/preddiction/predict (accessed on 15 June 2023), while potential antioxidant properties were evaluated using http://lin.uestc.edu.cn/server/antioxipred (accessed on 15 June 2023). Moreover, putative secondary structure models of selected peptides were examined using the PEP-FOLD3 web server (http://bioserv.rpbs.univ-paris-diderot.fr/services/PEP-FOLD3, accessed on 16 June 2023) as outlined by Lamiable et al. [40]. Following the selection of the optimal model, the 3D structure of each peptide was constructed using PyMOL.

4.4. Solid-Phase Chemical Synthesis of Selected Peptides

In this study, 12 peptides with potential antimicrobial and antioxidant activities (refer to Table 1) were synthesized using a solid-phase synthesis strategy, employing rink-amide resin with a substitution degree of 0.6 meq/g. Throughout the coupling stages, Fmoc amino acids were attached using HBTU (2-(1H-Benzotriazole-1-yl)-1,1,3,3-tetramethylaminium hexafluorophosphate) and TBTU (2-(1H-Benzotriazole-1-yl)-1,1,3,3-tetramethylaminium tetrafluoroborate) as activators.

Following synthesis, the peptides were cleaved from the resin using a trifluoroacetic acid/triisopropylhydrosilane (TIS)/water mixture in a 95:2.5:2.5 ratio. The resulting peptides were precipitated with diethyl ether, reconstituted in Milli-Q water, and subjected to lyophilization. Purification was achieved using a C18 column and an acetonitrile gradient from 0 to 60% in water.

The purity, exceeding 95%, and the molecular masses of the synthetic peptides were confirmed through reverse-phase high-performance liquid chromatography (RP-HPLC) and electrospray ionization mass spectrometry (ESI-MS), respectively.

The secondary structure analysis of the synthetic peptides was conducted via circular dichroism (CD) spectroscopy using a JASCO J-815 CD Spectrometer (Jasco Corp., Tokyo, Japan), following previously established procedures [4]. CD spectra of the peptides were acquired in both Milli-Q water and trifluoroethanol (TFE, 30% v/v in water) within the far ultraviolet (UV) range (190–250 nm). Quartz cuvettes with a path length of 0.1 cm and a bandwidth of 1 nm were utilized, with spectra recorded at a resolution of 0.1 nm. To obtain accurate measurements, the solvent contribution blank was subtracted from each sample spectrum. Molar ellipticity values were subsequently calculated for each peptide.

4.5. Antimicrobial Analysis

4.5.1. Antibacterial Activity

Three bacterial species, namely *Escherichia coli* ML35, *Vibrio anguillarum* 507, and *Vibrio ordalii* DSM 19621, were utilized in this study. *E. coli* was inoculated in Trypticase Soy Agar (TSA) and incubated for 24 h at 37 °C and then transferred to Trypticase Soy Broth (TSB) and incubated for an additional 2 h at 37 °C under agitation. Meanwhile, *V. anguillarum* and *V. ordalii* cells were cultured in TSA supplemented with 1.5% NaCl and incubated at 25 °C for 24 h. Subsequently, they were subcultured in TSB-1.5% NaCl and incubated with gentle agitation for an additional 16 h at 25 °C. Optical density (OD) of the cultures at 600 nm was measured and dilutions were made to achieve a concentration of 1×10^7 colony-forming units per milliliter (CFU/mL).

Firstly, *E. coli* ML35 was utilized as a Gram-negative model to assess the antibacterial activity, following the methodology outlined by Santana et al. [23]. Briefly, cultures containing 1×10^7 CFU/mL were exposed to synthetic peptides at a concentration of 100 µM and incubated for 1 h under previously described bacterial growth conditions. Subsequently, the treated cells were spread onto TSA plates and then incubated for 12 h at 37 °C (for *E. coli*) or 16 h at 37 °C. The resulting colonies were counted and bacterial survival was determined by calculating the CFU/mL. Additionally, untreated *E. coli* cultures and those treated with gentamicin at a concentration of 200 µM were used as controls. Independent experiments were repeated three times.

Following the antibacterial activity screening, peptides showing noticeable activity were selected to determine the minimum inhibitory concentration (MIC). Serial dilutions of these peptides were prepared, starting from a maximum concentration of 100 µM, and the same antibacterial activity test protocol was followed. The minimum inhibitory concentration

(MIC) was determined following the protocol reported by Flóres-Castillo et al. [41]. For the microdilution method, 100 µL two-fold dilutions of synthetic peptides from 100 µM to 3.12 µM were added to 96-well polystyrene plates; 100 µL of bacteria inoculum (1×10^7 CFU/well) was subsequently added and incubated in TSB (supplemented with 1.5% NaCl in the case of Vibrio strains) for 18h at the optimal growth temperature of bacteria strains. Finally, the MIC was determined by direct observation and by reading at 620 nm on a spectrophotometer. Strains were tested in duplicate with its respective controls: untreated bacteria (positive growth control), bacteria-free TSB medium (negative control), and gentamicin (200 µM).

4.5.2. Antiparasitic Activity

As there is currently no established method for determining activity against parasites of the studied species, the ectoparasite copepod *Caligus rogerresseyi* was employed as a model. The antiparasitic activity was assessed following the protocol outlined by Montory et al. [42] at the CRC-Innovation Company in the city of Puerto Montt, Chile. For the in vitro determination, sensitivity bioassays were conducted using copepods grouped into a 120 µm mesh with a reduced volume of seawater. The parasite stock was distributed in 96-well-bottomed plates. Peptide effects were assessed at concentrations of 50 µm and 150 µm in seawater, with 200 µL inoculated into each of the 96 wells. Bioassays and plate maintenance were conducted at 12 °C and the effects were evaluated in eight repetitions. The larvae were exposed for up to 144 h at different peptide concentrations. This methodology aimed to determine the percentage of affected and/or dead individuals at each peptide concentration, as exposed by Montory et al. [42].

4.6. Antioxidant Activity

To assess the antioxidant capacity of the synthetic peptides, two methods, namely 2,2-diphenyl-1-picrylhydrazyl (DPPH) for radical scavenging and total antioxidant capacity (TRAP), were employed.

4.6.1. DPPH Method

The DPPH method followed the methodology reported by Madrid et al. [43]. A 50 µM DPPH solution was prepared in absolute ethanol, and peptides were prepared at 1 mg/mL in Milli-Q water (kept on ice). Glass cells for spectrometry were used, and 2.9 mL of the preprepared DPPH solution was added to each cell and the absorbance at 517 nm was recorded (T0). After this initial measurement, 100 µL of each peptide was added to the cells, and the mixture was incubated for 15 min, repeating this process three times. A cell containing only ethanol was used as the control. After 15 min, the cells' absorbance at 517 nm was measured, and the results were used to calculate the percentage of radical scavenging capacity (SRC%):

$$SRS\% = [(T0 - \text{sample absorbance})/T0] \times 100.$$

4.6.2. TRAP Method

The total antioxidant capacity was determined using the TRAP method, following the procedure described by Leyton et al. [44]. A 10 mM 2,2'azobis (2-amidopropane) dihydrochloride (AAPH) solution was prepared and mixed with 150 µM 2,2'-azino-bis(3-ethylbenzothiazoline-6-sulfonic acid) (ABTS) solution in 100 mM phosphate buffer saline (pH 7.4). The mixture was incubated at 45 °C for 30 min to generate the ABTS radical. Then, 10 µL of peptides (1 mg/mL) were mixed with 990 µL of the ABTS radical solution, and absorbance was measured kinetically over 50 s at 734 nm. The percentage of inhibition of the radical (IR) was calculated using the equation: $IR = [(A_0 - A_{50})/A_0] \times 100$, where A_0 is the absorbance at 0 s and A_{50} is the absorbance at 50 s. The IR percentages were then extrapolated onto a Trolox® curve and the results were expressed in millimolar (mM) of antioxidant capacity equivalents of Trolox® (TEAC mM). These TEAC results were compared to the antioxidant activity of 4340 peptide from marine origin [19].

4.7. Extraction of Head Kidney Leukocytes and Respiratory Burst Analysis

Two fish of 2 kg of total body mass (*S. lalandi*) at the Fish Laboratory of the Universidad Católica del Norte were chosen for the extraction of blood via flow puncture, followed by the extraction of the head kidney. The tissue was kept cold in L-15 medium supplemented with 2% serum and antibiotics (1% commercial solution of 100 U/mL of penicillin, 100 mg/mL of streptomycin, and 5 µg/mL of gentamycin). The extraction of macrophages was performed using the method described by Stolen et al. [45], with some modifications.

The kidneys were manually crushed using sterile and filtered plastic micropistols through a 100 µm nylon membrane with L-15 medium supplemented with serum and antibiotics. After centrifuging at $450 \times g$ for 10 min at 4 °C, the supernatant was removed and the cells were suspended in the medium and subjected to a Ficoll gradient (Lymphoprep; 1:1). Subsequently, it was centrifuged at $600 \times g$ without acceleration for 30 min at 4 °C and the interface containing the macrophages was carefully transferred with a sterile Pasteur pipette to a new glass tube. The cells were then diluted in 1 mL of L-15 medium without supplement and centrifuged ($450 \times g$, 10 min, 4 °C) to wash out the residual Ficoll. After resting for 10 min, the sample was centrifuged at $685 \times g$ for 10 min at 4 °C. The supernatant was removed, and another washing step was performed and then centrifugated. The cells were resuspended again in 1 mL of L-15 medium. Subsequently, viable cells were identified by vital Trypan Blue staining (10 µL cells and 40 µL staining) in a Neubauer's chamber. Finally, the concentration was adjusted to 1×10^6 cells/mL and the cultures were prepared in 96-well-bottomed plates with 1×10^5 macrophages per well, using L-15 medium without serum but with antibiotics to promote cell adhesion to the polystyrene plates. After a 2-h incubation at 22 °C, the unattached cells were removed by two washings with culture medium. The macrophage cultures were then incubated overnight at 22 °C with L-15 medium supplemented with serum and antibiotics.

The production of intracellular superoxides by phagocytes was assessed through the reduction of tetrazolium nitroblue tetrazolium (NBT) reagent (Sigma), following the protocols outlined by Stolen et al. [45,46] and Boesen et al. [46]. Initially, macrophage cultures in the 96-well plate were washed with nonsupplemented L-15 medium and Hanks' balanced salt solution (HBSS) to eliminate any residual antibiotic. Subsequently, 100 µL of NBT dissolved to a concentration of 1 mg/mL in HBS was added to each well. In the initial assessment, 1 µg/µL of the peptide extract was used but doses were subsequently adjusted based on prior studies [19]. The cultures were then incubated at 22 °C for 45 min. As a positive control, wells were inoculated with 1 µg/mL of phorbol myristate acetate (PMA; Sigma). To assess the specificity of the reaction, 300 µL of superoxide dismutase (SOD; Sigma) was added to one of the wells treated with PMA. After the incubation period, the supernatant was removed and 70% methanol in water was added. Methanol was allowed to evaporate under an extraction hood overnight. The phagocyte form was solubilized by adding 120 µL of 2 M KOH and 140 µL of dimethyl sulfoxide (DMSO; Sigma). Absorbance at 620 nm was then measured using an EPOCH spectrophotometer. Finally, the results were expressed as a stimulation index, obtained by dividing the value of each treatment by the control without stimulation.

4.8. Statistical Analysis

Statistical analysis was performed in R v4.3.1 The normal distribution of all data was assessed by Shapiro–Wilks test. Statistical significance of differences in antibacterial activity was determined with a one-way ANOVA test. For antiparasitic and respiratory burst activities, two-way ANOVA tests were employed, considering significance at $p = 0.05$.

For antioxidant activity, a Chi-squared test was carried out. For the TRAP and DPPH methods, a Kruskal–Wallis test was used for multiple independent samples with a significance level of $p = 0.01$.

5. Conclusions

The present study successfully identified and demonstrated the biological activity of nine peptides within the mucus secretions of marine fish native to Chile. Specifically, five of them were found in the mucus of juveniles of *S. violacea*, while the remaining four were identified in the mucus of *S. lalandi*.

All the characterized peptides exhibited a disordered or random coil secondary structure, indicating that their biological activity was closely related to their amino acid composition. Notably, those peptides displaying strong antimicrobial activity showcased a higher abundance of basic amino acids, like lysine and arginine, coupled with hydrophobic residues, such as phenylalanine and tryptophan. This amphipathic nature likely contributes to their efficacy in combating pathogens. Moreover, these peptides demonstrated the additional capability of stimulating respiratory burst in fish leukocytes.

Furthermore, the obtained results highlight the significance of aromatic amino acids, along with cysteine, in significantly enhancing the antioxidant activity of the peptides present in mucosal secretions. This dual role of certain peptides in antimicrobial defense and antioxidant protection underscores their multifunctional nature.

While the present study has provided valuable insights, it is imperative to conduct further investigations to assess additional biological activities of these peptides, such as their potential antifungal and antiviral functions. This research is ongoing, being essential for expanding the understanding of the peptides' broader roles and their relevance in determining the health status of cultured fish.

Supplementary Materials: The following supporting information can be downloaded at: https://www.mdpi.com/article/10.3390/md22060248/s1, Figure S1: RP-HPLC chromatogram of synthetic peptides; Figure S2: ESI MS/MS spectrum of the [M]$^+$ molecular ion of synthetic peptides; Figure S3: 3D-structure model of peptides.

Author Contributions: Conceptualization, C.A.Á., C.C., P.A.S. and F.G.; Formal analysis, C.A.Á., C.C., C.J.-G., P.A.S. and F.G.; Investigation, C.A.Á., T.T.-A., J.P.C., B.V., M.J.T., V.C.-A. and T.R.; Methodology, C.A.Á., T.T.-A., J.P.C., B.V., M.J.T., T.R., V.C.-A. and C.J.-G.; Project administration, F.G., P.A.S. and C.A.Á.; Resources, C.A.Á., P.A.S. and F.G.; Validation, C.A.Á., J.P.C., C.C., C.J.-G., P.A.S. and F.G.; Writing—original draft, all authors; Writing—review and editing, C.A.Á., C.C., P.A.S. and F.G. All authors have read and agreed to the published version of the manuscript.

Funding: This work was supported by grants from ANID-Chile, FONDECYT 1210056 to F.G., FONDECYT 1230712 and FOVI230160 to C.A.A., and FOVI230188 to P.A.S.

Institutional Review Board Statement: This study was conducted in accordance with the Declaration of Helsinki and approved by the Ethics Committee of the Pontificia Universidad Católica de Valparaíso (Permit Number) (protocol code BIOEPUCV-B 626-2023 with the date of approval 23 May 2023).

Data Availability Statement: The original data presented in the study are included in the article/Supplementary Material; further inquiries can be directed to the corresponding author.

Conflicts of Interest: The authors declare no conflicts of interest.

References

1. Nerici, C.; Merino, G.; Silva, A. Effects of Two Temperatures on the Oxygen Consumption Rates of *Seriolella violacea* (Palm Fish) Juveniles under Rearing Conditions. *Aquac. Eng.* **2012**, *48*, 40–46. [CrossRef]
2. Alveal, K.; Silva, A.; Lohrmann, K.B.; Viana, M.T. Morphofunctional Characterization of the Digestive System in the Palm Ruff Larvae, *Seriolella violacea* under Culture Conditions. *Aquaculture* **2019**, *501*, 51–61. [CrossRef]
3. Allen, P.J.; Brokordt, K.; Oliva, M.; Alveal, K.; Flores, H.; Álvarez, C.A. Physiological Insights for Aquaculture Diversification: Swimming Capacity and Efficiency, and Metabolic Scope for Activity in Cojinoba *Seriolella violacea*. *Aquaculture* **2021**, *531*, 735968. [CrossRef]
4. Álvarez, C.A.; Alvarado, J.F.; Farías, M.; Cárcamo, C.B.; Flores, H.; Guzmán, F.; Martín, S.S.; Varas, J.; Messina, S.; Acosta, F.; et al. First Insights about Orexigenic Activity and Gastrointestinal Tissue Localization of Ghrelin from Corvina Drum (*Cilus gilberti*). *Aquaculture* **2023**, *571*, 739468. [CrossRef]
5. Miccoli, A.; Saraceni, P.R.; Scapigliati, G. Vaccines and Immune Protection of Principal Mediterranean Marine Fish Species. *Fish Shellfish Immunol.* **2019**, *94*, 800–809. [CrossRef] [PubMed]

6. Sicuro, B.; Luzzana, U. The State of Seriola Spp. Other Than Yellowtail (*S. quinqueradiata*) Farming in the World. *Rev. Fish. Sci. Aquac.* **2016**, *24*, 314–325. [CrossRef]
7. Ji, Q.; Wang, S.; Ma, J.; Liu, Q. A Review: Progress in the Development of Fish Vibrio Spp. Vaccines. *Immunol. Lett.* **2020**, *226*, 46–54. [CrossRef] [PubMed]
8. Miranda, C.D.; Rojas, R. Vibriosis in the Flouder *Paralichithys adspersus* (Steindachner, 1867) in Captivity. *Rev. Biol. Mar.* **1996**, *12*, 1536.
9. Rubio-Godoy, M. Inmunología de Los Peces Óseos: Revisión Teleost Fish Immunology: Review. *Rev. Mex. Cienc. Pecu.* **2010**, *1*, 47–57.
10. Concha, K.; Olivares, P.; Fonseca-Salamanca, F.; Sanchez, R.; Serrano, F.; Parodi, J. Mucogenic Additives for the Control of Caligus Rogercresseyi in Atlantic Salmon (*Salmo salar*). *Rev. Investig. Vet. Peru* **2017**, *28*, 477–489. [CrossRef]
11. Benhamed, S.; Guardiola, F.A.; Mars, M.; Esteban, M.Á. Pathogen Bacteria Adhesion to Skin Mucus of Fishes. *Vet. Microbiol.* **2014**, *171*, 1–12. [CrossRef] [PubMed]
12. Aranishi, F.; Nakane, M. Epidermal proteases of the Japanese eel. *Fish Physiol. Biochem.* **1997**, *16*, 471–478. [CrossRef]
13. Sanahuja, I.; Fernández-Alacid, L.; Ordóñez-Grande, B.; Sánchez-Nuño, S.; Ramos, A.; Araujo, R.M.; Ibarz, A. Comparison of Several Non-Specific Skin Mucus Immune Defences in Three Piscine Species of Aquaculture Interest. *Fish Shellfish Immunol.* **2019**, *89*, 428–436. [CrossRef] [PubMed]
14. Zhang, L.; Falla, T.J. Cosmeceuticals and Peptides. *Clin. Dermatol.* **2009**, *27*, 485–494. [CrossRef] [PubMed]
15. Shabir, U.; Ali, S.; Magray, A.R.; Ganai, B.A.; Firdous, P.; Hassan, T.; Nazir, R. Fish Antimicrobial Peptides (AMP's) as Essential and Promising Molecular Therapeutic Agents: A Review. *Microb. Pathog.* **2018**, *114*, 50–56. [CrossRef] [PubMed]
16. Valero, Y.; Saraiva-Fraga, M.; Costas, B.; Guardiola, F.A. Antimicrobial Peptides from Fish: Beyond the Fight against Pathogens. *Rev. Aquac.* **2020**, *12*, 224–253. [CrossRef]
17. Reddy, K.V.R.; Yedery, R.D.; Aranha, C. Antimicrobial Peptides: Premises and Promises. *Int. J. Antimicrob. Agents* **2004**, *24*, 536–547. [CrossRef] [PubMed]
18. Medina, M.; Prado-Barragán, B.; Martínez-Hernández, A.; Ruíz, H.A.A.; Rodríguez, R.M.; Contreras-Esquivel, A.; Aguilar, C.N. Péptidos Bio-Funcionales: Bioactividad, Producción y Aplicaciones. Bio-Functional Peptides: Bioactivity, Production and Applications. *Rev. Científica Univ. Autónoma Coahuila* **2019**, *11*, 1–7.
19. Zhou, X.; Wang, C.; Jiang, A. Antioxidant Peptides Isolated from Sea Cucumber *Stichopus japonicus*. *Eur. Food Res. Technol.* **2012**, *234*, 441–447. [CrossRef]
20. Li, Z.; Zhang, S.; Gao, J.; Guang, H.; Tian, Y.; Zhao, Z.; Wang, Y.; Yu, H. Structural and Functional Characterization of CATH_BRALE, the Defense Molecule in the Ancient Salmonoid, *Brachymystax lenok*. *Fish Shellfish Immunol.* **2013**, *34*, 1–7. [CrossRef]
21. Guo, Z.; Qiao, X.; Cheng, R.; Shi, N.; Wang, A.; Feng, T.; Chen, Y.; Zhang, F.; Yu, H.; Wang, Y. As-CATH4 and 5, Two Vertebrate-Derived Natural Host Defense Peptides, Enhance the Immuno-Resistance Efficiency against Bacterial Infections in Chinese Mitten Crab, *Eriocheir sinensis*. *Fish Shellfish Immunol.* **2017**, *71*, 202–209. [CrossRef] [PubMed]
22. Carvajal-Rondanelli, P.; Aróstica, M.; Marshall, S.H.; Albericio, F.; Álvarez, C.A.; Ojeda, C.; Aguilar, L.F.; Guzmán, F. Inhibitory Effect of Short Cationic Homopeptides against Gram-Negative Bacteria. *Amino Acids* **2016**, *48*, 1445–1456. [CrossRef] [PubMed]
23. Santana, P.A.; Salinas, N.; Álvarez, C.A.; Mercado, L.A.; Guzmán, F. Alpha-Helical Domain from IL-8 of Salmonids: Mechanism of Action and Identification of a Novel Antimicrobial Function. *Biochem. Biophys. Res. Commun.* **2018**, *498*, 803–809. [CrossRef] [PubMed]
24. Álvarez, C.A.; Guzmán, F.; Cárdenas, C.; Marshall, S.H.; Mercado, L. Antimicrobial Activity of Trout Hepcidin. *Fish Shellfish Immunol.* **2014**, *41*, 93–101. [CrossRef] [PubMed]
25. Zhang, J.; Yu, L.p.; Li, M.f.; Sun, L. Turbot (*Scophthalmus maximus*) Hepcidin-1 and Hepcidin-2 Possess Antimicrobial Activity and Promote Resistance against Bacterial and Viral Infection. *Fish Shellfish Immunol.* **2014**, *38*, 127–134. [CrossRef] [PubMed]
26. Lorenzon, E.N.; Piccoli, J.P.; Santos-Filho, N.A.; Cilli, E.M. Dimerization of Antimicrobial Peptides: A Promising Strategy to Enhance Antimicrobial Peptide Activity. *Protein Pept. Lett.* **2019**, *26*, 98–107. [CrossRef] [PubMed]
27. Ohno, M.K.; Kirikae, T.; Yoshihara, E.; Kirikae, F.; Ishida, I. Addition of L-Cysteine to the N- or C-Terminus of the All-D-Enantiomer [D(KLAKLAK)2] Increases Antimicrobial Activities against Multidrug-Resistant *Pseudomonas aeruginosa*, *Acinetobacter baumannii* and *Escherichia coli*. *PeerJ* **2020**, *8*, e10176. [CrossRef] [PubMed]
28. Fernandes, J.M.O.; Ruangsri, J.; Kiron, V. Atlantic Cod Piscidin and Its Diversification through Positive Selection. *PLoS ONE* **2010**, *5*, e9501. [CrossRef] [PubMed]
29. Colorni, A.; Ullal, A.; Heinisch, G.; Noga, E.J. Activity of the Antimicrobial Polypeptide Piscidin 2 against Fish Ectoparasites. *J. Fish. Dis.* **2008**, *31*, 423–432. [CrossRef]
30. Zughaier, S.M.; Shafer, W.M.; Stephens, D.S. Antimicrobial Peptides and Endotoxin Inhibit Cytokine and Nitric Oxide Release but Amplify Respiratory Burst Response in Human and Murine Macrophages. *Cell Microbiol.* **2005**, *7*, 1251–1262. [CrossRef]
31. Chen, J.; Lin, Y.F.; Chen, J.H.; Chen, X.; Lin, Z.H. Molecular Characterization of Cathelicidin in Tiger Frog (*Hoplobatrachus rugulosus*): Antimicrobial Activity and Immunomodulatory Activity. *Comp. Biochem. Physiol. Part—C Toxicol. Pharmacol.* **2021**, *247*, 109072. [CrossRef] [PubMed]

32. Wang, C.b.; Yan, X.; Wang, G.h.; Liu, W.q.; Wang, Y.; Hao, D.f.; Liu, H.m.; Zhang, M. NKHs27, a Sevenband Grouper NK-Lysin Peptide That Possesses Immunoregulatory and Antimicrobial Activity. *Fish Shellfish Immunol.* **2023**, *136*, 108715. [CrossRef] [PubMed]
33. Chen, J.; Lv, Y.P.; Dai, Q.M.; Hu, Z.H.; Liu, Z.M.; Li, J.H. Host Defense Peptide LEAP-2 Contributes to Monocyte/Macrophage Polarization in Barbel Steed (*Hemibarbus labeo*). *Fish Shellfish Immunol.* **2019**, *87*, 184–192. [CrossRef]
34. Jiang, B.; Zhang, X.; Yuan, Y.; Qu, Y.; Feng, Z. Separation of Antioxidant Peptides from Pepsin Hydrolysate of Whey Protein Isolate by ATPS of EOPO Co-Polymer (UCON)/Phosphate. *Sci. Rep.* **2017**, *7*, 13320. [CrossRef] [PubMed]
35. Kalyanaraman, B. Teaching the Basics of Redox Biology to Medical and Graduate Students: Oxidants, Antioxidants and Disease Mechanisms. *Redox Biol.* **2013**, *1*, 244–257. [CrossRef] [PubMed]
36. Sampath Kumar, N.S.; Nazeer, R.A.; Jaiganesh, R. Purification and Identification of Antioxidant Peptides from the Skin Protein Hydrolysate of Two Marine Fishes, Horse Mackerel (*Magalaspis cordyla*) and Croaker (*Otolithes ruber*). *Amino Acids* **2012**, *42*, 1641–1649. [CrossRef] [PubMed]
37. Ngo, D.H.; Ryu, B.M.; Vo, T.S.; Himaya, S.W.A.; Wijesekara, I.; Kim, S.K. Free Radical Scavenging and Angiotensin-I Converting Enzyme Inhibitory Peptides from Pacific Cod (*Gadus macrocephalus*) Skin Gelatin. *Int. J. Biol. Macromol.* **2011**, *49*, 1110–1116. [CrossRef]
38. Jiang, H.; Tong, T.; Sun, J.; Xu, Y.; Zhao, Z.; Liao, D. Purification and Characterization of Antioxidative Peptides from Round Scad (*Decapterus maruadsi*) Muscle Protein Hydrolysate. *Food Chem.* **2014**, *154*, 158–163. [CrossRef] [PubMed]
39. Guzmán, F.; Gauna, A.; Roman, T.; Luna, O.; Álvarez, C.; Pareja-Barrueto, C.; Mercado, L.; Albericio, F.; Cárdenas, C. Tea Bags for Fmoc Solid-Phase Peptide Synthesis: An Example of Circular Economy. *Molecules* **2021**, *26*, 5035. [CrossRef]
40. Lamiable, A.; Thévenet, P.; Rey, J.; Vavrusa, M.; Derreumaux, P.; Tufféry, P. PEP-FOLD3: Faster de Novo Structure Prediction for Linear Peptides in Solution and in Complex. *Nucleic Acids Res.* **2016**, *44*, W449–W454. [CrossRef]
41. Flórez-Castillo, J.M.; Rondón-Villareal, P.; Ropero-Vega, J.L.; Mendoza-Espinel, S.Y.; Moreno-Amézquita, J.A.; Méndez-Jaimes, K.D.; Farfán-García, A.E.; Gómez-Rangel, S.Y.; Gómez-Duarte, O.G. Ib-M6 Antimicrobial Peptide: Antibacterial Activity against Clinical Isolates of Escherichia Coli and Molecular Docking. *Antibiotics* **2020**, *9*, 79. [CrossRef]
42. Montory, J.A.; Chaparro, O.R.; Averbuj, A.; Salas-Yanquin, L.P.; Büchner-Miranda, J.A.; Gebauer, P.; Cumillaf, J.P.; Cruces, E. The Filter-Feeding Bivalve *Mytilus chilensis* Capture Pelagic Stages of *Caligus rogercresseyi*: A Potential Controller of the Sea Lice Fish Parasites. *J. Fish. Dis.* **2020**, *43*, 475–484. [CrossRef]
43. Madrid, A.M.; Espinoza, L.J.; Mellado, M.A.; Osorio, M.E.; Montenegro, I.J.; Jara, C.E. Evaluation of the Antioxidant Capacity of *Psoralea glandulosa* L. (*Fabaceae*) EXTRACTS. *J. Chil. Chem. Soc.* **2012**, *57*, 1328–1332. [CrossRef]
44. Leyton, M.; Mellado, M.; Jara, C.; Montenegro, I.; González, S.; Madrid, A. Free Radical-Scavenging Activity of Sequential Leaf Extracts of *Embothrium coccineum*. *Open Life Sci.* **2015**, *10*, 260–268. [CrossRef]
45. Stolen, J.S.; Fletcher, T.C.; Anderson, D.P.; Roberson, B.S.; van Muiswinkel, W.B. *Techniques in Fish Immunology*; SOS Publications: Fair Haven, NJ, USA, 1990; pp. 1–220.
46. Boesen, H.T.; Larsen, M.H.; Larsen, J.L.; Ellis, A.E. In Vitro Interactions between Rainbow Trout (*Oncorhynchus mykiss*) Macrophages and Vibrio *Anguillarum* serogroup O2a. *Fish Shellfish Immunol.* **2001**, *11*, 415–431. [CrossRef]

Disclaimer/Publisher's Note: The statements, opinions and data contained in all publications are solely those of the individual author(s) and contributor(s) and not of MDPI and/or the editor(s). MDPI and/or the editor(s) disclaim responsibility for any injury to people or property resulting from any ideas, methods, instructions or products referred to in the content.

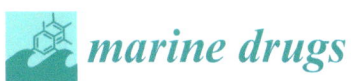

Article

Systematical Investigation on Anti-Fatigue Function and Underlying Mechanism of High Fischer Ratio Oligopeptides from Antarctic Krill on Exercise-Induced Fatigue in Mice

Sha-Yi Mao [1], Shi-Kun Suo [1], Yu-Mei Wang [1], Chang-Feng Chi [2,*] and Bin Wang [1,*]

[1] Zhejiang Provincial Engineering Technology Research Center of Marine Biomedical Products, School of Food and Pharmacy, Zhejiang Ocean University, Zhoushan 316022, China; msy1361209282@163.com (S.-Y.M.); 13275896859@163.com (S.-K.S.); wangyumei731@163.com (Y.-M.W.)

[2] National and Provincial Joint Engineering Research Centre for Marine Germplasm Resources Exploration and Utilization, School of Marine Science and Technology, Zhejiang Ocean University, Zhoushan 316022, China

* Correspondence: chichangfeng@hotmail.com (C.-F.C.); wangbin@zjou.edu.cn (B.W.); Tel./Fax: +86-580-2554818 (C.-F.C. & B.W.)

Abstract: High Fischer ratio oligopeptides (HFOs) have a variety of biological activities, but their mechanisms of action for anti-fatigue are less systematically studied at present. This study aimed to systematically evaluate the anti-fatigue efficacy of HFOs from Antarctic krill (HFOs-AK) and explore its mechanism of action through establishing the fatigue model of endurance swimming in mice. Therefore, according to the comparison with the endurance swimming model group, HFOs-AK were able to dose-dependently prolong the endurance swimming time, reduce the levels of the metabolites (lactic acid, blood urea nitrogen, and blood ammonia), increase the content of blood glucose, muscle glycogen, and liver glycogen, reduce lactate dehydrogenase and creatine kinase extravasation, and protect muscle tissue from damage in the endurance swimming mice. HFOs-AK were shown to enhance Na^+-K^+-ATPase and Ca^{2+}-Mg^{2+}-ATPase activities and increase ATP content in muscle tissue. Meanwhile, HFOs-AK also showed significantly antioxidant ability by increasing the activities of superoxide dismutase and glutathione peroxidase in the liver and decreasing the level of malondialdehyde. Further studies showed that HFOs-AK could regulate the body's energy metabolism and thus exert its anti-fatigue effects by activating the AMPK signaling pathway and up-regulating the expression of p-AMPK and PGC-α proteins. Therefore, HFOs-AK can be used as an auxiliary functional dietary molecules to exert its good anti-fatigue activity and be applied to anti-fatigue functional foods.

Keywords: high Fischer ratio oligopeptides (HFO); Antarctic krill (*Euphausia superba*); anti-fatigue; in vivo metabolites; oxidative stress

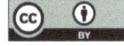

1. Introduction

Marine resources are used as a source of various health foods, and protein hydrolysates and peptides extracted from marine organisms have a variety of bioactive functions as well as pharmaceutical effects, like metal-chelating, antioxidant, anti-inflammatory, anti-hypertensive, antimicrobial, anticancer, and immunomodulatory activities [1,2]. Bioactive peptides are specific small amino acid fragments (usually 3 to 20 amino acids) obtained from natural sources that are capable of causing physicochemical changes in normal bodily processes, and these physicochemical effects arise from their unique amino acid composition, sequence, and molecular weights [3,4]. Peptides typically comprise a variety of amino acids, among which branched-chain amino acids (BCAAs) and aromatic amino acids (AAAs) are present in a molar ratio known as the Fischer ratio (or F-value). High Fischer ratio oligopeptides (HFOs) are mixed small-molecule peptides with a BCAA/AAA ratio greater than 20, whose oligopeptides have molecular weights between 200 and 1000 Da and are composed of 2 to 9 amino acids [5]. Thanks to their distinct amino acid and peptide makeup, HFO exhibit a range of impressive biological properties, such as serving as an adjunct therapy for hepatic encephalopathy [6], sobering and anti-intoxication activity [7], antioxidant activity [5,8], adjunctive therapy for phenylketonuria [9], anti-fatigue activity [10], and some clinical surgical treatments [11]. Every year, low-valuable protein resources from both land and sea go untapped in significant quantities. Transforming these resources into bioactive oligopeptides, marked by an HFO, promises substantial economic, nutritional, and medical benefits. Therefore, HFO have received widespread attention, and there have been successful cases ranging from hard-shell mussels [12], whey proteins [13], corn [14], Antarctic krill [5], flaxseed [15,16], gluten [17], goat's milk whey protein [18], bonito [7], oyster (*Pinctada martensii*) meat [19], and *Aspergillus niger* [20]. Hence, HFOs hold great promise for practical use in clinical settings because of their impressive bioactive properties. Comprehensive research into the physiological functions and underlying mechanisms of HFOs is crucial in unlocking their potential for integration into pharmaceutical and health-enhancing products.

Fatigue is usually divided into physiological or pathological causes which can lead to various discomforts and are related to various diseases. However, some studies have shown that exercise leads to fatigue, and the fatigue caused by high-intensity exercise is related to injury, the working ability and liver glycogen level, resulting in energy source [21]. Concurrently, the buildup of blood lactic acid (BLA) and blood urea nitrogen (BUN) while exercising results in the accumulation and threshold of metabolites, culminating in physical exhaustion [22]. During physical activity, the body extensively utilizes energy storage molecules, such as adenosine triphosphate (ATP), glucose, and fat. This depletion ultimately results in diminished skeletal muscle function, rendering individuals unable to sustain the intended exercise intensity. Consequently, this can lead to injury and increases in creatine kinase (CK) level [23]. In recent years, some related studies have been carried out to find natural substances with anti-fatigue activity to avoid the damage caused by ingesting chemical drugs, and these investigations have shown that the active peptides extracted from natural foods are safe and effective in preventing and relieving fatigue. For example, Corn peptides (CPs) are rich in amino acids, including glutamic acid, so that it has a significant ability to relieve exercise-induced fatigue. Moreover, they have significant anti-fatigue properties that help mitigate damage caused by synthetic drugs [21]. Soybean peptides, known as FSPPs, play a crucial role in facilitating protein synthesis and contributing to the energy provision for cells within skeletal muscle. Consequently, they trigger an anti-fatigue response [24]. On the other hand, the anti-fatigue properties of sea cucumber peptide (SCP) are attributed to its ability to restore normal energy metabolism while mitigating oxidative stress and inflammatory responses [23]. Moreover, oligopeptides with a high F value have a unique amino acid composition, which can increases the AAA content of the body's blood [12]. Therefore, compared with normal oligopeptides, HFO may have better anti-fatigue effects because of their unique amino acid composition, so as to develop anti-fatigue functional foods. However, the anti-fatigue mechanism of HFO still needs to be studied systematically.

Antarctic krill (*Euphausia superba*), which mainly lives in Antarctica, is the world's richest animal protein resource, with high nutritional value [25]. Antarctic krill protein contains all the essential amino acids required by the human body, and its bioactivity was evaluated to be higher than that of other animal and plant proteins and dairy proteins (casein) [26], so peptides with significant bioactivities were prepared from hydrolysates of Antarctic krill protein [27]. For example, Antarctic krill peptides not only significantly attenuates CCl_4-induced hepatic injury by activating the Nrf2/HO-1 pathway [28], but also ameliorates hepatic fibrosis by improving gut microbiota-mediated bile acid-NLRP3 pathway [29]. According to behavioral experiments, SSDAFFPFR and SNVDFMF from Antarctic krill can ameliorate scopolamine-induced memory deficits by altering the behavior of mice [30]. Ca-EEEFDATR chelate has effects on MC3T3-E1 cells with osteoblast proliferation, differentiation, and mineralization [31]. Peptides of VW and LKY have antihypertensive effects in spontaneously hypertensive rats [32]. In our previous research, HFO from Antarctic krill (HFOs-AK) was enzymatically prepared with alcalase and flavorzyme, and it showcased promising antioxidant properties in vitro [5]. However, more in-depth functional evaluation and mechanism studies on HFOs-AK, especially the anti fatigue function closely related to oxidative stress, are still lacking. Hence, the aim of this research was to methodically assess the effectiveness of HFOs-AK in combating fatigue and delve into its mechanism of operation by establishing a vigorous swimming-induced fatigue model in mice. This study provides experimental evidence and a theoretical basis for the application of Antarctic krill oligopeptides in fatigue reduction related functional foods.

2. Results

2.1. Effect of HFOs-AK on Body Weight and Organ Index of Fatigue Model of Mice

As depicted in Table 1, following gavage for 30 days, mice increased their body weight in all groups, but there was no significant difference in the body weight of mice among the blank, model, positive control, and HFOs-AK groups. It demonstrates that gavage of HFOs-AK does not negatively affect the growth and development of mice, and the mice in all groups were in a normal growth and feeding environment.

Table 1. Changes in the body weight of the mice in each group (n = 15).

Groups	Body Weight (g)		
	Starting Weight	Final Weight	Weight Change
Blank	22.85 ± 1.00	37.81 ± 2.45	13.33 ± 1.73 [b]
Model	22.96 ± 0.82	37.97 ± 3.17	15.01 ± 2.35 [a,b]
Whey peptides	23.31 ± 0.72	37.71 ± 1.86	14.40 ± 1.14 [a,b]
Low-dose HFOs-AK	22.91 ± 0.97	37.92 ± 1.22	15.01 ± 0.25 [a,b]
Mid-dose HFOs-AK	21.53 ± 0.94	37.57 ± 0.66	16.03 ± 0.28 [a,b]
High-dose HFOs-AK	22.38 ± 0.99	38.67 ± 2.60	16.29 ± 1.61 [a]

All data are presented as the mean ± SD (n = 15). [a,b] Values with the same letters indicate no significant difference in each column ($p > 0.05$).

According to the organ indices expressed in Table 2, the coefficients of the liver, spleen, kidney, and thymus of mice in the low-, medium-, and high-dose groups of HFOs-AK were not significantly different ($p > 0.05$) compared to those of the model group. Experimental data indicated that gavage of HFOs-AK did not produce adverse effects on the growth of mice.

Table 2. Organ indices of mice in each group (n = 15).

Groups	Liver (%)	Spleen (%)	Gallbladder (%)	Thymus Gland (%)
Blank	5.95 ± 0.41 [a]	0.32 ± 0.05 [a]	1.59 ± 0.14 [a]	0.15 ± 0.01 [a]
Model	5.85 ± 0.12 [a,b]	0.32 ± 0.01 [a]	1.56 ± 0.04 [a]	0.14 ± 0.01 [a]
Whey peptides	5.59 ± 0.05 [a,b]	0.31 ± 0.02 [a]	1.55 ± 0.04 [a]	0.13 ± 0.04 [a]
Low-dose HFOs-AK	5.88 ± 0.13 [a]	0.29 ± 0.02 [a]	1.56 ± 0.09 [a]	0.15 ± 0.06 [a]
Mid-dose HFOs-AK	5.59 ± 0.23 [b]	0.29 ± 0.01 [a]	1.51 ± 0.05 [a]	0.14 ± 0.04 [a]
High-dose HFOs-AK	5.69 ± 0.03 [a,b]	0.30 ± 0.03 [a]	1.55 ± 0.03 [a]	0.14 ± 0.05 [a]

All data are presented as the mean ± SD (n = 15). [a,b] Values with the same letters indicate no significant difference in each column ($p > 0.05$).

2.2. Effect of HFOs-AK on Tissue Morphology of Fatigue Model of Mice

The liver nuclei of mice in the blank group (Figure 1A) appeared intact and the hepatocytes showed no signs of necrosis in the H&E staining results. The hepatic blood sinusoids (yellow arrows) and hepatic cords (red arrowheads) were neatly aligned, and the hepatic lobules were clear in outline. Compared with the blank control group, the structure of the liver lobules in the model group (Figure 1B), positive control group (Figure 1C), and HFOs-AK groups (Figure 1D–F) was in a normal state, and the arrangement of the hepatic blood sinusoids (yellow arrowheads) and the hepatic cords (red arrowheads) did not undergo any alteration of the pathological state. It indicates that HFOs-AK do not cause damage to the mouse liver.

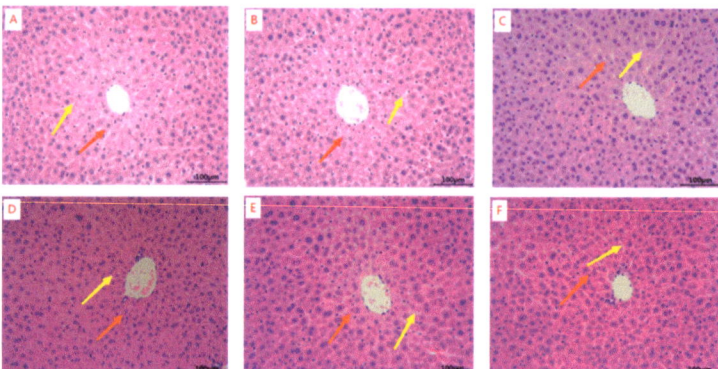

Figure 1. H&E staining of mouse liver tissue samples. The fatigue model of mice was established by an endurance swimming method. Whey peptides (0.5 mg/g·bw/d) served as a positive control. (**A**) Blank; (**B**) Model; (**C**) Whey peptides (0.5 mg/g·bw/d); (**D**) Low-dose of HFOs-AK (0.1 mg/g·bw/d); (**E**) Mid-dose of HFOs-AK (0.3 mg/g·bw/d); (**F**) High-dose of HFOs-AK (0.5 mg/g·bw/d). The yellow arrow indicates the hepatic sinusoids, and the red arrow indicates the hepatic cord.

The results of H&E staining of muscle tissues are shown in Figure 2. The muscle fibers of the gastrocnemius muscle of mice in the blank group (Figure 2A) were uniformly aligned with clear transverse striations. Compared with the blank group, the gastrocnemius muscles of mice in the model group (Figure 2B) showed damage (red arrow) and irregular arrangement. Compared with the model group, the low-, medium-, and high-dose HFOs-AK groups of HFOs-AK (Figure 2D–F) showed a reduction in the degree of damage appearing in the fibers of the mouse gastrocnemius muscle, indicating that HFOs-AK could effectively ameliorate the muscle damage in mice.

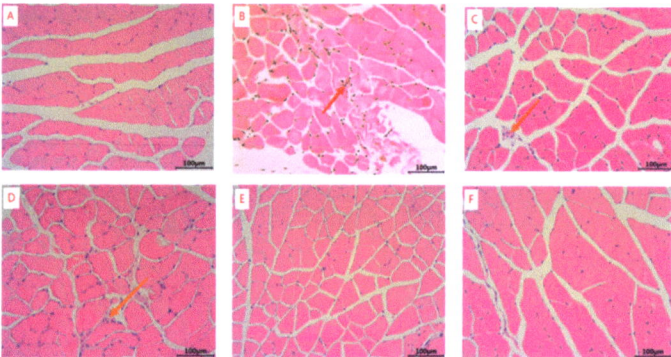

Figure 2. H&E staining of mouse muscle tissue samples. Whey peptides (0.5 g/g·bw/d) served as a positive control. (**A**) Blank; (**B**) Model; (**C**) Whey peptides (0.5 mg/g·bw/d); (**D**) Low-dose of HFOs-AK (0.1 mg/g·bw/d); (**E**) Mid-dose of HFOs-AK (0.3 mg/g·bw/d); (**F**) High-dose of HFOs-AK (0.5 mg/g·bw/d). The red arrows in the diagram indicate damage and irregular alignment of the gastrocnemius muscles of mice.

2.3. Effect of HFOs-AK on Exercise Capacity and Metabolite Levels of BUN, Lactic Acid (LA), and Blood Ammonia (BA) in Fatigue Model of Mice

Fatigue is the feeling of exhaustion that sets in following extended or intense physical activity, indicating a decline in physiological capacity and the body's ability to sustain its functions [10], so it can be measured by increased exercise endurance to measure the effect of fatigue resistance [23]. The effect of HFOs-AK on the exercise capacity of fatigue model of mice is shown in Figure 3A. The model group showed a time to exhaustion of 10.35 min, but the time to exhaustion was prolonged in all the HFOs-AK-administered groups by 20.64 ± 13.05% (low), 72.84 ± 25.63% (medium), and 154.14 ± 40.34% (high). In addition, there was a significant difference between the medium (17.89 ± 2.65 min) and high (26.31 ± 4.18 min-dose HFOs-AK groups compared to the model group ($p < 0.01$). Also, as the dose of HFOs-AK was increased, the endurance swimming time of the mice increased, showing a dose-dependent pattern. These data suggest that HFOs-AK have an anti-fatigue effect on mice, and the higher the dose, the more obvious the effect.

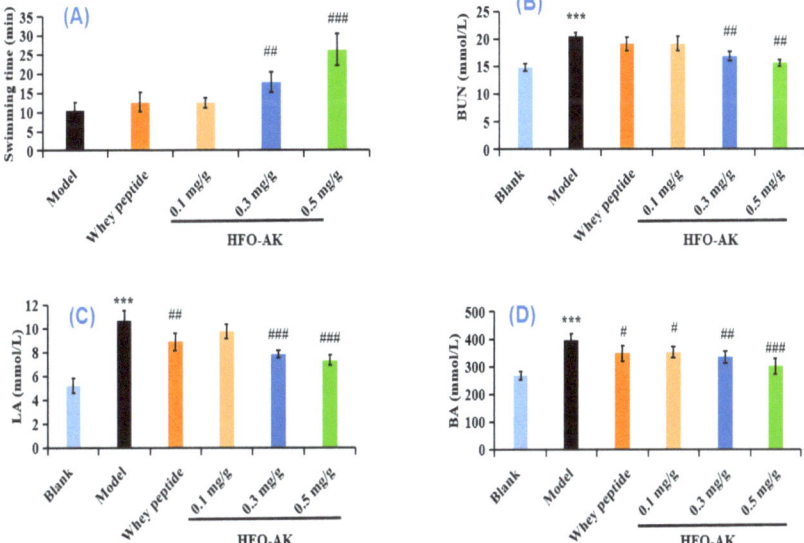

Figure 3. Effect of HFOs-AK on exercise capacity (**A**) and in vivo metabolites of BUN (**B**), LA (**C**), and BA (**D**) in fatigue model of mice. Whey peptides (0.5 g/g·bw/d) served as a positive control. *** $p < 0.001$ compared to blank control group. ### $p < 0.001$, ## $p < 0.01$ and # $p < 0.05$ compared to model group.

Metabolic waste is negatively correlated with exercise endurance [33]. When the energy supply in the body is insufficient, the energy needed by the body can be provided by protein metabolism. The process of protein catabolism produces large amounts of NH_3 and CO_2, and these metabolic wastes are synthesized into urea in the liver of the organism, which is excreted via the humoral circulation. The effect of HFOs-AK on BUN in the fatigue model of mice is shown in Figure 3B. Compared with the blank group (14.85 ± 0.71 mmol/L), the model group of mice, which had been subjected to swimming and had not been gavaged with HFOs-AK, had the highest BUN levels of 20.49 ± 0.71 mmol/L, indicating successful modeling of low exercise tolerance in mice. The BUN levels in low-, medium-, and high-dose HFOs-AK groups were dose-dependently decreased by 6.74% ± 6.55%, 17.68% ± 3.82%, and 23.85% ± 2.93%, respectively. Moreover, the BUN level in the high-dose HFOs-AK group of HFOs-AK was 15.60 ± 0.60 mmol/L, which was highly significant ($p < 0.001$) compared with the model group. It indicates that HFOs-AK participate in the process of collective energy metabolism and reduce the original protein metabolism to effectively reduce the BUN content in the body.

Glycolysis is the main source of energy for high-intensity exercise in a short period of time. Lactic acid (LA) is produced under anaerobic conditions by glycolysis. As glycolysis accelerates, LA increases in muscle and accumulates in the body, lowering the pH of the body and leading to fatigue as well as reduced exercise capacity [34]. The effects of HFOs-AK on LA in fatigue model of mice are shown in Figure 3C. After endurance swimming exercise in mice, the LA levels in low, medium and high-dose HFOs-AK groups were 9.74 ± 0.61, 7.83 ± 0.34, and 7.32 ± 0.43 mmol/L, respectively, which were significantly decreased ($p < 0.001$) compared to the model group (10.67 ± 0.87 mmol/L). It shows that HFOs-AK have certain anti-fatigue activity by reducing the accumulation of LA in the muscle and body of mice.

Adenosine triphosphate (ATP) is the direct source of energy for all vital activities in the body, and nutrients, such as creatine phosphate, glycogen, glucose, fat, and protein, provide indirect energy for exercise [35]. When proteins and amino acids are degraded to provide energy for the body, a large amount of ammonia enters the bloodstream, and the high concentration of NH_3 in the body affects the energy metabolism and motor balance of the body, causing fatigue [36]. The effects of HFOs-AK on blood ammonia (BA) in the fatigue model of mice are shown in Figure 3D. Compared with the model group (395.19 ± 22.41 mmol/L), the BA contents in the low-dose HFOs-AK (352.09 ± 19.76 mmol/L), medium-dose HFOs-AK (334.46 ± 21.08 mmol/L), high-dose HFOs-AK (301.81 ± 27.66 mmol/L), and the positive control (347.52 ± 28.72 mmol/L) groups were significantly decreased ($p < 0.001$). It indicates that HFOs-AK play its anti-fatigue activity through reducing the energy metabolism and exercise homeostasis of the body.

2.4. Effect of HFOs-AK on Lactate Dehydrogenase (LDH) and CK of Fatigue Model of Mice

LDH mainly catalyzes the mutual conversion between acetone and LA, indicating the degree of lactate metabolism. Increases in LDH concentrations caused by high-intensity exercise can lead to muscle damage. Therefore, LDH is also considered to be one of the specific markers for assessing physical fatigue [37]. The effects of HFOs-AK on LDH in fatigue mice are shown in Figure 4A. LDH levels in the low, medium and high-dose HFOs-AK groups were 490.30 ± 40.28, 458.08 ± 60.21, and 412.35 ± 69.76 U/L, respectively, significantly lower than that in the model group (552.53 ± 50.74 U/L). It suggests that HFOs-AK can alleviate exercise fatigue and protect muscles by reducing LDH content.

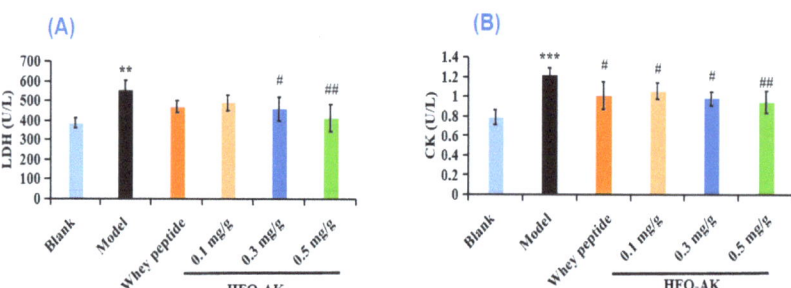

Figure 4. Effect of HFOs-AK on LDH (**A**) and CK (**B**) activity in fatigue model of mice. Whey peptides (0.5 g/g·bw/d) served as a positive control. *** $p < 0.001$ and ** $p < 0.01$ compared to blank control group. ## $p < 0.01$ and # $p < 0.05$ compared to model group.

CK, mainly found in the cytoplasm and mitochondria, is an important kinase and involved in intracellular energy conversion, ATP production, and muscle contraction. Serum CK is mainly derived from skeletal muscle in the organism; therefore, changes in serum CK activity can be used as an indicator to assess skeletal muscle injury and recovery after exercise in the organism, and the higher the CK activity, the more severe the skeletal muscle injury and fatigue [37]. The effect of HFOs-AK on CK in fatigue mice is shown in Figure 4B. Compared with the blank group (0.79 ± 0.08 U/L), the CK activity in the model group (1.22 ± 0.07 U/L) was significantly increased, indicating successful modeling of fatigued mice. However, the CK levels in the low-, medium-, and high dose groups of HFOs-AK were 1.06 ± 0.08, 0.98 ± 0.07, and 0.94 ± 0.11 U/L, respectively, and were reduced by 12.89% ± 6.82%, 19.48% ± 5.74%, and 22.50% ± 9.01%, respectively, in comparison with the model group. These results indicate that HFOs-AK are able to attenuate muscle damage caused by strenuous exercise.

2.5. Effect of HFOs-AK on Blood Glucose (BG), Muscle Glycogen (MG), and Liver Glycogen (LG) of Fatigue Model of Mice

Glycogen are used for long-term energy storage, which can be rapidly consumed when fatigue occurs to meet the urgent need for glucose, and increased glycogen levels in the liver and muscles can enhance endurance during intense exercise. During strenuous exercise, the organism enhances glycogen metabolism and lowers BG levels to maintain them in the normal physiological range [37]. Therefore, glycogen content is an important test indicator for fatigue resistance [38].

As shown in Figure 5A, the level of BG in model group (7.69 ± 0.51 mmol/L) was significantly lower than that in the blank group (9.06 ± 0.56 mmol/L) ($p < 0.05$). Furthermore, the medium (7.33 ± 0.90 mmol/L) and high (7.39 ± 1.00 mmol/L-dosage groups of HFOs-AK exhibited notably elevated blood glucose levels compared to the model group ($p < 0.05$). This suggests that HFOs-AK have the potential to enhance blood glucose utilization and modulate energy metabolism within the exhausted mice's bodies, which could improve the organism's exercise tolerance.

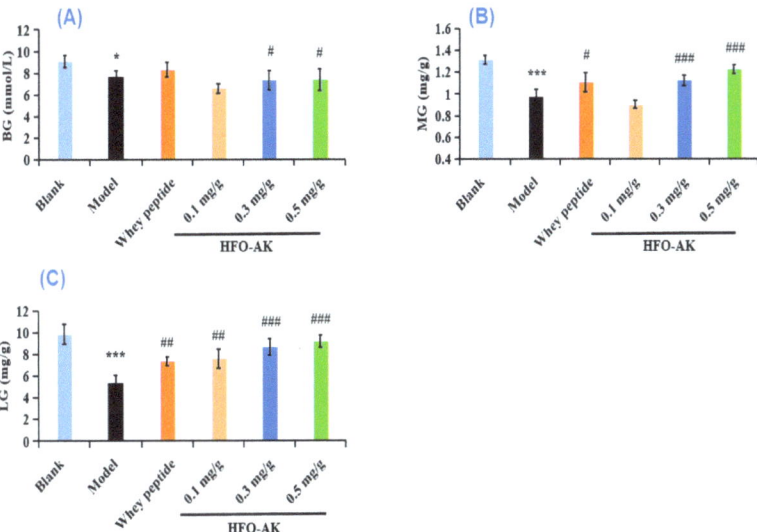

Figure 5. Effect of HFOs-AK on the contents of BG (**A**), MG (**B**), and LG (**C**) in fatigue model of mice. Whey peptides (0.5 g/g·bw/d) served as a positive control. *** $p < 0.001$ and * $p < 0.05$ compared to blank control group. ### $p < 0.001$, ## $p < 0.01$ and # $p < 0.05$ compared to model group.

Figure 5B,C showed the effect of HFOs-AK on MG and LG levels in the fatigue mice. The data indicated that the MG levels of the HFOs-AK groups, especially the medium-dose group (1.12 ± 0.05 mg/g) and the high-dose group (1.22 ± 0.04 mg/g), were significantly higher (0.97 ± 0.07 mg/g) than that model group ($p < 0.001$) (Figure 5B).

The results in Figure 5C showed that the LG level of the model group (5.40 ± 0.67 mg/g) was significantly lower ($p < 0.001$) than that (9.85 ± 0.89 mg/g) of the blank group. Treatment with HFOs-AK, the LG levels of fatigue mice in the low, medium and high-dose HFOs-AK groups were 7.58 ± 0.89, 8.66 ± 0.78, and 9.21 ± 0.55 mg/g, respectively. The findings revealed markedly elevated levels of MG and LG in the experimental group compared to those in the control group ($p < 0.01$). Consequently, as the dosage increased, there was a notable rise in the average concentrations of MG and LG within the mouse system ($p < 0.05$). In conclusion, gavage of HFOs-AK can increase glycogen content, regulate energy metabolism, and enhance exercise tolerance in mice.

2.6. Effect of HFOs-AK on ATP Content and Activities of Na^+-K^+-ATPase and Ca^{2+}-Mg^{2+}-ATPase of Fatigue Model of Mice

The most basic carrier of energy conversion in an organism is ATP. Usually, ATP levels decrease when the cell is apoptotic, necrotic, or in some pathological state, which indicates that the mitochondria have impaired functionality with decreased viability. The impact of HFOs-AK on ATP levels in fatigued mice is illustrated in Figure 6A. In comparison to the control group (3013.48 ± 241.92 µmol/g prot), mice in the model group (1785.31 ± 148.19 µmol/g prot) exhibited a notable decline in ATP content ($p < 0.001$). Conversely, mice administered with low, medium, and high doses of HFOs-AK demonstrated ATP levels of 2546.10 ± 125.33, 2606.62 ± 87.05, and 2879.27 ± 197.19 µmol/g prot, respectively, indicating a significant rise and a marked disparity in comparison to the model group ($p < 0.001$). These findings suggest that HFOs-AK directly enhance energy provision in vivo, thereby sustaining organismal energy metabolism and enhancing the fatigue resistance of the mice.

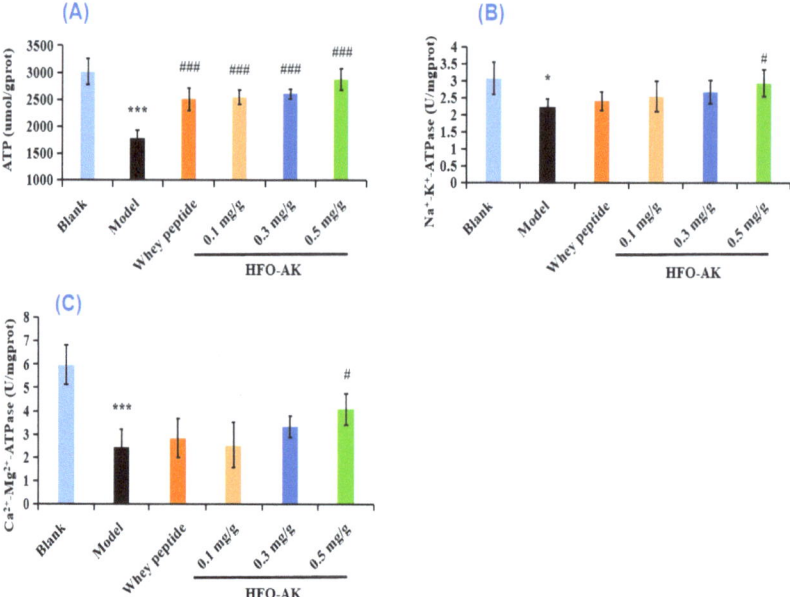

Figure 6. Effect of HFOs-AK on ATP content (**A**), Na^+-K^+-ATPase (**B**) and Ca^{2+}-Mg^{2+}-ATPase (**C**) activities in fatigue mice. Whey peptides (0.5 g/g·bw/d) served as a positive control. *** $p < 0.001$ and * $p < 0.05$ compared to blank control group. ### $p < 0.001$ and # $p < 0.05$ compared to model group.

Na^+-K^+-ATPase and Ca^{2+}-Mg^{2+}-ATPase play crucial roles in the physiological processes of material transfer, energy conversion, and information transfer, and are the key enzymes in degrading ATP [39]. When their activity decreases, the level of reactive oxygen species (ROS) in the mitochondria increases, which results in impaired mitochondrial function and impaired energy synthesis, producing fatigue. Figure 6B,C showed the effect of HFOs-AK on Na^+-K^+-ATPase and Ca^{2+}-Mg^{2+}-ATPase activity in fatigue mice. After endurance swimming, the Na^+-K^+-ATPase activity in mice decreased from 3.06 ± 0.47 U/mg prot to 2.22 ± 0.24 U/mg prot, but the Na$^+$-K$^+$-ATPase activity was significantly increased to 2.94 ± 0.39 U/mg prot after administration of 0.5 mg/g HFOs-AK ($p < 0.001$) (Figure 6A). The Na$^+$-K$^+$-ATPase activity showed the similar trend. The Ca^{2+}-Mg^{2+}-ATPase decreased from 5.97 ± 0.85 U/mg prot to 2.45 ± 0.77 U/mg prot in mice after endurance swimming, but the Ca^{2+}-Mg^{2+}-ATPase activity was significantly increased to 4.08 ± 0.66 U/mg prot after administration of 0.5 mg/g HFOs-AK ($p < 0.001$) (Figure 6C). Therefore, the administration of HFOs-AK can improve mitochondrial function, enhance the breakdown of ATP in skeletal muscle cells, fuel muscle cells with energy, and enhance the body's capacity to combat fatigue.

2.7. Effect of HFOs-AK on Antioxidant Capacity of Fatigue Model of Mice

It has been shown that superfluous ROS are produced during strenuous exercise, which can lead to fatigue and lipid peroxidation damage. Antioxidant enzymes like superoxide dismutase (SOD) and glutathione peroxidase (GSH-Px) play a key role in eliminating surplus ROS produced during intense physical activity in order to avert oxidative harm, thereby sidestepping cellular injury and muscle depletion [40,41].

Malondialdehyde (MDA), a byproduct of cell membrane breakdown due to lipid peroxidation, increases as fatigue intensifies. Figure 7A illustrates a significant rise in MDA levels in fatigued mice, jumping from 1.36 ± 0.05 nmol/mg prot to 2.05 ± 0.03 nmol/mg prot post exhaustive swimming. Comparatively, the MDA concentrations in groups administered with varying doses of HFOs-AK were notably decreased by 16.76% ± 2.56%, 18.35% ± 1.08%, and 32.53% ± 5.04%, respectively ($p < 0.05$) when contrasted with the control group. These findings suggest that HFOs-AK have the potential to diminish liver injury by alleviating oxidative stress, as evidenced by reduced MDA formation in the livers of fatigued mice.

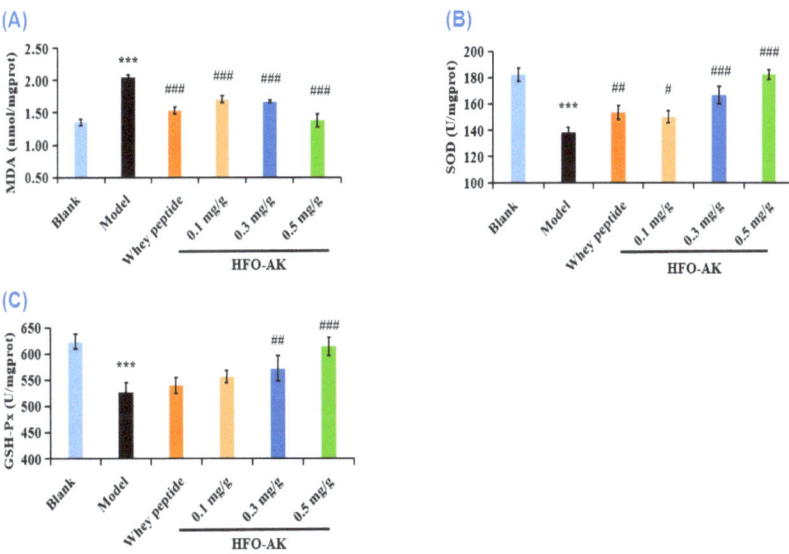

Figure 7. Effect of HFOs-AK on MDA (**A**) content, and SOD (**B**) and GSH-Px (**C**) activities in fatigue model of mice. Whey peptides (0.5 g/g·bw/d) served as a positive control. *** $p < 0.001$ compared to blank control group. ### $p < 0.001$, ## $p < 0.01$ and # $p < 0.05$ compared to model group.

SOD is an antioxidant enzyme that helps to improve cellular resistance to oxidative stress. Figure 7B represents the effect of HFOs-AK on SOD activity in fatigue mice. According to the data, the SOD activity in the model group (138.51 ± 3.62 U/mg prot) is significantly lower compared to the blank group (182.45 ± 4.74 U/mg prot). Furthermore, in the medium- and high-dose groups of HFOs-AK, there was a noticeable increase in SOD activity in the liver tissue of fatigued mice, with increments of 20.36% ± 4.62% and 31.71% ± 2.61%, respectively, significantly higher than that of the model group. Additionally, the SOD activity in the medium- (166.71 ± 6.39 U/mg prot) and high-dose groups (182.43 ± 3.62 U/mg prot) of HFOs-AK is slightly higher than that of the positive control group (153.49 ± 5.25 U/mg prot). This indicates that HFOs-AK have a protective effect on the mouse liver, and this effect is dose-dependent.

GSH-Px is a widely recognized antioxidant known for its ability to combat ROS and is frequently utilized as a biomarker for gauging the level of oxidative stress-induced damage. According to the data presented in Figure 7C, the concentration of GSH-Px in the model group presented a noteworthy reduction to 526.67 ± 18.04 U/mg prot, a figure significantly below that of the control group (623.20 ± 14.25 U/mg prot) ($p < 0.001$). In addition, the GSH-Px levels in the medium- and high dosage of HFOs-AK groups stood at 572 ± 23.78 and 614 ± 17.74 U/mg prot, respectively, while the GSH-Px content in the high dosage of HFOs-AK group was significantly elevated compared to that of the model group ($p < 0.001$). These findings indicated that HFOs-AK was able to increase GSH-Px levels in liver tissues of fatigue mice, suggesting that HFOs-AK could increase liver antioxidant levels and reduce injury.

In summary, referring to the related literatures [42], it could be theorized that HFOs-AK could help alleviate fatigue by enhancing the functioning of antioxidant enzymes within the body and limiting the generation of lipid peroxides in cellular membranes.

2.8. Effect of HFOs-AK on Protein Expression of the AMPK/PGC-1α/Nrf2 Signaling Pathways in Fatigue Model of Mice

Mitochondria are pivotal in energy metabolism, with mitochondrial dysfunction and structural irregularities being potential culprits behind fatigue. AMP-activated protein kinase (AMPK) is instrumental in regulating glucose and lipid metabolism, aiding in the maintenance of ATP levels across diverse conditions. The AMPK signaling pathway is triggered during sustained physical activity, enhancing basal glucose uptake. Peroxisome proliferator-activated receptor gamma coactivator-1 alpha (PGC-1α) emerges as a vital player in mitochondrial biogenesis and other physiological functions, predominantly observed in skeletal muscle tissues rich in mitochondria [43,44]. AMPK-1α and PGC-1α are key regulators of metabolism, and they increase resistance mainly by increasing the degradation of glucogenesis, glucose enzymes, sugar intake, and fatty acid oxidation. During exercise, AMPK is activated and electro-stimulated to shrink, thereby promoting the intake of basic glucose. In our study, HFOs-AK was found to enhance the expression of the phosphorus form of AMPK in the liver and bone muscle of mouse motors through analysis of protein traces. In addition, we also found an enhancement expression of PGC-1α (transcript co-activating factor), which activates the metabolic and biological processes in fibroblasts, thereby converting type II muscle fibers into type I muscle fiber. They can use oxygen and synthesize more ATP for continuous muscle contractions and become more fatigued.

Figure 8B shows the effect of HFOs-AK on the p-AMPK protein expression level in fatigue mice. The p-AMPK protein expression level in the model group (0.53 ± 0.03 GAPDH) was significantly reduced ($p < 0.001$) compared with the blank group. The study revealed a notable increase ($p < 0.001$) in the p-AMPK protein levels in the liver tissue of mice treated with 0.3 and 0.5 mg/g of HFOs-AK, elevating them to 0.62 ± 0.03 GAPDH and 0.67 ± 0.03 GAPDH, respectively. These findings indicate that HFOs-AK play a role in modulating energy metabolism and demonstrating anti-fatigue properties by activating the AMPK pathway.

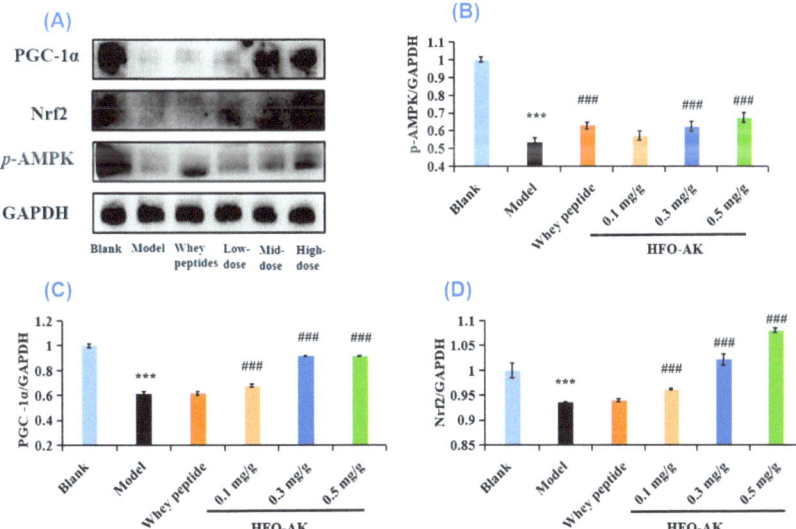

Figure 8. Protein map of HFOs-AK on anti-fatigue signaling pathway in mice (**A**). Effect of HFOs-AK on expression levels of *p*-AMPK (**B**), PGC-1α (**C**), and Nrf2 (**D**) protein in mice. Whey peptides (0.5 g/g·bw/d) served as a positive control. *** $p < 0.001$ compared to blank control group. ### $p < 0.001$ compared to model group.

Figure 8C shows the effect of HFOs-AK on the protein expression level of PGC-1α in fatigue mice. Compared with the blank group, the expression level of the PGC-1α protein was measured at 0.61 ± 0.02 GAPDH in the control group and showed a significant decrease ($p < 0.001$). In contrast, the liver tissue of the mouse model exhibited a noteworthy increase in PGC-1α protein levels to 0.92 ± 0.002 GAPDH and 0.92 ± 0.003 GAPDH after being treated with 0.3 and 0.5 mg/g of HFOs-AK, respectively. These findings indicate that HFOs-AK can influence energy metabolism and reduce fatigue by stimulating the PGC-1α pathway.

Mitochondria and other organelles of skeletal muscle and liver are vulnerable to lipid peroxidation [45]. During intense swimming sessions, excessive ROS are generated and build up significantly in the mouse's body. This accumulation leads to harmful effects by attacking crucial organic molecules and cell structures, causing oxidative stress and the creation of lipid peroxidation byproducts like MDA [46]. The nuclear factor E2-related factor 2 (Nrf2) signaling pathway serves as a crucial target for combating fatigue and various diseases associated with oxidative stress [45]. This pathway primarily operates by triggering the production of phase II enzymes that aid in defending against oxidative stress and scavenging ROS. In essence, Nrf2 acts as a pivotal regulator of cellular oxidation on a transcriptional level, controlling the expression of key downstream factors [47]. The impact of HFOs-AK on Nrf2 protein expression levels in fatigued mice, as depicted in Figure 8D, is evident. In comparison to the control group, the model group exhibited a noteworthy decrease in Nrf2 protein expression levels (0.94 ± 0.022 GAPDH) ($p < 0.001$). Conversely, the Nrf2 protein levels in liver tissues of fatigued mice significantly increased ($p < 0.001$) to 0.96 ± 0.002, 1.02 ± 0.011, and 1.08 ± 0.005 GAPDH following the administration of 0.1, 0.3, and 0.5 mg/g HFOs-AK, respectively. Subsequently, HFOs-AK modulates energy metabolism and exerts anti-fatigue effects by activating the Nrf2 pathway.

3. Discussion

Recent research has demonstrated the vital role of branched-chain amino acids in HFO as essential nutrients for tissue synthesis, energy provision, and overall health. Specifically, leucine and isoleucine undergo transamination to acetyl coenzyme A (acetyl-CoA), which enters the citric acid cycle, enhancing energy production in active muscles. On the other hand, isoleucine and valine are transformed into α-keto acid through transamination, further metabolized into succinyl coenzyme A, malate, and pyruvate, and eventually converting into alanine. This alanine is then transported to the liver via the bloodstream, where it is converted into pyruvate and subsequently into glucose. This glucose is carried back to the muscle for energy utilization during physical exertion [48]. The addition of HFOs-AK supplementation, along with swimming training, has been shown to notably enhance glycogen storage in both the liver and muscle. As demonstrated in Figure 3A, these adaptations led to a considerable enhancement in exercise endurance performance, an extension of the duration prior to exhaustion during physical activity in mice, and the effective preservation of glycogen levels following swimming exercise [49].

Maintaining stable blood glucose levels is essential for the proper functioning of organs, as blood glucose serves as a primary energy source for the central nervous system and red blood cells. Vigorous physical activity over an extended period depletes carbohydrate stores and lowers blood glucose levels, typically stored as glycogen in the liver and muscles. Research indicates that glycogen stored in these areas serves as the primary energy source during prolonged endurance exercise of moderate to high intensity [50]. Simultaneously, intense physical activity results in a significant energy expenditure and the production of surplus free radicals in muscle tissue. The excessive buildup of these free radicals triggers lipid peroxidation in the cell membrane, altering the normal composition of cellular proteins and genetic material. Consequently, this disrupts the permeability of the mitochondria's internal membrane, leading to oxidative fatigue. Bioactive peptides have the ability to neutralize free radicals within lipids or impede the propagation of free radical chains, safeguarding cells against oxidative harm. This process enhances the body's antioxidant capabilities and boosts its resistance to fatigue. It has been found that a large number of free radicals are produced during exhaustive swimming, leading to fatigue, and are prone to lipid peroxidation damage to organelles such as mitochondria in liver and skeletal muscle tissue [45].

Among natural active substances, bioactive peptides have received attention for their ability to reduce fatigue-induced muscle damage to varying degrees. Short peptides extracted from deer blood were evaluated in swimming mice and not only increased hepatic glycogen (HG) stores to improve exercise endurance, but also helped to reduce muscle lactate (MLA) accumulation and HG increase, exerting anti-fatigue activity [51]. Supplementation with sea dragon peptides exerted anti-fatigue effects on exercise-fatigued mice, and its mechanism may be to inhibit oxidative stress, improve grip strength, and prolong the swimming time of mice by reducing the accumulation of metabolites LA, BUN, and MDA. It promotes the expression of proteins related to the AMPK/PGC-1α and Nrf2 signaling pathways and regulates gut microbial homeostasis [52]. Using a mouse model of endurance swimming, peptides from striped bass (*Trichiurus lepturus*) [22], tilapia (*Oreochromis nilotica* L.) [53], yak bone [54], hemp seed [15], ankylosing fish [55], seahorses [50], and sea cucumbers [23] can prolong endurance swimming time in mice, reduce metabolites and antioxidant activity in vivo, and increase glycogen reserves and energy metabolism while decreasing the levels of LDH and CK due to muscular fatigue, resulting in anti-fatigue effects.

The Figure 9 show that when the energy ATP supply in the body is insufficient, the levels of key enzymes, including Na^+-K^+-ATPase and Ca^{2+}-Mg^{2+}-ATPase, which degrade ATP, will also decrease. The result is that the contents of BUN, LA, and BA are decreased, while the levels of BG, MG, and LG will continue to increase. While the muscles will produce large amounts of LDH and CK, which will lead to muscle damage. An overabundance of ROS can trigger oxidative stress, thereby inhibiting the function of internal antioxidant enzymes like SOD, and GSH-Px.

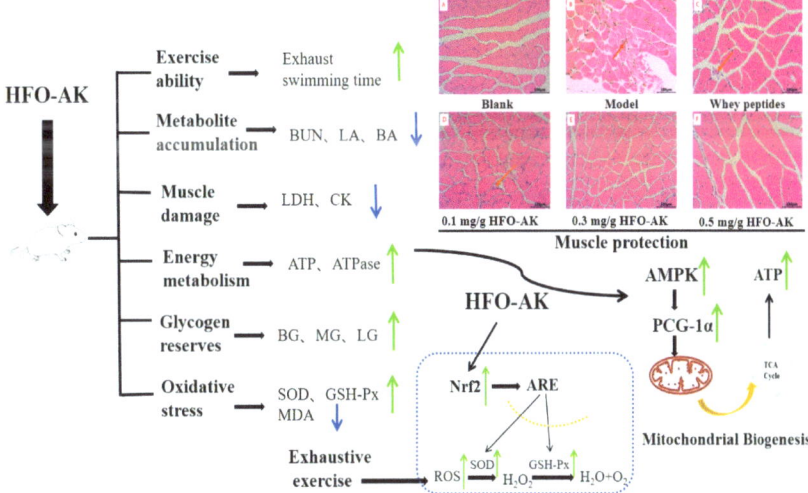

Figure 9. Anti-fatigue mechanisms of HFOs-AK on fatigue model of mice. The blue arrows in the chart indicate that the data is trending downward. The green arrows in the chart indicate that the data is trending upwards. The red arrows in the diagram indicate damage and irregular alignment of the gastrocnemius muscles of mice.

Typically, AMPK boosts the oxidation of fatty acids by inhibiting the formation of malonyl coenzyme A. Yet, during prolonged activation of AMPK, it governs the oxidation of fatty acids differently by activating peroxisome proliferator-activated Receptor α (PPARα) and PGC-1α. Additionally, it controls the uptake of glucose and the synthesis of mitochondria from scratch, which relies entirely on PGC-1α, whether in a living organism or in a laboratory setting [56]. The signaling cascade reactions of AMPK/PGC-1α are crucial across mammalian species, spanning from mice to humans, particularly in the skeletal muscles, where they contribute significantly to mitochondrial biosynthesis and maturation [57]. In the realm of muscle physiology, PGC-1α emerges as a pivotal player, igniting the process of mitochondrial biogenesis. This, in turn, bolsters both the quantity and quality of mitochondria within skeletal muscle fibers. Notably, skeletal muscle tissue showcases abundant expression of PGC-1α, orchestrating the synthesis of ATP to stave off muscle dysfunction. However, when PGC1-α veers off its typical course, metabolic disorders of an associative nature ensue. AMPK, in its active state, assumes a crucial role in this scenario, directly modulating the activity of PGC-1α through phosphorylation [58]. Thus, the tandem action of AMPK and PGC-1α emerges as the linchpin of the body's resilience against fatigue. In Figure 9, it is evident that there was a notable increase in the levels of AMPK/PGC-1α proteins in the liver tissue of tired mice following the administration of HFOs-AK ($p < 0.001$). The mechanism suggests that HFOs-AK can activate the AMPK pathway, up-regulate p-AMPK, stimulate the production of downstream PGC-1α proteins, and boost the functionality of the intracellular antioxidant enzymes SOD and GSH-Px, all the while diminishing the levels of MDA. Consequently, HFOs-AK regulates energy metabolism and delivers anti-fatigue benefits by stimulating the AMPK/PGC-1α pathway.

The Nrf2 protein plays a crucial role in regulating redox reactions within cells and controlling the expression of related factors downstream [59]. It is typically found in the cytoplasm, where it is bound to kelch-like ECH-associated protein 1 (Keap1) [60]. When ROS build up in the cell, Nrf2 separates from Keap1 and moves to the nucleus to bond with the antioxidant response element (ARE), which is overseen by the promoters of specific enzyme genes like heme oxygenase-1 (HO-1). Overall, the level of Nrf2 in cells is often inadequate to completely counteract the oxidative stress caused by physical exertion. Hence, the Keap1/Nrf2/ARE signaling pathway serves as a crucial target in combating fatigue and diseases related to oxidative stress. This pathway primarily operates by stimulating the production of phase II enzymes responsible for defending against oxidative stress and clearing ROS [45]. The results depicted in Figures 8 and 9 clearly demonstrate a significant increase in Nrf2 protein expression within liver tissues of fatigued mice treated with HFOs-AK, indicating the activation of the Nrf2 pathway. This suggests that HFOs-AK could potentially alleviate fatigue through Nrf2 pathway activation.

Some natural products show good anti-fatigue function by modulating mitochondrial biological functions. For example, flavonoids extracted from parsley (*Petroselinum crispum*) can repair mitochondrial dysfunction by regulating PGC-1α and have good anti-fatigue activity [61]. Astragalus polysaccharide has the ability to repair mitochondrial malfunction by addressing issues with the fusion and division processes, while also decreasing the presence of PGC-1α [62]. Various research has shown that herbal remedies containing antioxidants possess effective anti-fatigue properties. Administering luteolin-6-C-Neohesperidoside helped restore depleted levels of HO-1 and Nrf2 due to exhaustive swimming [60]. Therefore, from Figure 9, it can be shown that in this experiment, the oxidative stress in vivo caused by the exhaustive swimming experiment in mice can change the morphology and function of mitochondria. In the Western blot analysis, HFOs-AK demonstrates its ability to maintain ATP levels in vivo by triggering the AMPK/PGC-1α/Nrf2 pathways (Figure 8). Furthermore, it enhances the functioning of antioxidant enzymes (SOD and GSH-Px) and reduces the presence of lipid peroxidation MDA, highlighting its promising anti-fatigue properties.

4. Materials and Methods

4.1. Materials and Chemical Reagents

HFOs-AK were prepared in our laboratory according to the previous method [5]. Whey peptides were purchased from Shanxi Feimi Biotechnology Co., Ltd. (Taiyuan, China). Assay kits for determination of lactylic acid (LA), hydrouric nitrogen (BUN), lactic acid dehydrogenase (LDH), creatine enzyme (CK), superoxide dioxidase (SOD), glutathione peroxide (GSH-Px), malondialdehyde (MDA), liver/plasmodium, and ATP were purchased from Nanjing Jiancheng Bioengineering Institute (Nanjing, China). The activity assay kits of Na^+-K^+-ATPase, Ca^{2+}-Na^+-K^+-ATPase, and Ca^{2+}-ATPase were purchased from Hangzhou Leyi Bio-technology Co., Ltd. (Hangzhou, China). AMPK alpha 2 Polyclonal antibody (18167-1-AP), PGC-1α monoclonal antibody (66369-1-Ig), GAPDHH antibody (MP50049-1), mouse antibody (HRP-10283), and rabbit anti-rat (IgG) antibody (ab6703) were bought from Sanying Bio-Biological Antibody Co., Ltd. (Wuhan, China).

4.2. Experimental Methods

4.2.1. Animal Breeding and Experimental Design

Ninety male ICR mice (18–22 g) were purchased from Hangzhou Ziyuan Laboratory Animal Technology Co., Ltd. (Hangzhou, China). The animal experiments were standardized and approved by the Laboratory Animal Ethics Committee of Zhejiang Ocean University (certificate no. SYXK (Zhejiang) 2019–0031). The mice were kept at 25 ± 2 °C with $50 \pm 5\%$ relative humidity, following a 12-h light-dark cycle, and the mice had free access to food and water. After a week of acclimatization, male ICR mice were sorted into two groups: 10 mice in each of the 12 cages in group A and 5 mice in each of the 6 cages in group B. Blank group: mice were not gavaged. Model group: mice were injected with 0.2 mL distilled water for 30 days. Positive control group: male ICR mice received 0.2 mL whey peptides at a dose of 0.5 mg·g·bw/d for 30 days. HFOs-AK low-dose group: male ICR mice were treated with 0.2 mL HFOs-AK at a dose of 0.1 mg·g·bw/d for 30 days. HFOs-AK medium-dose group: Male ICR mice received 0.2 mL HFOs-AK at a dose of 0.3 mg·g·bw/d for 30 days. HFOs-AK high-dose group: male ICR mice received 0.2 mL HFOs-AK at a dose of 0.5 mg·g·bw/d for 30 days.

4.2.2. Establishment of a Fatigue Model of Endurance Swimming Mice

According to the described method [23,63], 30 min after the final gavage in group A, the mice were introduced into a controlled swimming environment, where the water was maintained at a stable temperature of 25 °C and a depth of 30 cm. They were tasked with navigating a submerged wire structure while carrying a weight equivalent to 5% of their body weight. The water in the pool was continuously circulated throughout the swimming session. Duration of swimming was measured from the onset of activity until the mice were unable to resurface within 8 s after their heads submerged. This duration was documented as their swimming time.

4.2.3. Measurement of Body Weight and Organ Index of Mice

After the beginning of the experiment, it was necessary to weigh and record the body weight of the mice at regular intervals every day, and all the mice were given mouse food daily according to the standard diet and free water. After the experiment, blood was removed from the mice's eyeballs, and the liver, leg muscles, kidney, spleen, and thymus of the mice were taken for dissection. Each group of mice was weighed accurately on an analytical balance to calculate their organ index. The formula for calculating the organ index was as follows (1):

$$\text{Organ index (\%)} = \text{Weight of organs (g)} / \text{The mass of a mouse (g)} \tag{1}$$

4.2.4. Histopathological Changes Observed

In male ICR mice, liver and muscle tissues were fixed overnight in 4% paraformaldehyde. Afterwards, paraffin is applied. Subsequently, H&E staining was performed on 4 mm sections of paraffin. A light microscope was used to observe the changes in histopathology.

4.2.5. Measurement of Biochemical Indexes among Mice

Upon completion of 30 days of intervention, group B mice with ICR were subjected to blood sampling from the eyeballs immediately 30 min after the end of swimming, and the supernatant was centrifuged at 4000 rpm for 10 min and stored for further use. After the serum was taken, the mice were executed, and the liver and muscle of the mice were accurately weighed, added to a 0.9% NaCl solution, ground in an ice bath under a tissue homogenizer to prepare a 10% homogenate of the liver and muscle tissues of the mice, and centrifuged at 4000 rpm for 20 min. In addition to the supernatant of the tissues, oxidative stress indicators and changes of LA, BUN, BA, BG, MG, LG, LDH, CK, Na^+-K^+-ATP, CA^{2+}-Mg^{2+}-ATP, SOD, and GSH-Px were measured by a kit.

4.2.6. Detecting the Expression of Relevant Signaling Pathway Proteins

A portion of liver tissue stored at −80 °C was used for Western blot analysis according to a previous method [64]. An RIPA lysis solution was used to homogenize and lyse liver tissue proteins, centrifuged at low temperature for 10 min at 12,000 rpm, and supernatants were taken, partitioned, and stored at −80 °C in a refrigerator for spare use. The total protein content in each group of samples was calculated by BCA protein assay according to the established method [63], and the calculated adjusted protein uploading volume was 5 µg/µL. Extracted proteins were uploaded onto a 12% SDS-acrylamide gel and then transferred onto a PVDF membrane. After incubation with primary and secondary antibodies, protein bands were visualized with an ECL luminescent solution. The quantitative analysis of the bands was performed by the Fluochem-FC3 system (Portsmouth, NH, USA) and statistically analyzed using SPSS (version 27.0).

4.3. Data Analysis

All data were expressed as means ± standard deviation (SD) (n = 15) and statistically analyzed using SPSS software for one-way ANOVA, LSD, and Duncan post hoc comparisons, and differences were considered statistically significant at $p < 0.05$.

5. Conclusions

In the study, we built an endurance swimming mice model to verify how HFOs-AK fights fatigue. The findings indicated that the HFOs-AK exhibited varying degrees of increased endurance during force exhaustion swimming, primarily attributable to two key factors. Regulating the AMPK signaling pathway induced a decrease in the levels of the metabolites LA, BUN, and BA and an increase in the contents of BG, MG, and LG in mice. Simultaneously, the decrease in LDH and CK leakage promoted the functions of Na^+-K^+-ATPase and Ca^{2+}-Mg^{2+}-ATPase, shielding the tissues from harm and boosting ATP levels within them. Regulatory of the Keap1/Nrf2/ARE signaling pathway led to a notable upsurge in SOD and GSH-Px functions and a drop in MDA concentrations in the hepatic tissue of mice, indicating the potential antioxidant properties of HFOs-AK. Therefore, HFOs-AK presented remarkable anti-fatigue function and can be used as a functional peptide applied in anti-fatigue food.

In addition, some relevant indicators, such as hemoglobin level, fecal SCFA content (propionic acid and butyric acid content), and intestinal flora changes, have not been comprehensively detected after force exhaustion swimming in mice, and the mechanism of HFOs-AK on attenuating muscle damage needs further study. More importantly, the efficacy and potential side effects of long-term use of HFOs-AK need to study in our follow-up experiments.

Author Contributions: S.-Y.M. and S.-K.S.: data curation, investigation, validation, and writing —original draft. Y.-M.W.: investigation and methodology. C.-F.C.: resources, supervision, & writing —review&editing. B.W.: conceptualization, funding acquisition, resources, supervision, & writing —review & editing. All authors have read and agreed to the published version of the manuscript.

Funding: This work was funded by the National Natural Science Foundation of China (No. 82073764), the Ten-thousand Talents Plan of Zhejiang Province (No. 2019R52026), and the Innovation and Entrepreneurship Training Program for College Students of China (No. 202210340034).

Institutional Review Board Statement: Not applicable.

Data Availability Statement: Data are contained within the article.

Conflicts of Interest: The authors declare no conflicts of interest.

Abbreviations

AAA: aromatic amino acids; ALT, alanine aminotransferase; AMPK, adenosine monophosphate activated protein kinase; ARE, antioxidant response element; AST, aspartate aminotransferase; ANOVA, analysis of variance; AMPK, Adenosine 5′-monophosphate (AMP)-activated protein kinase; BA, blood ammonia; BCAA, branched chain amino acid; BCA, bicinchoninic acid; BG, blood glucose; BUN, blood urea nitrogen; CK, creatine kinase; Da, dalton; ELISA, enzyme-linked immunosorbent assay; ECL, enhanced chemiluminescence; GSH-Px, glutathione peroxidase; HDL-C, high density lipoprotein cholesterol; H&E, hematoxylin-eosin staining; HFOs-AK, high Fischer ratio oligopeptides from Antarctic krill; HO-1, heme oxygenase-1; IκBα, Inhibitor Kappa Bα; LA, lactic acid; LDH, lactate dehydrogenase; LDL-C, low-density lipoprotein cholesterol; LG, liver glycogen; MDA, Malondialdehyde; MG, muscle glycogen; MW, molecular weight; NQO1, NAD(P)H: quinine oxidoreductase 1; Nrf2, nuclear factor erythroid 2-related factor 2; PPARα, peroxisome proliferator-activated receptor-α; PVDF, polyvinylidene difluoride; PGC-α, Peroxisome proliferator-activated receptor-γ coactivator; ROS, reactive oxygen species; SOD, superoxide dismutase; SREBP-1C, sterol regulatory element binding proteins-1c; SDS, Sodium dodecyl sulfate; SD, stable disease; SPSS, Statistical Package for the Social Sciences; SDS-PAGE sodium dodecyl sulfate polyacrylamide gel electrophoresis; TC, total cholesterol; TG, Triglyceride; TNF-α, tumour necrosis factor-α; TBS, Tris buffered saline; TBST, Tris buffered saline with Tween 20.

References

1. Abachi, S.; Offret, C.; Fliss, I.; Marette, A.; Bazinet, L.; Beaulieu, L. Isolation of immunomodulatory biopeptides from Atlantic Mackerel (*Scomber scombrus*) protein hydrolysate based on molecular weight, charge, and hydrophobicity. *Food Bioprocess Technol.* **2022**, *15*, 852–874. [CrossRef]
2. Hu, Y.D.; Xi, Q.H.; Kong, J.; Zhao, Y.Q.; Chi, C.F.; Wang, B. Angiotensin-I-converting enzyme (ACE)-inhibitory peptides from the collagens of monkfish (*Lophius litulon*) swim bladders: Isolation, characterization, molecular docking analysis and activity evaluation. *Mar. Drugs* **2023**, *21*, 516. [CrossRef] [PubMed]
3. Quintal-Bojórquez, N.; Segura-Campos, M.R. Bioactive peptides as therapeutic adjuvants for cancer. *Nutr. Cancer* **2021**, *73*, 1309–1321. [CrossRef] [PubMed]
4. Wang, Y.M.; Zhang, Z.; Sheng, Y.; Chi, C.F.; Wang, B. A systematic review on marine umami peptides: Biological sources, preparation methods, structure-umami relationship, mechanism of action and biological activities. *Food Biosci.* **2024**, *57*, 103637. [CrossRef]
5. Lan, C.; Zhao, Y.Q.; Li, X.R.; Wang, B. High Fischer ratio oligopeptides determination from Antarctic krill: Preparation, peptides profiles, and in vitro antioxidant activity. *J. Food Biochem.* **2019**, *43*, e12827. [CrossRef] [PubMed]
6. Tanabe, S.; Tanimoto, S.Y.; Watanabe, M.; Arai, S. Nutritional effects of an oligopeptide mixture with a very high Fischer ratio on the amino acid absorption and cerebral amine metabolism in rats suffering from galactosamine-induced liver injury. *Agric. Biol. Chem.* **1991**, *55*, 2585–2590.
7. Wang, Z.G.; Ying, X.G.; Wang, Y.F.; Yu, X.W.; Luo, H.Y. Structural analysis and activity evaluation of high Fischer ratio oligopeptides from minced meat of skipjack (*Katsuwonus pelamis*). *J. Aquat. Food Prod. Technol.* **2019**, *28*, 1063–1075. [CrossRef]
8. Wang, L.; Sun, J.; Ding, S.; Qi, B. Isolation and identification of novel antioxidant and antimicrobial oligopeptides from enzymatically hydrolyzed anchovy fish meal. *Process Biochem.* **2018**, *74*, 148–155. [CrossRef]
9. Niu, R.; Feng, W. Research progress of phenylketonuria and its relevavent treatment. *Chin. New Drugs J.* **2018**, *27*, 154–158.
10. Liu, R.; Li, Z.; Yu, X.-C.; Hu, J.-N.; Zhu, N.; Liu, X.-R.; Hao, Y.-T.; Kang, J.-W.; Li, Y. The effects of peanut oligopeptides on exercise-induced fatigue in mice and its underlying mechanism. *Nutrients* **2023**, *15*, 1743. [CrossRef]
11. Li, D.; Ren, J.-W.; Xu, T.; Li, L.; Liu, P.; Li, Y. Effect of bovine bone collagen oligopeptides on wound healing in mice. *Aging* **2021**, *13*, 9028. [CrossRef] [PubMed]
12. Zheng, S.L.; Wang, Y.Z.; Zhao, Y.Q.; Chi, C.F.; Zhu, W.Y.; Wang, B. High Fischer ratio oligopeptides from hard-shelled mussel: Preparation and hepatoprotective effect against acetaminophen-induced liver injury in mice. *Food Biosci.* **2023**, *53*, 102638. [CrossRef]
13. Zhang, X.; Li, S.; Li, M.; Hemar, Y. Study of the in vitro properties of oligopeptides from whey protein isolate with high Fisher's ratio and their ability to prevent allergic response to β-lactoglobulin in vivo. *Food Chem.* **2023**, *405*, 134841. [CrossRef]
14. Wang, Y.; Song, X.; Feng, Y.; Cui, Q. Changes in peptidomes and Fischer ratios of corn-derived oligopeptides depending on enzyme hydrolysis approaches. *Food Chem.* **2019**, *297*, 124931. [CrossRef]
15. Ying, Z.; Yuyang, H.; Meiying, L.; Bingyu, S.; Linlin, L.; Mingshou, L.; Min, Q.; Huanan, G.; Xiuqing, Z. High Fischer ratio peptide of hemp seed: Preparation and anti-fatigue evaluation in vivo and in vitro. *Food Res. Int.* **2023**, *165*, 112534. [CrossRef] [PubMed]
16. Salma, N.U.; Govindaraju, K.; Kumar, B.S.G.; Muthukumar, S.P.; Lakshmi, A.J. Ameliorative effect of enhanced Fischer ratio flaxseed protein hydrolysate in combination with antioxidant micronutrients on ethanol-induced hepatic damage in a rat model. *Br. J. Nutr.* **2022**, *127*, 696–710. [CrossRef] [PubMed]
17. Zhao, P.; Hou, Y.; Chen, X.; Zhang, M.; Hu, Z.; Chen, L.; Huang, J. High Fischer ratio oligopeptides of gluten alleviate alcohol-induced liver damage by regulating lipid metabolism and oxidative stress in rats. *Foods* **2024**, *13*, 436. [CrossRef]
18. Qin, Y.; Cheng, M.; Fan, X.; Shao, X.; Wang, C.; Jiang, H.; Zhang, X. Preparation and antioxidant activities of high Fischer's ratio oligopeptides from goat whey. *Food Sci. Anim. Resour.* **2022**, *42*, 800. [CrossRef] [PubMed]
19. Zheng, H.; Zhang, C.; Cao, W.; Liu, S.; Ji, H. Preparation and characterisation of the pearl oyster (*Pinctada martensii*) meat protein hydrolysates with a high Fischer ratio. *Int. J. Food Sci. Technol.* **2009**, *44*, 1183–1191. [CrossRef]
20. Xiong, K.; Liu, J.; Wang, X.; Sun, B.; Zhang, Y.; Zhao, Z.; Pei, P.; Li, X. Engineering a carboxypeptidase from *Aspergillus niger* M00988 by mutation to increase its ability in high Fischer ratio oligopeptide preparation. *J. Biotechnol.* **2021**, *330*, 1–8. [CrossRef]
21. Feng, Z.; Wei, Y.; Xu, Y.; Zhang, R.; Li, M.; Qin, H.; Gu, R.; Cai, M. The anti-fatigue activity of corn peptides and their effect on gut bacteria. *J. Sci. Food Agric.* **2022**, *102*, 3456–3466. [CrossRef] [PubMed]
22. Wang, P.; Zeng, H.; Lin, S.; Zhang, Z.; Zhang, Y.; Hu, J. Anti-fatigue activities of hairtail (*Trichiurus lepturus*) hydrolysate in an endurance swimming mice model. *J. Funct. Foods* **2020**, *74*, 104207. [CrossRef]
23. Ye, J.; Shen, C.H.; Huang, Y.Y.; Zhang, X.Q.; Xiao, M.T. Anti-fatigue activity of sea cucumber peptides prepared from *Stichopus japonicus* in an endurance swimming rat model. *J. Sci. Food Agric.* **2017**, *97*, 4548–4556. [CrossRef] [PubMed]
24. Fang, L.; Zhang, R.X.; Wei, Y.; Ling, K.; Lu, L.; Wang, J.; Pan, X.C.; Cai, M.Y. Anti-fatigue effects of fermented soybean protein peptides in mice. *J. Sci. Food Agric.* **2022**, *102*, 2693–2703. [CrossRef]
25. Ge, M.-X.; Chen, R.-P.; Zhang, L.; Wang, Y.-M.; Chi, C.-F.; Wang, B. Novel Ca-chelating peptides from protein hydrolysate of Antarctic krill (*Euphausia superba*): Preparation, characterization, and calcium absorption efficiency in Caco-2 cell monolayer model. *Mar. Drugs* **2023**, *21*, 579. [CrossRef] [PubMed]
26. Li, Y.; Tan, L.; Liu, F.; Li, M.; Zeng, S.; Gui, Y.; Zhao, Y.; Wang, J.J. Effects of soluble Antarctic krill protein-curcumin complex combined with photodynamic inactivation on the storage quality of shrimp. *Food Chem.* **2023**, *403*, 134388. [CrossRef]

27. Wang, Y.Z.; Zhao, Y.Q.; Wang, Y.M.; Zhao, W.H.; Wang, P.; Chi, C.F.; Wang, B. Antioxidant peptides from Antarctic Krill (*Euphausia superba*) hydrolysate: Preparation, identification and cytoprotection on H_2O_2-induced oxidative stress. *J. Funct. Foods* **2021**, *86*, 104701. [CrossRef]
28. Wang, M.; Zhang, L.; Yue, H.; Cai, W.; Yin, H.; Tian, Y.; Dong, P.; Wang, J. Peptides from Antarctic krill (*Euphausia superba*) ameliorate acute liver injury in mice induced by carbon tetrachloride via activating the Nrf2/HO-1 pathway. *Food Funct.* **2023**, *14*, 3526–3537. [CrossRef]
29. Yue, H.; Li, Y.; Cai, W.; Bai, X.; Dong, P.; Wang, J. Antarctic krill peptide alleviates liver fibrosis via downregulating the secondary bile acid mediated NLRP3 signaling pathway. *Food Funct.* **2022**, *13*, 7740–7749. [CrossRef]
30. Zheng, J.; Gao, Y.; Ding, J.; Sun, N.; Lin, S. Antarctic krill peptides improve scopolamine-induced memory impairment in mice. *Food Biosci.* **2022**, *49*, 101987. [CrossRef]
31. Liu, Y.; Lin, S.; Hu, S.; Wang, D.; Yao, H.; Sun, N. Co-administration of Antarctic krill peptide EEEFDATR and calcium shows superior osteogenetic activity. *Food Biosci.* **2022**, *48*, 101728. [CrossRef]
32. Hatanaka, A.; Miyahara, H.; Suzuki, K.I.; Sato, S. Isolation and identification of antihypertensive peptides from Antarctic krill tail meat hydrolysate. *J. Food Sci.* **2009**, *74*, H116–H120. [CrossRef] [PubMed]
33. Li, X.; Zhang, H.; Xu, H. Analysis of chemical components of shiitake polysaccharides and its anti-fatigue effect under vibration. *Int. J. Biol. Macromol.* **2009**, *45*, 377–380. [CrossRef] [PubMed]
34. Glancy, B.; Kane, D.A.; Kavazis, A.N.; Goodwin, M.L.; Willis, W.T.; Gladden, L.B. Mitochondrial lactate metabolism: History and implications for exercise and disease. *J. Physiol.* **2021**, *599*, 863–888. [CrossRef] [PubMed]
35. Zhao, R.; Wu, R.; Jin, J.; Ning, K.; Wang, Z.; Yi, X.; Kapilevich, L.; Liu, J. Signaling pathways regulated by natural active ingredients in the fight against exercise fatigue—A review. *Front. Pharmacol.* **2023**, *14*, 1269878. [CrossRef]
36. Liu, R.; Wu, L.; Du, Q.; Ren, J.W.; Chen, Q.H.; Li, D.; Mao, R.X.; Liu, X.R.; Li, Y. Small molecule oligopeptides isolated from walnut (*Juglans regia* L.) and their anti-fatigue effects in mice. *Molecules* **2018**, *24*, 45. [CrossRef]
37. Zhong, L.; Zhao, L.; Yang, F.; Yang, W.; Sun, Y.; Hu, Q. Evaluation of anti-fatigue property of the extruded product of cereal grains mixed with *Cordyceps militaris* on mice. *J. Int. Soc. Sports Nutr.* **2017**, *14*, 15. [CrossRef]
38. Lu, X.; Chen, J.; Huang, L.; Ou, Y.; Wu, J.; Guo, Z.; Zheng, B. The anti-fatigue effect of glycoprotein from Hairtail fish (*Trichiurus lepturus*) on BALB/c mice. *Foods* **2023**, *12*, 1245. [CrossRef]
39. Yu, Y.; Wu, G.; Jiang, Y.; Li, B.; Feng, C.; Ge, Y.; Le, H.; Jiang, L.; Liu, H.; Shi, Y.; et al. Sea cucumber peptides improved the mitochondrial capacity of mice: A potential mechanism to enhance gluconeogenesis and fat catabolism during exercise for improved antifatigue property. *Oxidative Med. Cell. Longev.* **2020**, *2020*, 4604387. [CrossRef]
40. Kozakowska, M.; Pietraszek-Gremplewicz, K.; Jozkowicz, A.; Dulak, J. The role of oxidative stress in skeletal muscle injury and regeneration: Focus on antioxidant enzymes. *J. Muscle Res. Cell Motil.* **2015**, *36*, 377–393. [CrossRef]
41. Suo, S.K.; Zheng, S.L.; Chi, C.F.; Luo, H.Y.; Wang, B. Novel angiotensin-converting enzyme inhibitory peptides from tuna byproducts-milts: Preparation, characterization, molecular docking study, and antioxidant function on H_2O_2-damaged human umbilical vein endothelial cells. *Front. Nutr.* **2022**, *9*, 957778. [CrossRef] [PubMed]
42. Liu, S.; Wang, M.Y.; Xing, Y.B.; Wang, X.R.; Cui, C.B. Anti-oxidation and anti-fatigue effects of the total flavonoids of *Sedum aizoon* L. *J. Agric. Food Res.* **2023**, *12*, 100560. [CrossRef]
43. Zou, D.; Liu, P.; Chen, K.; Xie, Q.; Liang, X.; Bai, Q.; Zhou, Q.; Liu, K.; Zhang, T.; Zhu, J.; et al. Protective effects of myricetin on acute hypoxia-induced exercise intolerance and mitochondrial impairments in rats. *PLoS ONE* **2015**, *10*, e0124727.
44. Zou, D.; Chen, K.; Liu, P.; Chang, H.; Zhu, J.; Mi, M. Dihydromyricetin improves physical performance under simulated high altitude. *Med. Sci. Sports Exerc.* **2014**, *46*, 2077–2084. [CrossRef]
45. Wang, X.; Qu, Y.; Zhang, Y.; Li, S.; Sun, Y.; Chen, Z.; Teng, L.; Wang, D. Antifatigue potential activity of *Sarcodon imbricatus* in acute excise-treated and chronic fatigue syndrome in mice via regulation of Nrf2-mediated oxidative stress. *Oxidative Med. Cell. Longev.* **2018**, *2018*, 9140896. [CrossRef] [PubMed]
46. Fu, X.; Ji, R.; Dam, J. Antifatigue effect of coenzyme Q10 in mice. *J. Med. Food* **2010**, *13*, 211–215. [CrossRef] [PubMed]
47. Osman, W.N.W.; Mohamed, S. Standardized *Morinda citrifolia* L. and *Morinda elliptica* L. leaf extracts alleviated fatigue by improving glycogen storage and lipid/carbohydrate metabolism. *Phytother. Res.* **2018**, *32*, 2078–2085. [CrossRef] [PubMed]
48. Lee, M.C.; Hsu, Y.J.; Lin, Y.Q.; Chen, L.N.; Chen, M.T.; Huang, C.C. Effects of perch essence supplementation on improving exercise performance and anti-fatigue in mice. *Int. J. Environ. Res. Public Health* **2022**, *19*, 1155. [CrossRef]
49. Falavigna, G.; Junior, J.A.D.A.; Rogero, M.M.; Pires, I.S.D.O.; Pedrosa, R.G.; Junior, E.M.; de Castro, I.A.; Tirapegui, J. Effects of diets supplemented with branched-chain amino acids on the performance and fatigue mechanisms of rats submitted to prolonged physical exercise. *Nutrients* **2012**, *4*, 1767–1780. [CrossRef]
50. Guo, Z.; Lin, D.; Guo, J.; Zhang, Y.; Zheng, B. In vitro antioxidant activity and in vivo anti-fatigue effect of sea horse (*Hippocampus*) peptides. *Molecules* **2017**, *22*, 482. [CrossRef]
51. Lv, J.J.; Liu, Y.; Zeng, X.Y.; Yu, J.; Li, Y.; Du, X.Q.; Wu, Z.B.; Hao, S.L.; Wang, B.C. Anti-fatigue peptides from the enzymatic hydrolysates of *Cervus elaphus* blood. *Molecules* **2021**, *26*, 7614. [CrossRef]
52. Cai, B.; Yi, X.; Wang, Z.; Zhao, X.; Duan, A.; Chen, H.; Wan, P.; Chen, D.; Huang, J.; Pan, J. Anti-fatigue effects and mechanism of *Syngnathus schlegeli* peptides supplementation on exercise-fatigued mice. *J. Funct. Foods* **2023**, *110*, 105846. [CrossRef]
53. Ren, Y.; Wu, H.; Chi, Y.; Deng, R.; He, Q. Structural characterization, erythrocyte protection, and antifatigue effect of antioxidant collagen peptides from tilapia (*Oreochromis nilotica* L.) skin. *Food Funct.* **2020**, *11*, 10149–10160. [CrossRef] [PubMed]

54. Feng, R.; Zou, X.; Wang, K.; Liu, H.; Hong, H.; Luo, Y.; Tan, Y. Antifatigue and microbiome reshaping effects of yak bone collagen peptides on Balb/c mice. *Food Biosci.* **2023**, *52*, 102447. [CrossRef]
55. Wang, X.Q.; Yu, H.H.; Xing, R.G.; Liu, S.; Chen, X.L.; Li, P.C. Structural properties, anti-fatigue and immunological effect of low molecular weight peptide from monkfish. *J. Funct. Foods* **2023**, *105*, 105546. [CrossRef]
56. Ke, R.; Xu, Q.; Li, C.; Luo, L.; Huang, D. Mechanisms of AMPK in the maintenance of ATP balance during energy metabolism. *Cell Biol. Int.* **2018**, *42*, 384–392. [CrossRef] [PubMed]
57. Shrikanth, C.B.; Nandini, C.D. AMPK in microvascular complications of diabetes and the beneficial effects of AMPK activators from plants. *Phytomedicine* **2020**, *73*, 152808. [CrossRef] [PubMed]
58. Zhang, L.; Zhou, Y.; Wu, W.; Hou, L.; Chen, H.; Zuo, B.O.; Xiong, Y.; Yang, J. Skeletal muscle-specific overexpression of PGC-1α induces fiber-type conversion through enhanced mitochondrial respiration and fatty acid oxidation in mice and pigs. *Int. J. Biol. Sci.* **2017**, *13*, 1152. [CrossRef]
59. Cai, W.-W.; Hu, X.-M.; Wang, Y.-M.; Chi, C.-F.; Wang, B. Bioactive peptides from Skipjack tuna cardiac arterial bulbs: Preparation, identification, antioxidant activity, and stability against thermal, pH, and simulated gastrointestinal digestion treatments. *Mar. Drugs* **2022**, *20*, 626. [CrossRef]
60. Duan, F.F.; Guo, Y.; Li, J.W.; Yuan, K. Antifatigue effect of luteolin-6-C-neohesperidoside on oxidative stress injury induced by forced swimming of rats through modulation of Nrf2/ARE signaling pathways. *Oxidative Med. Cell. Longev.* **2017**, 3159358. [CrossRef]
61. Wang, Y.; Zhang, Y.; Hou, M.; Han, W. Anti-fatigue activity of parsley (*Petroselinum crispum*) flavonoids via regulation of oxidative stress and gut microbiota in mice. *J. Funct. Foods* **2022**, *89*, 104963. [CrossRef]
62. Huang, Y.F.; Lu, L.; Zhu, D.J.; Wang, M.; Yin, Y.; Chen, D.X.; Wei, L.B. Effects of astragalus polysaccharides on dysfunction of mitochondrial dynamics induced by oxidative stress. *Oxidative Med. Cell. Longev.* **2016**, 9573291.
63. Zhao, C.; Gong, Y.; Zheng, L.; Zhao, M. Whey protein hydrolysate enhances exercise endurance, regulates energy metabolism, and attenuates muscle damage in exercise mice. *Food Biosci.* **2023**, *52*, 102453. [CrossRef]
64. Zheng, S.L.; Wang, Y.M.; Chi, C.F.; Wang, B. Chemical characterization of honeysuckle polyphenols and their alleviating function on ultraviolet B-damaged HaCaT cells by modulating the Nrf2/NF-κB signaling pathways. *Antioxidants* **2024**, *13*, 294. [CrossRef] [PubMed]

Disclaimer/Publisher's Note: The statements, opinions and data contained in all publications are solely those of the individual author(s) and contributor(s) and not of MDPI and/or the editor(s). MDPI and/or the editor(s) disclaim responsibility for any injury to people or property resulting from any ideas, methods, instructions or products referred to in the content.

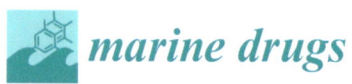 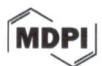

Article

In Silico Identification and Molecular Mechanism of Novel Tyrosinase Inhibitory Peptides Derived from Nacre of *Pinctada martensii*

Fei Li [1], Haisheng Lin [1,2,3,*], Xiaoming Qin [1,2,3], Jialong Gao [1,2,3], Zhongqin Chen [1,2,3], Wenhong Cao [1,2,3], Huina Zheng [1,2,3] and Shaohe Xie [4]

[1] College of Food Science and Technology, National Research and Development Branch Center for Shellfish Processing (Zhanjiang), Guangdong Provincial Key Laboratory of Aquatic Products Processing and Safety, Guangdong Provincial Engineering Technology Research Center of Seafood, Guangdong Province Engineering Laboratory for Marine Biological Products, Guangdong Ocean University, Zhanjiang 524088, China; 2112203055@stu.gdou.edu.cn (F.L.); qinxm@gdou.edu.cn (X.Q.); gaojl@gdou.edu.cn (J.G.); chenzhongqin@gdou.edu.cn (Z.C.); cwenhong@gdou.edu.cn (W.C.); zhenghn@gdou.edu.cn (H.Z.)

[2] Shenzhen Institute of Guangdong Ocean University, Shenzhen 518108, China

[3] Collaborative Innovation Center of Seafood Deep Processing, Dalian Polytechnic University, Dalian 116034, China

[4] Guangdong Shaohe Pearl Co., Ltd., Shantou 515041, China; xsh5760288@126.com

* Correspondence: linhs@gdou.edu.cn

Abstract: Pearl and nacre powders have been valuable traditional Chinese medicines with whitening properties for thousands of years. We utilized a high-temperature and high-pressure method along with compound enzyme digestion to prepare the enzymatic hydrolysates of nacre powder of *Pinctada martensii* (NP-PMH). The peptides were identified using LC–MS/MS and screened through molecular docking and molecular dynamics simulations. The interactions between peptides and tyrosinase were elucidated through enzyme kinetics, circular dichroism spectropolarimetry, and isothermal titration calorimetry. Additionally, their inhibitory effects on B16F10 cells were explored. The results showed that a tyrosinase-inhibitory peptide (Ala-His-Tyr-Tyr-Asp, AHYYD) was identified, which inhibited tyrosinase with an IC_{50} value of 2.012 ± 0.088 mM. The results of the in vitro interactions showed that AHYYD exhibited a mixed-type inhibition of tyrosinase and also led to a more compact enzyme structure. The binding reactions of AHYYD with tyrosinase were spontaneous, leading to the formation of a new set of binding sites on the tyrosinase. The B16F10 cell-whitening assay revealed that AHYYD could reduce the melanin content of the cells by directly inhibiting the activity of intracellular tyrosinase. Additionally, it indirectly affects melanin production by acting as an antioxidant. These results suggest that AHYYD could be widely used as a tyrosinase inhibitor in whitening foods and pharmaceuticals.

Keywords: *Pinctada martensii*; molecular docking; B16F10 cells; melanogenesis; antioxidant

Citation: Li, F.; Lin, H.; Qin, X.; Gao, J.; Chen, Z.; Cao, W.; Zheng, H.; Xie, S. In Silico Identification and Molecular Mechanism of Novel Tyrosinase Inhibitory Peptides Derived from Nacre of *Pinctada martensii*. *Mar. Drugs* 2024, 22, 359. https://doi.org/10.3390/md22080359

Academic Editors: Chang-Feng Chi and Bin Wang

Received: 15 July 2024
Revised: 5 August 2024
Accepted: 5 August 2024
Published: 7 August 2024

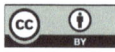

Copyright: © 2024 by the authors. Licensee MDPI, Basel, Switzerland. This article is an open access article distributed under the terms and conditions of the Creative Commons Attribution (CC BY) license (https://creativecommons.org/licenses/by/4.0/).

1. Introduction

Pinctada martensii is found in mainland China and the South China Sea. Its primary use is in pearl production, making it a significant marine cultural shellfish resource in China [1]. Shells and pearls are similar in structure and material composition. Both are biominerals formed under the regulation of an organic matrix secreted by the outer coat membrane tissue [2]. The nacre is secreted by the outer mantle tissue and consists of a lustrous material that gradually envelops the foreign matter to form a pearl over time [3]. The Chinese Pharmacopoeia 2020 stipulates that the source of medicinal pearls is from the pearl shellfish family, which includes pearl shellfish and other bivalves stimulated by the formation of pearls, and it has been recorded to have the effect of calming the mind and nerves, detoxifying the muscles, moisturizing the skin, and removing blemishes [4]. Pearls and nacre are rich sources of calcium, as well as shell proteins, small amounts of trace metals, hydrophobic amino acids, and aromatic amino acids. Calcium constitutes more than 90% of the weight of the pearl and nacre [5]. Studies have indicated that peptides inhibiting tyrosinase typically consist of these amino acids [6]. Therefore, nacre peptides are considered to have the potential of being tyrosinase-inhibiting peptides. Studies have shown that the main components of nacre powder are extremely similar to those of pearl powder and exhibit a variety of biological activities. Sedative-hypnotic [5], anti-photoaging [6], antioxidant [7], trauma repair [8], are some of the functional activities of pearl powder as supported by modern medicine. However, the specific whitening ingredients and mechanisms remain unclear.

Excessive melanin deposition can lead to a range of skin problems. Melanin is a phenolic polymer widely distributed in plants and animals [9]. It is the main factor in determining the color of the skin and hair and can inhibit ultraviolet rays and free radicals that stimulate damage to the skin cells [10]. However, when melanin is over-synthesized, excessive deposition of melanin in the surface layer of the skin may result in a series of skin diseases such as dark spots, brown spots, and further promote skin aging; ultimately, this excessive melanin production could lead to melanoma and other skin cancers. Tyrosinase is a copper-containing metal oxidase and is the key enzyme that regulates melanin production. Tyrosinase oxidizes tyrosine to produce dopamine quinone, which reacts with amino acids or proteins, ultimately resulting in melanin production [11]. Therefore, tyrosinase inhibition and antioxidants are particularly crucial. There are two main ways to inhibit tyrosinase: one involves direct inhibition of tyrosinase, while the other involves indirect regulation of the antioxidant system to inhibit tyrosinase production [12,13]. Currently proven effective whitening ingredients, such as Kojic acid and its derivatives, Resveratrol and Arbutin, have been found to have a stronger inhibitory effect on tyrosinase [14–16]. However, they are also prone to side effects such as skin redness, itching, ulcers, and even toxicity to the body [17,18]. The current whitening products available on the market, while commonly used, still carry a higher risk of causing allergic reactions or other adverse effects on the user's skin [19,20]. Therefore, safe and stable whitening preparations are receiving increasing attention. A large number of by-products, such as shells, are produced during the pearl harvest from the *Pinctada martensii* [21]. The main ways of utilization include decoration, building paint, feed, and other purposes. Shell meat, as well as other tissues, has been the main focus of existing studies, while the active peptides in the inner nacre of the shell have been less studied. Previous studies have shown that peptides extracted from the shell flesh tissues of pearl oysters and their related tissues have demonstrated a variety of biological activities, such as antioxidant [22], anti-photoaging [23], and blood pressure-lowering effects [24]. Zhou et al. simulated gastrointestinal hydrolysis to prepare peptides from the meat of *Pinctada martensii* and verified the antioxidant activity of the peptides using HepG$_2$ cells [22]. A study successfully predicted potential tyrosinase-inhibitory peptides from abalone proteins using an anti-tyrosinase prediction tool [25]. However, there has been limited research on potential whitening peptides within the shell of pearl oysters.

In the present study, peptides derived from the nacre powder of *Pinctada martensii* after undergoing high temperature and pressure treatment. Neutral proteases have been used in the enzymatic digestion of shellfish. To break down the insoluble proteins in the pearl layer, we conducted a combination of neutral proteases and pineapple protease for enzymatic digestion, and then characterized them using LC–MS/MS. The potential tyrosinase-inhibitory peptides were then screened through molecular docking. Subsequently, they were synthesized in solid phase and examined for their tyrosinase-inhibitory mechanism and antioxidant capacity at both in vitro and cellular levels. These findings could contribute to the development of new cosmetic ingredients and natural food-based functional foods.

2. Results and Discussion

2.1. Inhibition of Tyrosinase and Antioxidant Activity of the Enzymatic Hydrolysis Product

A preliminary investigation of tyrosinase activity and antioxidant activity was conducted on the enzymatic hydrolysis product obtained from nacre powder after high-temperature and high-pressure treatment and complex enzymatic digestion. The results, as presented in Table 1, indicate that the nacre peptide digest exhibits a certain inhibitory effect on tyrosinase and possesses antioxidant properties. These findings suggest that it holds promise for the development of tyrosinase-inhibiting peptides.

Table 1. Tyrosinase-inhibitory activity and antioxidant activity of Enzymatic hydrolysis product NP-PMH.

Enzymatic Hydrolysis Product	Tyrosinase Inhibitory Activity (IC_{50}, mg/mL)	DPPH Free Radical Scavenging (1 mg/mL, %)	ABTS Free Radical Scavenging (1 mg/mL, %)
NP-PMH	6.743 ± 0.067	1.139 ± 0.232	85.050 ± 2.770

2.2. Identification and Molecular Docking

The mass spectrometry data were analyzed using the software PEAKS Studio 8.5. The identification results were compared using the UniProt database. For efficient screening, peptides with amino acid residues < 10 and score > 20 were selected to docking with tyrosinase (2Y9X) [26].

Molecular docking is a commonly used method to simulate the way molecules interact with each other and predict their binding modes and affinities using a computerized platform [27]. The method is widely used to probe the binding ability of small molecules interacting with large molecules [28]. A lower intermolecular binding energy indicates better peptide–protein affinity and theoretically more tyrosinase-inhibitory activity of the peptides.

As shown in Table 2, molecular docking of 32 peptides was performed using Autodock vina, and the receptor was tyrosinase [29]. In terms of amino acid composition, hydrophobic amino acids, aromatic ring-containing amino acids, and polar amino acids play a crucial role in protein–ligand interactions [30]. Additionally, the amino acid composition also influences the water solubility of peptides. Taking into account the peptide's GRAVY score < −0.5, amino acid composition, and binding energy, three peptides—AHYYD, KPIWT, and TFSGNYP—were finally selected for the subsequent study. The predicted binding energies of AHYYD, KPIWT, and TFSGNYP were −8.0 kcal/mol, −7.4 kcal/mol, and −7.3 kcal/mol, respectively. Docking binding was slightly lower than the results for peptides extracted from *Atrina pectinata* Mantle, where a lower binding energy indicates a more favorable binding effect [31]. To visually demonstrate how the peptides bind to tyrosinase, a visual analysis was conducted using the Discovery Studio 2019 client tool. As shown in Table 3 and Figure 1, Docking results showed that the peptide formed interactions with residues such as HIS263, ASN260, and VAL283 near the active site pocket of tyrosinase [32]. AHYYD formed four hydrogen bonds with SER282, CYS83, GLU322, and ASN260 of tyrosinase. The bond lengths ranged from 2.10 Å to 3.18 Å. KPIWT formed two hydrogen bonds with MET280 and ASN81 of tyrosinase, with bond lengths of 2.62 Å and 3.36 Å. TFSGNYP formed six hydrogen bonds with ASN81, SER282, GLY281, VAL283, ALA246, and GLY245 of tyrosinase, and the bond lengths ranged from 2.13 to 5.26 Å. The shorter the hydrogen bond, the greater the bond energy, indicating that the ligand and receptor form a more stable bond [26]. In the hydrophobic interactions with tyrosinase, all three peptides form hydrophobic interactions with PRO284 and HIS263. KPIWT and AHYYD form hydrophobic interactions with VAL283. KPIWT and TFSGNYP form hydrophobic interactions with ALA286. On the basis of the amino acid residues where the three peptides form hydrophobic interactions, most of the amino acids they interact with are similar to each other. Due to the similarity of the hydrophobic interactions, we infer that the difference in binding energies is primarily due to variations in hydrogen bonding. Hydrogen bonding is identified as the main driving force.

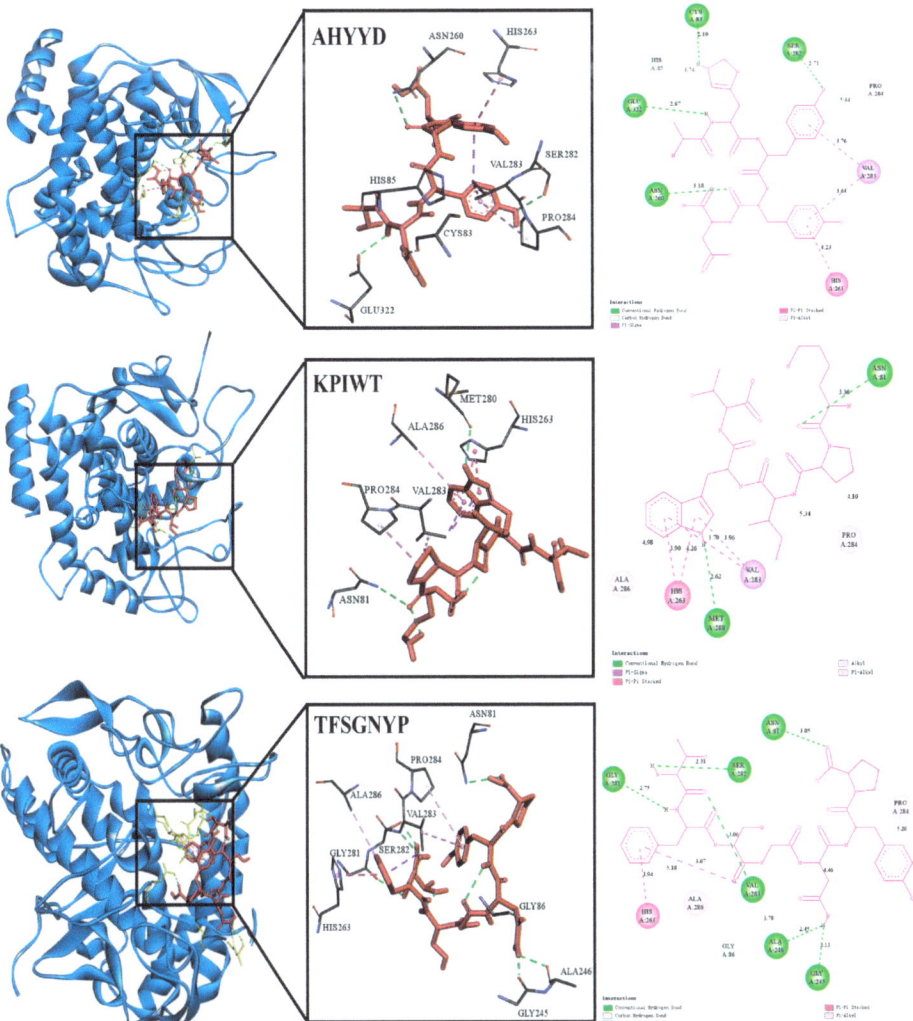

Figure 1. The 3D and 2D visualizations of molecular docking of AHYYD, KPIWT, and TFSGNYP with tyrosinase (2Y9X).

Table 2. Potential tyrosinase-inhibitory peptide sequences: screening by mass spectrometry and molecular docking.

NO.	Sequences	Length	Score	Toxicity	Affinity	Gravy
1	AHYYD	5	27.12	Non	−8.0	−1.5
2	GGFGNW	6	30.94	Non	−7.8	−0.47
3	KPIWT	5	20.49	Non	−7.4	−0.52
4	TFSGNYP	7	21.74	Non	−7.3	−0.79
5	ATFDAI	6	27.86	Non	−7.2	1.12
6	NRIPN	5	25.39	Non	−7.2	−1.72
7	KRSLE	5	21.85	Non	−7.0	−1.78
8	HKDGY	5	26.84	Non	−6.9	−2.46
9	ERHLGY	6	24.12	Non	−6.9	−1.52
10	SIIDEVVA	8	23.32	Non	−6.9	1.43

Table 2. Cont.

NO.	Sequences	Length	Score	Toxicity	Affinity	Gravy
11	KDLFF	5	20.31	Non	−6.9	0.4
12	GHSLTQF	7	35.06	Non	−6.8	−0.29
13	FGSLSF	6	24.8	Non	−6.8	1.23
14	GGSFSVR	7	26	Non	−6.8	0.01
15	TNNFT	5	20.4	Non	−6.7	−1.12
16	LPEEV	5	23	Non	−6.7	−0.12
17	SASTTLEE	8	22.84	Non	−6.6	−0.55
18	VTANPANT	8	21	Non	−6.6	−0.28
19	HSSAHS	6	20.36	Non	−6.5	−1.17
20	TNTSNP	6	23.65	Non	−6.5	−1.8
21	SDLGGI	6	21.62	Non	−6.5	0.53
22	MVSLEG	6	20.69	Non	−6.5	0.87
23	LKGHEDL	7	20.01	Non	−6.4	−0.99
24	SIDLYK	6	20.7	Non	−6.4	−0.2
25	MDLSHA	6	21.73	Non	−6.3	0
26	DYQLP	5	21.75	Non	−6.2	−1.22
27	KEMQGG	6	20.62	Non	−6.2	−1.63
28	HTLESKPNPD	10	22.99	Non	−5.9	−1.85
29	KEPNK	5	20.77	Non	−5.9	−3.28
30	TDIIDG	6	24.25	Non	−5.8	0.15
31	KKQLM	5	20.39	Non	−5.8	−1.12
32	MQVTPASA	8	22.86	Non	−5.8	0.39

Table 3. Molecular docking sites of AHYYD, KPIWT, and TFSGNYP with tyrosinase (2Y9X).

Peptides	Hydrogen Bonds	Hydrophobic Interaction	Electrostatic Interaction
AHYYD	Ser282,Cys83 Glu322,Asn260	Val283,Pro284,His263	
KPIWT	Met280,Asn81	Ala286,His263Val283,Pro284	
TFSGNYP	Asn81,Ser282,Gly281,Val283,Ala246,Gly245	His263,Ala286,Pro284	

2.3. Molecular Dynamics Simulation

The stability and binding affinity between tyrosinase and the three small molecules were further investigated using the GROMACS program, with the three complex docked systems as the initial structure. The 100 ns molecular dynamics (MD) simulation method was used to obtain stable complex systems for further comparison of the three small molecules at the molecular level. The trajectory data obtained from the 100 ns were analyzed to derive the kinetic properties of the three complexes. Root mean square deviation (RMSD), radius of gyration (Rg), solvent accessible surface area (SASA), root mean square fluctuation (RMSF), and Hbond number were utilized to assess each system in the MD study, and the results are presented. As shown in Figure 2, a graph of each parameter of the dynamics is plotted.

Root mean square deviation (RMSD) is a metric used to assess structural changes in proteins [33]. The results show that the RMSD between proteins and small molecules is large in the first 30 ns of the simulation. Tyrosinase with AHYYD stabilizes the fastest, the RMSD value remains within a small range, indicating that the binding of proteins to small molecules is relatively stable. Root mean square fluctuation (RMSF) is a metric used to assess the dynamics of proteins [34]. The results show that the residues in the key regions increase in flexibility, and the RMSF values are larger in the binding portion in the 300–400 region. Tyrosinase with AHYYD and tyrosinase with TFSGNYP were more variable. The RMSF of tyrosinase with AHYYD reaches a maximum value of 0.5 nm, while it is smaller in the unbound portion. The RMSF values are all below 1 Å. The minimal fluctuation indicates that these atoms create stable complexes with tyrosinase because of robust intermolecular interactions, restricting their movement in molecular dynamics simulations [35]. Gyrate is an indicator of the overall compactness of a protein and characterizes the distribution of system atoms along a specific axis [28]. The results indicate that after the binding of the protein with the three small molecules, the gyrate value of tyrosinase with AHYYD tends to stabilize after 20 ns, while the gyrate value of tyrosinase with TFSGNYP tends to decrease after 60 ns. This suggests that the binding of small molecules leads to a more compact protein structure. KPIWT, on the other hand, kept fluctuating within a small range repeatedly. SASA is a metric used to assess the surface area of proteins. The results indicate that the amplitude of the tyrosinase with AHYYD curve fluctuates slightly between 170 and 180 and then decreases slightly. This suggests that protein–protein interactions have little effect on the stability of protein molecules. The amplitudes of the tyrosinase with TFSGNYP and tyrosinase with KPIWT curves are similar, but they exhibit opposite trends. The SASA value of tyrosinase with TFSGNYP shows a decreasing trend after 60 ns, indicating that the binding of small molecules causes the protein molecule to become more compact, aligning with the results of gyrate analysis. A hydrogen bond is a metric used to assess hydrogen bonding between proteins and small molecules. The results show that many hydrogen bonds are formed between proteins and small molecules during the simulation. These bonds are dominated by interactions between key residues in tyrosinase and peptides in the molecular docking results.

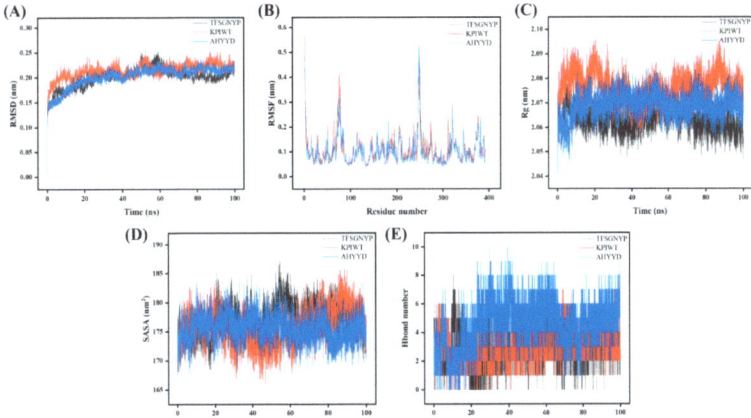

Figure 2. Molecular dynamics results of tyrosinase with AHYYD, KPIWT, and TFSGNYP. (**A**) RMSD; (**B**) RMSF; (**C**) Rg; (**D**) SASA; (**E**) Hbond number.

Analyzing the RMSD, RMSF, Gyrate, SASA, and Hbond number results of the three peptide–enzyme complexes mentioned above, it can be concluded that AHYYD and TF-SGNYP interact with tyrosinase more effectively than KPIWT, protein–small molecule interaction appears stable, and the binding of small molecules leads to a more compact protein structure.

2.4. Tyrosinase-Inhibitory Activity and Antioxidant Capacity of Synthetic Peptides

In terms of amino acid composition, AHYYD contains two repetitive benzene-ring-containing amino acid residues, Tyr, and a hydrophobic amino acid, Ala. It has been shown that the repetitive amino acid sequence enhances tyrosinase inhibition [36]. TFSGNYP contains the polar amino acid Ser, a benzene-ring-containing amino acid residue, Phe, and a hydrophobic amino acid, Pro. KPIWT has the benzene-ring-containing amino acid residue Trp and the hydrophobic amino acid Pro. It has been reported that hydrophobic amino acids, benzene-ring-containing amino acid residues, and polar amino acids contribute to tyrosinase inhibition. As shown in Table 4, the synthetic peptides AHYYD, KPIWT, and TFSGNYP derived from *Pinctada martensii* exhibited varying degrees of inhibitory activity against tyrosinase, with Kojic acid serving as a positive control. From the molecular docking visualization results, it can be seen that although the hydrophobic interactions between the three peptides and the enzyme are relatively similar, their distinct hydrogen-bonding interactions may affect the inhibition of tyrosinase activity in vitro. Among these, AHYYD demonstrated a significant inhibitory effect, its IC_{50} value is 2.012 ± 0.088 mM, consistent with the findings of molecular docking screening; this result is similar to the peptides activity identified in the mantle of *Atrina pectinata* [31].

Table 4. Effects of AHYYD, TFSGNYP, KPIWT, and positive control Kojic acid on tyrosinase activity.

Samples	IC_{50} (mM)
AHYYD	2.012 ± 0.088
TFSGNYP	>5
KPIWT	>10
Kojic acid	0.01 ± 0.003

As depicted in Figure 3, there was no significant difference in DPPH clearance between AHYYD and TFSGNYP at any of the five concentrations ($p > 0.05$). However, KPIWT showed a significant difference from both AHYYD and TFSGNYP at concentrations of 0.1–2 mg/mL; AHYYD and TFSGNYP exhibited a stronger DPPH clearance effect than KPIWT ($p < 0.05$) at the corresponding concentrations. There was no significant difference in the clearance of DPPH by the three peptides at a concentration of 4 mg/mL. The IC_{50} values for ABTS clearance by AHYYD, KPIWT, and TFSGNYP were 1.416 mg/mL, 0.7955 mg/mL, and 0.2785 mg/mL, respectively, with a significant difference between the three peptides ($p < 0.05$). A smaller IC_{50} value indicates a better scavenging effect. It can be observed that TFSGNYP exhibits the strongest scavenging ability for ABTS radicals, followed by KPIWT and AHYYD. Vitamin C (Vc) was utilized as a positive control.

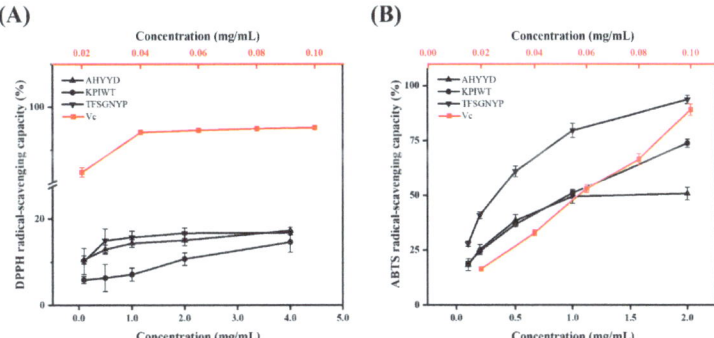

Figure 3. Scavenging capacity of peptides for DPPH free radicals (**A**); Scavenging capacity of peptides for ABTS free radicals (**B**).

2.5. Inhibition Dynamics Analysis

Based on the observation that the inhibition of tyrosinase by the synthetic peptide AHYYD was reversible, the type of inhibition was further elucidated by constructing a Lineweaver–Burk double inverse plot of the enzymatic reaction rate against the concentration of the substrate (L-tyrosine). In this plot, the intercept with the Y-axis represents 1/Vmax, while the intercept with the X-axis represents $-1/K_m$. As depicted in Figure 4, when the concentration of tyrosinase, the concentration of synthetic peptide (0, 0.3, 0.6, 1.2 mM, respectively), and the concentration of substrate L-tyrosine remained constant, the reciprocal of the enzymatic reaction rate exhibited a linear correlation with the reciprocal of the substrate concentration. The slope of the line increased with the rise in synthetic peptide concentration, indicating a mixed type of inhibition [37]. By using the quadratic plotting method, the slopes of the four straight lines in the Lineweaver–Burk double inverse plot were plotted against the synthetic peptide concentration [38]. The inhibition constants of AHYYD on the free enzyme were calculated as K_i = 0.601 mmol/L, and as K_{is} = 38.375 mmol/L on the enzyme–substrate complex. The smaller the inhibition constants, the higher the binding affinity of the inhibitor to the enzyme, $K_i \ll K_{is}$ indicates that AHYYD clearly favors the binding site with the free enzyme.

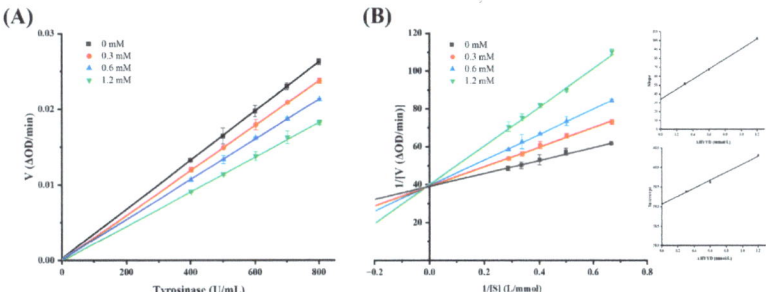

Figure 4. (**A**) Plots of enzymatic reaction rate versus tyrosinase concentration. (**B**) Plots of Lineweaver–Burk; the secondary plots of slope and Y-intercept versus concentration of AHYYD are shown in the inset.

2.6. CD Spectra Analysis

CD spectroscopy is a precise method used to study the secondary structure of biomolecules, including proteins. It allows for the rapid analysis of protein conformational changes caused by the addition of ligands [39]. The addition of AHYYD caused changes in the secondary structure of tyrosinase (Figure 5). In the spectrum of free tyrosinase, there are two negative bands near 208 nm and 222 nm, which are characteristic peaks of the α-helical structure in the secondary structure [40]. The content of α-helix, β-folding, and β-turning increased from 32.53%, 16.27%, and 18.20% to 36.8%, 23.77%, and 21.93% and the random coil content decreased from 30.83% to 18.33%, respectively. The rise in the α-helix content suggests that the interaction between the peptide and tyrosinase caused the tyrosinase structure to become more compact. This finding contrasts with the interaction between tretinoin and tyrosinase, suggesting that it leads to a change in the tyrosinase conformation to some extent [37].

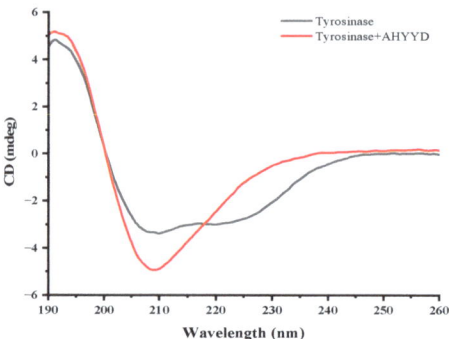

Figure 5. The CD spectra of tyrosinase in the absence and presence of AHYYD. c (tyrosinase) = 0.4 mg/mL, and c (AHYYD) = 0.6 mM.

2.7. Isothermal Titration Calorimetry Analysis

ITC can measure the binding strength of protein–protein interactions by quantifying the thermodynamic changes in complex reactions [41]. The titration of tyrosinase by AHYYD exhibited significant heat changes, indicating binding (Figure 6). The data were analyzed using the independent model, and the thermodynamic binding parameters were calculated. The results showed that the enthalpy (ΔH) was -7.282 kJ/mol, the binding constant (Ka) was 2.495×10^4 M^{-1}, the entropy change (ΔS) was 60.7 J/mol·K, and the standard free energy change (ΔG) was -1.883×10^4 kJ/mol. Negative values of ΔG indicate that the bimolecular reaction is spontaneous. The change in enthalpy indicates that the process is essentially exothermic, which is consistent with the findings of Yu et al [34]. The titration curves are more consistent with the "one set of binding sites" model [42]. The mechanism of inhibition categorizes AHYYD as competitive inhibition, indicating that AHYYD binds to the active site of tyrosinase. This finding further confirms the proposed mechanism of inhibition based on inhibition kinetics.

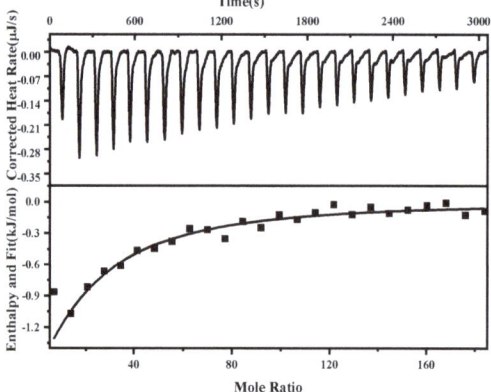

Figure 6. Interaction of AHYYD with tyrosinase studied by ITC at 37 °C showed the thermogram and binding isotherm (tyrosinase) = 0.001 mM, and c (AHYYD) = 1 mM.

2.8. Study on the Whitening Effect of Peptides Based on B16F10 Cells

2.8.1. Cell Viability

As depicted in Figure 7A, there was no significant difference in the viability of B16F10 cells within the concentration range of 15–1200 μM concentration of the synthetic peptide AHYYD compared to the control group ($p > 0.05$). This suggests that the synthetic peptide AHYYD did not exhibit any cytotoxic effects. Consequently, the concentrations of 15, 37.5, and 75 μM were chosen for the subsequent experiments.

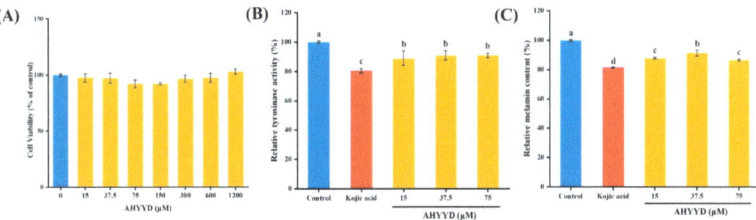

Figure 7. (**A**) Effects of AHYYD on cell viability. (**B**) Effects of AHYYD and Kojic acid on tyrosinase activity in B16F10 cells. (**C**) Effects of AHYYD and Kojic acid on melanin production in B16F10 cells. c (Kojic acid) = 350 μM. Different letters indicate that there are significant differences in data ($p < 0.05$).

2.8.2. Effect of AHYYD on the Tyrosinase Activity and Melanin Content of B16F10 Cells

As shown in Figure 7B,C, compared with the control group, AHYYD significantly inhibited the tyrosinase activity of B16F10 cells in the concentration range of 15–75 μM ($p < 0.05$). Additionally, the intracellular melanin content was significantly reduced by AHYYD in the concentration range of 15–75 μM ($p < 0.05$). The trend in tyrosinase activity and melanin content mirrored that of the peptides extracted from pearl shell meat [26]. At the maximum treatment concentration, the intracellular tyrosinase activity and melanin content were reduced by 9.08% and 13.48%, respectively. Kojic acid caused a reduction of 19.51% in tyrosinase activity and 18.54% in melanin content.

2.8.3. Effect of AHYYD on the Antioxidant Enzyme Activity and ROS Content of B16F10 Cells

SOD, CAT, and GSH-Px are antioxidant enzymes that collaborate to regulate antioxidant processes and safeguard cells from oxidative stress damage [43]. As can be seen from Figure 8, the activities of GSH-Px and SOD enzymes exhibited a concentration-dependent relationship with increasing concentrations of AHYYD. The activities of CAT, GSH-Px, and SOD increased by 73.05%, 139.08%, and 41.25%, respectively, under the maximum treatment concentration, and by 24.55%, 52.85%, and 68.92%, respectively. At the maximum treatment concentration, the CAT and GSH-Px activities were superior ($p < 0.05$) compared to Kojic acid. However, both of them were still far away from Kojic acid in terms of SOD activity ($p < 0.05$). Therefore, AHYYD exhibited a protective effect on the antioxidant system by enhancing the activity of antioxidant enzymes in B16F10 cells, thereby preventing melanin production. Reactive oxygen species (ROS) serve as a crucial indicator of antioxidant connectivity in the organism. As shown in Figure 8G, at a concentration of 75 μM, the intracellular ROS levels were reduced to 52.61% and 65.44% of the untreated group after AHYYD and tretinoin treatment, respectively.

GSH, GSSG, and MDA are crucial metabolic regulators in the cell [44]. GSH helps maintain normal immune system function and has antioxidant effects. It exists in two forms: reduced glutathione (GSH) and oxidized glutathione (GSSG). MDA content is a significant parameter that reflects the body's antioxidant potential, indicating the rate and intensity of lipid peroxidation and indirectly reflecting the extent of tissue peroxidation damage. Under the maximum treatment concentration, the content of GSH increased by 44.07%, while the content of GSSG and MDA decreased by 52.86% and 56.56%, respectively. These changes were not significantly different from those observed in the positive control group treated with Kojic acid ($p > 0.05$). This suggests that AHYYD demonstrates a superior ability in regulating GSH, GSSG, and MDA levels. Along with the antioxidant enzymes mentioned above, it effectively protects B16F10 cells from oxidative damage.

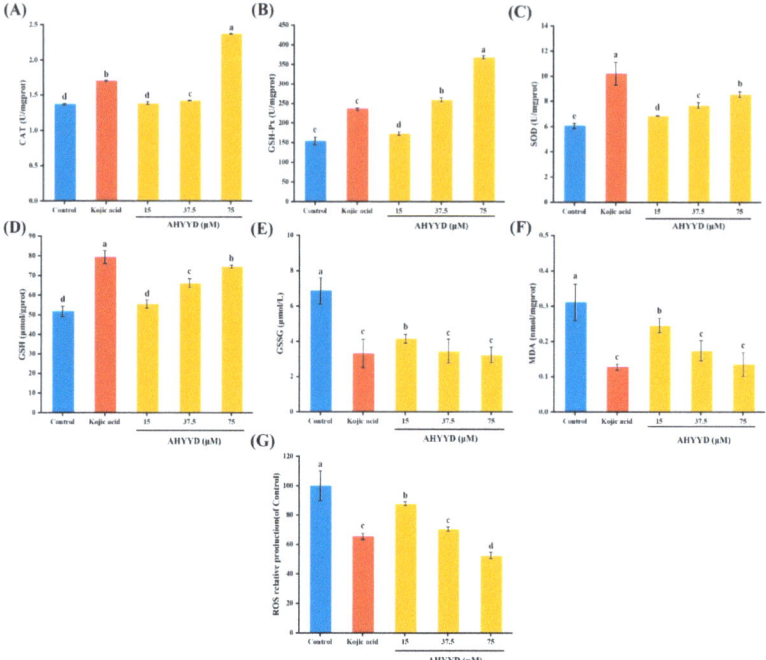

Figure 8. Effect of AHYYD on the intracellular antioxidant capacity in B16F10 cells; (**A**) CAT; (**B**) GSH-Px; (**C**) SOD; (**D**) GSH; (**E**) GSSG; (**F**) MDA; (**G**) ROS. c (Kojic acid) = 350 μM. Different letters indicate that there are significant differences in data ($p < 0.05$).

3. Materials and Methods

3.1. Materials

The nacre powder of the *Pinctada martensii* was purchased from Guangdong Shaohe Pearl Co., Ltd. (Shantou, China). The tyrosinase (from Mushroom, 500 U/mg) and PBS buffer were purchased from Shanghai Yuanye Biotechnology Co., Ltd. (Shanghai, China). The L-tyrosine was obtained from Shanghai Macklin Biochemical Technology Co., Ltd. (Shanghai, China). The fetal bovine serum (FBS) was purchased from Serana Europe GmbH (Dorfstrasse 17A, Pessin, Brandenburg, Germany), and the penicillin–streptomycin mixture was purchased from Beijing Soleberg Biotechnology Co., Ltd. (Beijing, China). The DMEM/F−12 medium and trypsin-EDTA digest were purchased from Thermo Fisher Scientific (Shanghai, China).

3.2. Preparation of Enzymatic Digests of Nacre Peptides

A total of 50 g of nacre powder from *Pinctada martensii* was dissolved in 250 mL ($v:w$ = 5:1) of water and heated at high temperature (121 °C) and pressure for 20 min. Then, 0.1250 g of pineapple protease (0.25% by mass of nacre powder) and 0.2500 g of neutral protease (0.5% by mass of nacre powder) were added to the pre-treated nacre powder solution, and the enzyme digestion was conducted at a temperature of 50 °C for 4 h. Finally, the mixture was heated at 100 °C for 20 min. The supernatant was centrifuged at 8000 rpm for 20 min at 4 °C to obtain the pearl peptide solution after vacuum concentration.

3.3. Tyrosinase-Inhibitory Activity and Antioxidant Activity Assay of Enzyme Digests

We followed the method of Yu [37], with a slight modification. L-tyrosine solution (0.5 mg/mL), sample solution, and PBS buffer were sequentially added into the 96-well plate, thoroughly mixed, and then incubated at 37 °C for 10 min, then 20 µL of tyrosinase solution (500 U/mL) was added into each well, followed by immediate placement into the enzyme marker after the reaction at 37 °C for (10 min ± 5 s). The results were analyzed at 475 nm. DPPH and ABTS free-radical-scavenging capacity assays were conducted using kits from Grace Biotechnology Co., Ltd. (Jiangsu, China).

$$\text{Tyrosinase inhibition rate\%} = \left(1 - \frac{A_4 - A_3}{A_2 - A_1}\right) \times 100\% \quad (1)$$

where A_4 is the absorption value of the reaction well, A_3 is the absorption value of the Sample Background well, A_2 is the absorption value of the Solvent reaction well, and A_1 is the absorption value of the Solvent base well.

3.4. Protein Sequence Identification

The amino acid sequence was identified by using the Bio-Tech Pack Technology Co. (Beijing, China). The nacre peptides were reduced and alkylated separately as samples, an Easy-nLC 1200 system coupled with a Q Exactive™ Hybrid Quadrupole-Orbitrap™ Mass Spectrometer (Thermo Fisher Scientific, Waltham, MA, USA) with an ESI nanospray source. Then, they were analyzed by liquid chromatography–mass spectrometry (LC–MS/MS) to generate a raw file of the mass spectrometry results. The total ion chromatograms were obtained using Xcalibur 4.0 software. The mass spectrometry data were analyzed using the software PEAKS Studio 8.5, and the identification results were compared with the UniProt database.

3.5. Molecular Docking Studies

Studying the peptides and tyrosinase using molecular docking methods, we referred to the method of Wang [31]. The ligands and proteins required for molecular docking were prepared using AutoDock Vina 1.1.2 software. Tyrosinase (PDB: 2Y9X) was utilized as the receptor, and a peptide was employed as the ligand. The peptides were designed using ChemDraw and energy-minimized using Chem3D. The crystal structure of the target protein was obtained from the PDB database (https://www.rcsb.org/structure/2Y9X, accessed on 25 November 2023). Autodock Vina 1.1.2 software was used to perform molecular docking with default parameters to calculate the binding energy of the peptide sequence to the enzyme. The binding-free energy (kcal/mol) of the target structure represents the binding ability of the two molecules, and the lower the binding-free energy, the more stable the binding between the ligand and the receptor. Pymol (https://pymol.org/2/, accessed on 3 December 2023) was used for visual analysis, while Discovery Studio 2019 was utilized for further exploration. Discovery Studio 2019 (https://www.3ds.com/products/biovia/discovery-studio/visualization, accessed on 3 December 2023) was used for visual analysis of the 2D images. The tyrosinase docking centers were X = −10.09, Y = −28.03, and Z = −43.14.

3.6. Molecular Dynamics Simulations

GROMACS 2022.3 software was used for the molecular dynamics simulation [45,46]. For small molecule preprocessing, AmberTools22 was employed to apply the GAFF force field to small molecules, while Gaussian 16W was used for hydrogenating small molecules and calculating the RESP potential. Potential data will be added to the topology file of molecular dynamics system. Following the completion of the simulation, the software's built-in tool was utilized to analyze the trajectory. The root mean square variance (RMSD), root mean square fluctuation (RMSF), solvent accessible surface area (SASA), radius of gyration (Rg), and hydrogen bond were calculated for each amino acid trajectory.

3.7. Peptides Synthesis

The peptide was obtained through solid-phase synthesis and synthesized by Aminolink Biotechnology Co., Ltd. (Shanghai, China). Three peptides with purity above 98% (w/w) were detected by HPLC: Ala-His-Tyr-Tyr-Asp (AHYYD), Thr-Phe-Ser-Gly-Asn-Tyr-Pro (TFSGNYP), and Lys-Pro-Ile-Trp-Thr (KPIWT). Mobile phase A, 0.1% trifluoroacetic in 100% water; mobile phase B, 0.1% trifluoroacetic in 100% acetonitrile; flow rate, 1 mL/min; column, Inertsil ODS-SP (4.6 × 250 mm × 5 μm), with a detection wavelength of 220 nm. Eventually, the purified peptides were identified by ESI–MS spectroscopy.

3.8. Determination of Inhibition Type

Keeping the L-tyrosine concentration constant at 0.5 mg/mL, the concentrations of the synthetic peptide and tyrosinase were varied. The change in the OD_{475} absorbance value was continuously monitored at 37 °C after mixing. The enzyme concentration is plotted on the horizontal axis, while the rate of absorbance change is plotted on the vertical axis. Under the conditions of varying the peptide concentration and substrate concentration while keeping the tyrosinase solution constant, the reciprocal of the substrate concentration was plotted on the horizontal axis, and the reciprocal of the rate of absorbance change was plotted on the vertical ax.

3.9. CD Measurements

We used circular dichroism to study peptide–enzyme interactions, referring to the method of Yu [47]. The concentration of AHYYD was 0.6 mM, and the concentration of tyrosinase was 0.4 mg/mL. The reaction system comprised 100 μL of tyrosinase solution mixed with 20 μL of AHYYD solution, which reacted for over 30 min at 37 °C. All data were collected three times. The changes in the secondary structure were analyzed using CDNN 2.1 software.

3.10. Isothermal Titration Calorimetry Analysis

Peptide (1 mM) was used to titrate tyrosinase (0.001 mM) to study thermodynamic changes. The initial volume of the peptide solution for titration was 50 μL (inhaled into the syringe); the initial volume of the tyrosinase solution for titration was 300 μL (added to the cuvette). The reaction conditions included adding 25 drops of 2 μL each with a 120 s interval between drops at 37 °C and a stirring speed of 350 r/min; the experimental group involved titrating the peptide with tyrosinase, while the control group involved titrating the peptide with a solvent buffer. We calculated the binding constant (Ka), enthalpy change (ΔH), and entropy change (ΔS) during the Gibbs free energy (ΔG) changes [39].

$$\Delta G = \Delta H - T \cdot \Delta S \qquad (2)$$

3.11. Cytotoxicity of AHYYD to B16F10 Cells

The B16F10 cells were obtained from FengHui Biotechnology Co., Ltd. (Hunan, China). B16F10 cell cultures from generations 10–25 were grown in medium (DMEM supplemented with 10% fetal bovine serum, 1% antibiotic–antifungal solution) in a 5% CO_2 incubator at 37 °C.

Cell viability was assessed using the Cell Counting Kit-8 (CCK-8) assay. During the logarithmic growth phase, 100 μL of cell suspension was dispensed into 96-well plates, with 3000 cells per well, and the supernatant was removed after incubation at 37 °C for 24 h. Wells containing 100 μL of medium served as blank controls. Determination of viability after 48 h of sample treatment.

3.12. Effect of AHYYD on Melanin and Tyrosinase Synthesis in B16F10 Melanoma Cells

The cells in the logarithmic growth phase were seeded at a density of 2×10^5 cells per well in 6-well plates. After 24 h of culture, the supernatant was removed. The control group, positive control group for Kojic acid (350 μM) [48], and peptide-treated groups

(15, 37.5, 75 µM) were established. After 48 h of incubation, the cells were lysed, and the cell lysates were centrifuged at 12,000 rpm for 10 min. The reaction mixture consisted of 50 µL of cell lysate supernatant, 50 µL of 1 mg/mL L-DOPA, and 50 µL of PBS buffer. The mixture was incubated at 37 °C for 1 h. The dopamine formation level was then measured spectrophotometrically at 475 nm. Tyrosinase activity was expressed as a percentage of the blank control [49].

The cell culture stage for melanin content determination was as follows: the cells were washed twice with PBS buffer after 48 h of peptide treatment. Trypsin digestion was performed, and the cells were collected. The lower precipitate was removed by centrifugation for 5 min and the precipitate was lysed by dissolving it in 1 mol/L NaOH containing 10% DMSO for 1 h at 80 °C. Subsequently, the cell lysate was centrifuged at 12,000 rpm for 10 min. A total of 200 µL of the supernatant was transferred to a 96-well plate, and the absorbance was measured at 405 nm. The melanin content was then expressed as a percentage of the control group [49].

3.13. Effect of AHYYD on Antioxidant Enzyme Activity and ROS in B16F10 Cells

The cell culture and treatment methods were the same as those described in Section 3.12. The activities of catalase (CAT), glutathione peroxidase (GSH-Px), and superoxide dismutase (SOD) were determined using the assay kit from Nanjing Jianjian Bioengineering Research Institute (Nanjing, China). The ROS content was determined using the method provided by Biyuntian Bio-Technology Company Limited (Shanghai, China).

3.14. Statistical Analysis

All data are expressed as the mean ± standard deviation (SD) of at least three different experiments. Multiple group comparisons were conducted using one-way analysis of variance (ANOVA) and Duncan's multiple-range test in IBM SPSS Statistics 27. A *p*-value less than 0.05 was considered statistically significant. The molecular docking was performed using AutoDock Vina, and the molecular dynamics simulations were performed by GROMACS 2022.3. The graphical abstracts were created using Figdraw 2.0.

4. Conclusions

In the present study, we found that peptides derived from the nacre powder of the *Pinctada martensii* exhibit significant potential for inhibiting tyrosinase. The inhibitory peptide AHYYD was identified from nacre powder peptide by LC–MS/MS and molecular docking screening. It exhibited tyrosinase inhibition with an IC_{50} value of 2.012 ± 0.088 mM. Inhibition kinetics and isothermal titration results showed that AHYYD was a reversible competitive inhibitor. Molecular docking and molecular dynamics simulations indicated that AHYYD had a strong binding affinity, with a binding energy of −8.0 kcal/mol. The effects of AHYYD on tyrosinase activity, melanin production, and antioxidant enzyme activities were investigated in mouse B16F10 melanoma cells. The results showed that AHYYD significantly inhibited intracellular tyrosinase activity and melanin content, and had a positive effect on the intracellular antioxidant enzyme system. It can be concluded that the peptide AHYYD extracted from *Pinctada martensii* has good therapeutic efficacy. This can be further confirmed through animal experiments and utilized for the development of food or cosmetic products.

Author Contributions: Conceptualization, F.L.; methodology, F.L. and H.L.; software, validation, and formal analysis, F.L. and H.L.; investigation, F.L. and H.L.; resources, H.L. and S.X.; data curation and writing—original draft preparation, F.L. and H.L.; writing—review and editing, X.Q., J.G., Z.C., W.C. and H.Z.; visualization, F.L.; supervision, project administration, and funding acquisition, H.L., X.Q., H.Z. and S.X. All authors have read and agreed to the published version of the manuscript.

Funding: This work was supported by the earmarked fund for China Agriculture Research System (CARS-49), Doctoral Startup Project of Guangdong Ocean University (R17082), the Guangdong Province Modern Agricultural Industry Technology System Innovation Team Construction Project

(Grant No. 2023KJ146), the Innovative Team Program of High Education of Guangdong Province (2021KCXTD021).

Data Availability Statement: The data shown in this study are contained within the article.

Conflicts of Interest: Shaohe Xie is employed by Guangdong Shaohe Pearl Co., Ltd., and the other authors declare that there are no potential conflicts of interest. Guangdong Shaohe Pearl Co., Ltd. has no role in the study design, collection, analysis, interpretation of data, the writing of this article or the decision to submit it for publication.

References

1. Deng, Z.; Sun, J.; Wei, H.; Zhao, W.; Chen, M.; Li, Y.; Yu, G.; Wang, Y. Shell colors and microstructures of four pearl oyster species in the South China Sea. *Aquac. Rep.* **2022**, *25*, 101214. [CrossRef]
2. Marie, B.; Joubert, C.; Tayale, A.; Zanella-Cleon, I.; Belliard, C.; Piquemal, D.; Cochennec-Laureau, N.; Marin, F.; Gueguen, Y.; Montagnani, C. Different secretory repertoires control the biomineralization processes of prism and nacre deposition of the pearl oyster shell. *Proc. Natl. Acad. Sci. USA* **2012**, *109*, 20986–20991. [CrossRef] [PubMed]
3. Mariom; Take, S.; Igarashi, Y.; Yoshitake, K.; Asakawa, S.; Maeyama, K.; Nagai, K.; Watabe, S.; Kinoshita, S. Gene expression profiles at different stages for formation of pearl sac and pearl in the pearl oyster *Pinctada fucata*. *BMC Genom.* **2019**, *20*, 240. [CrossRef] [PubMed]
4. Committee, C.P. *Pharmacopoeia of the People's Republic of China*; China Medical Science and Technology Press: Beijing, China, 2020.
5. Zhang, J.-X.; Li, S.-R.; Yao, S.; Bi, Q.-R.; Hou, J.-J.; Cai, L.-Y.; Han, S.-M.; Wu, W.-Y.; Guo, D.-A. Anticonvulsant and sedative-hypnotic activity screening of pearl and nacre (mother of pearl). *J. Ethnopharmacol.* **2016**, *181*, 229–235. [CrossRef] [PubMed]
6. Song, Y.; Chen, S.; Li, L.; Zeng, Y.; Hu, X. The Hypopigmentation Mechanism of Tyrosinase Inhibitory Peptides Derived from Food Proteins: An Overview. *Molecules* **2022**, *27*, 2710. [CrossRef] [PubMed]
7. Zhang, Z.; Xu, Y.; Lai, R.; Deng, H.; Zhou, F.; Wang, P.; Pang, X.; Huang, G.; Chen, X.; Lin, H.; et al. Protective Effect of the Pearl Extract from Pinctada fucata martensii Dunker on UV-Induced Photoaging in Mice. *Chem. Biodivers.* **2022**, *19*, e202100876. [CrossRef] [PubMed]
8. Chiu, H.-F.; Hsiao, S.-C.; Lu, Y.-Y.; Han, Y.-C.; Shen, Y.-C.; Venkatakrishnan, K.; Wang, C.-K. Efficacy of protein rich pearl powder on antioxidant status in a randomized placebo-controlled trial. *J. Food Drug Anal.* **2018**, *26*, 309–317. [CrossRef] [PubMed]
9. Loh, X.J.; Young, D.J.; Guo, H.; Tang, L.; Wu, Y.; Zhang, G.; Tang, C.; Ruan, H. Pearl Powder-An Emerging Material for Biomedical Applications: A Review. *Materials* **2021**, *14*, 2797. [CrossRef] [PubMed]
10. Cordero, R.J.B.; Casadevall, A. Melanin. *Curr. Biol.* **2020**, *30*, R142–R143. [CrossRef] [PubMed]
11. Slominski, R.M.; Sarna, T.; Plonka, P.M.; Raman, C.; Brozyna, A.A.; Slominski, A.T. Melanoma, Melanin, and Melanogenesis: The Yin and Yang Relationship. *Front. Oncol.* **2022**, *12*, 842496. [CrossRef] [PubMed]
12. Wang, Y.; Xiong, B.; Xing, S.; Chen, Y.; Liao, Q.; Mo, J.; Chen, Y.; Li, Q.; Sun, H. Medicinal Prospects of Targeting Tyrosinase: A Feature Review. *Curr. Med. Chem.* **2023**, *30*, 2638–2671. [CrossRef] [PubMed]
13. Fu, W.; Wu, Z.; Zheng, R.; Yin, N.; Han, F.; Zhao, Z.; Dai, M.; Han, D.; Wang, W.; Niu, L. Inhibition mechanism of melanin formation based on antioxidant scavenging of reactive oxygen species. *Analyst* **2022**, *147*, 2703–2711. [CrossRef] [PubMed]
14. Liu, F.; Qu, L.; Li, H.; He, J.; Wang, L.; Fang, Y.; Yan, X.; Yang, Q.; Peng, B.; Wu, W.; et al. Advances in Biomedical Functions of Natural Whitening Substances in the Treatment of Skin Pigmentation Diseases. *Pharmaceutics* **2022**, *14*, 3154. [CrossRef] [PubMed]
15. Saeedi, M.; Eslamifar, M.; Khezri, K. Kojic acid applications in cosmetic and pharmaceutical preparations. *Biomed. Pharmacother.* **2019**, *110*, 582–593. [CrossRef] [PubMed]
16. He, M.; Fan, M.; Yang, W.; Peng, Z.; Wang, G. Novel kojic acid-1,2,4-triazine hybrids as anti-tyrosinase agents: Synthesis, biological evaluation, mode of action, and anti-browning studies. *Food Chem.* **2023**, *419*, 136047. [CrossRef] [PubMed]
17. Shaito, A.; Posadino, A.M.; Younes, N.; Hasan, H.; Halabi, S.; Alhababi, D.; Al-Mohannadi, A.; Abdel-Rahman, W.M.; Eid, A.H.; Nasrallah, G.K.; et al. Potential Adverse Effects of Resveratrol: A Literature Review. *Int. J. Mol. Sci.* **2020**, *21*, 2084. [CrossRef] [PubMed]
18. Zilles, J.C.; dos Santos, F.L.; Kulkamp-Guerreiro, I.C.; Contri, R.V. Biological activities and safety data of kojic acid and its derivatives: A review. *Exp. Dermatol.* **2022**, *31*, 1500–1521. [CrossRef] [PubMed]
19. Masub, N.; Khachemoune, A. Cosmetic skin lightening use and side effects. *J. Dermatol. Treat.* **2022**, *33*, 1287–1292. [CrossRef]
20. Hu, S.; Laughter, M.R.; Anderson, J.B.; Sadeghpour, M. Emerging topical therapies to treat pigmentary disorders: An evidence-based approach. *J. Dermatol. Treat.* **2022**, *33*, 1931–1937. [CrossRef] [PubMed]
21. Reboucas, J.S.A.; Oliveira, F.P.S.; Araujo, A.C.D.S.; Gouveia, H.L.; Latorres, J.M.; Martins, V.G.; Prentice Hernandez, C.; Tesser, M.B. Shellfish industrial waste reuse. *Crit. Rev. Biotechnol.* **2023**, *43*, 50–66. [CrossRef] [PubMed]
22. Zhou, J.; Wei, M.; You, L. Protective Effect of Peptides from Pinctada Martensii Meat on the H_2O_2-Induced Oxidative Injured HepG2 Cells. *Antioxidants* **2023**, *12*, 535. [CrossRef] [PubMed]
23. Wei, M.; Qiu, H.; Zhou, J.; Yang, C.; Chen, Y.; You, L. The Anti-Photoaging Activity of Peptides from Pinctada martensii Meat. *Mar. Drugs* **2022**, *20*, 770. [CrossRef] [PubMed]

24. Sasaki, C.; Tamura, S.; Tohse, R.; Fujita, S.; Kikuchi, M.; Asada, C.; Nakamura, Y. Isolation and identification of an angiotensin I-converting enzyme inhibitory peptide from pearl oyster (*Pinctada fucata*) shell protein hydrolysate. *Process Biochem.* **2019**, *77*, 137–142. [CrossRef]
25. Kongsompong, S.; E-Kobon, T.; Taengphan, W.; Sangkhawasi, M.; Khongkow, M.; Chumnanpuen, P. Computer-Aided Virtual Screening and In Vitro Validation of Biomimetic Tyrosinase Inhibitory Peptides from Abalone Peptidome. *Int. J. Mol. Sci.* **2023**, *24*, 3154. [CrossRef] [PubMed]
26. Huang, P.; Miao, J.; Liao, W.; Huang, C.; Chen, B.; Li, Y.; Wang, X.; Yu, Y.; Liang, X.; Zhao, H.; et al. Rapid screening of novel tyrosinase inhibitory peptides from a pearl shell meat hydrolysate by molecular docking and the anti-melanin mechanism. *Food Funct.* **2023**, *14*, 1446–1458. [CrossRef] [PubMed]
27. Jin, Z.; Wei, Z. Molecular simulation for food protein-ligand interactions: A comprehensive review on principles, current applications, and emerging trends. *Compr. Rev. Food Sci. Food Saf.* **2024**, *23*, e13280. [CrossRef] [PubMed]
28. Li, X.; Guo, J.; Lian, J.; Gao, F.; Khan, A.J.; Wang, T.; Zhang, F. Molecular Simulation Study on the Interaction between Tyrosinase and Flavonoids from Sea Buckthorn. *Acs Omega* **2021**, *6*, 21579–21585. [CrossRef] [PubMed]
29. Trott, O.; Olson, A.J. Software News and Update AutoDock Vina: Improving the Speed and Accuracy of Docking with a New Scoring Function, Efficient Optimization, and Multithreading. *J. Comput. Chem.* **2010**, *31*, 455–461. [CrossRef] [PubMed]
30. Skolnick, J.; Zhou, H. Implications of the Essential Role of Small Molecule Ligand Binding Pockets in Protein-Protein Interactions. *J. Phys. Chem. B* **2022**, *126*, 6853–6867. [CrossRef] [PubMed]
31. Wang, W.; Lin, H.; Shen, W.; Qin, X.; Gao, J.; Cao, W.; Zheng, H.; Chen, Z.; Zhang, Z. Optimization of a Novel Tyrosinase Inhibitory Peptide from Atrina pectinata Mantle and Its Molecular Inhibitory Mechanism. *Foods* **2023**, *12*, 3884. [CrossRef] [PubMed]
32. Xiong, S.-L.; Lim, G.T.; Yin, S.-J.; Lee, J.; Si, Y.-X.; Yang, J.-M.; Park, Y.-D.; Qian, G.-Y. The inhibitory effect of pyrogallol on tyrosinase activity and structure: Integration study of inhibition kinetics with molecular dynamics simulation. *Int. J. Biol. Macromol.* **2019**, *121*, 463–471. [CrossRef] [PubMed]
33. Zhao, W.; Tan, L.; Zhang, Q.; Chen, F.; Yu, Z. In silico identification and mechanistic evaluation of novel tyrosinase inhibitory peptides derived from coconut proteins. *Food Biosci.* **2024**, *61*, 104595. [CrossRef]
34. Yu, Z.; Fu, L.; Zhang, Q.; Zhao, W. In silico identification and molecular mechanism of novel egg white-derived tyrosinase inhibitory peptides. *Food Biosci.* **2024**, *57*, 103567. [CrossRef]
35. Najafi, Z.; Haramabadi, M.Z.; Chehardoli, G.; Ebadi, A.; Iraji, A. Design, synthesis, and molecular dynamics simulation studies of some novel kojic acid fused 2-amino-3-cyano-4H-pyran derivatives as tyrosinase inhibitors. *BMC Chem.* **2024**, *18*, 41. [CrossRef] [PubMed]
36. Lee, Y.-C.; Hsiao, N.-W.; Tseng, T.-S.; Chen, W.-C.; Lin, H.-H.; Leu, S.-J.; Yang, E.-W.; Tsai, K.-C. Phage Display-Mediated Discovery of Novel Tyrosinase-Targeting Tetrapeptide Inhibitors Reveals the Significance of N-Terminal Preference of Cysteine Residues and Their Functional Sulfur Atom. *Mol. Pharmacol.* **2015**, *87*, 218–230. [CrossRef] [PubMed]
37. Yu, S.; He, M.; Zhai, Y.; Xie, Z.; Xu, S.; Yu, S.; Xiao, H.; Song, Y. Inhibitory activity and mechanism of trilobatin on tyrosinase: Kinetics, interaction mechanism and molecular docking. *Food Funct.* **2021**, *12*, 2569–2579. [CrossRef] [PubMed]
38. Yoshino, M.; Murakami, K. A graphical method for determining inhibition constants. *J. Enzym. Inhib. Med. Chem.* **2009**, *24*, 1288–1290. [CrossRef] [PubMed]
39. Whitmore, L.; Mavridis, L.; Wallace, B.A.; Janes, R.W. DichroMatch at the protein circular dichroism data bank (DM@PCDDB): A web-based tool for identifying protein nearest neighbors using circular dichroism spectroscopy. *Protein Sci.* **2018**, *27*, 10–13. [CrossRef] [PubMed]
40. Paudyal, S.; Sharma, S.K.; da Silva, R.L.C.G.; Mintz, K.J.; Liyanage, P.Y.; Al-Youbi, A.O.; Bashammakh, A.S.; El-Shahawi, M.S.; Leblanc, R.M. Tyrosinase enzyme Langmuir monolayer: Surface chemistry and spectroscopic study. *J. Colloid Interface Sci.* **2020**, *564*, 254–263. [CrossRef] [PubMed]
41. Ott, F.; Rabe, K.S.; Niemeyer, C.M.; Gygli, G. Toward Reproducible Enzyme Modeling with Isothermal Titration Calorimetry. *Acs Catal.* **2021**, *11*, 10695–10704. [CrossRef]
42. Liu, J.; Liu, Y.; He, X.; Teng, B.; McRae, J.M. Valonea Tannin: Tyrosinase Inhibition Activity, Structural Elucidation and Insights into the Inhibition Mechanism. *Molecules* **2021**, *26*, 2747. [CrossRef] [PubMed]
43. Hu, Z.; Sha, X.; Zhang, L.; Huang, S.; Tu, Z. Effect of Grass Carp Scale Collagen Peptide FTGML on cAMP-PI3K/Akt and MAPK Signaling Pathways in B16F10 Melanoma Cells and Correlation between Anti-Melanin and Antioxidant Properties. *Foods* **2022**, *11*, 391. [CrossRef] [PubMed]
44. Soares de Castro, R.J.; Sato, H.H. Biologically active peptides: Processes for their generation, purification and identification and applications as natural additives in the food and pharmaceutical industries. *Food Res. Int.* **2015**, *74*, 185–198. [CrossRef] [PubMed]
45. Van der Spoel, D.; Lindahl, E.; Hess, B.; Groenhof, G.; Mark, A.E.; Berendsen, H.J.C. GROMACS: Fast, flexible, and free. *J. Comput. Chem.* **2005**, *26*, 1701–1718. [CrossRef] [PubMed]
46. Abraham, M.J.; Murtola, T.; Schulz, R.; Páll, S.; Smith, J.C.; Hess, B.; Lindahl, E. GROMACS: High performance molecular simulations through multi-level parallelism from laptops to supercomputers. *SoftwareX* **2015**, *1*, 19–25. [CrossRef]
47. Yu, Q.; Fan, L.; Ding, Z. The inhibition mechanisms between asparagus polyphenols after hydrothermal treatment and tyrosinase: A circular dichroism spectrum, fluorescence, and molecular docking study. *Food Biosci.* **2022**, *48*, 101790. [CrossRef]

48. Wang, W.; Gao, Y.; Wang, W.; Zhang, J.; Yin, J.; Le, T.; Xue, J.; Engelhardt, U.H.; Jiang, H. Kojic Acid Showed Consistent Inhibitory Activity on Tyrosinase from Mushroom and in Cultured B16F10 Cells Compared with Arbutins. *Antioxidants* **2022**, *11*, 502. [CrossRef]
49. Zhang, X.; Li, J.; Li, Y.; Liu, Z.; Lin, Y.; Huang, J.-A. Anti-melanogenic effects of epigallocatechin-3-gallate (EGCG), epicatechin-3-gallate (ECG) and gallocatechin-3-gallate (GCG) via down-regulation of cAMP/CREB/MITF signaling pathway in B16F10 melanoma cells. *Fitoterapia* **2020**, *145*, 104634. [CrossRef] [PubMed]

Disclaimer/Publisher's Note: The statements, opinions and data contained in all publications are solely those of the individual author(s) and contributor(s) and not of MDPI and/or the editor(s). MDPI and/or the editor(s) disclaim responsibility for any injury to people or property resulting from any ideas, methods, instructions or products referred to in the content.

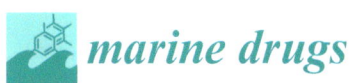

Article

Preparation and Vasodilation Mechanism of Angiotensin-I-Converting Enzyme Inhibitory Peptide from *Ulva prolifera* Protein

Zhiyong Li [1,2,†], Hongyan He [1,†], Jiasi Liu [1], Huiyue Gu [1], Caiwei Fu [1], Aurang Zeb [1], Tuanjie Che [3] and Songdong Shen [1,*]

1. School of Biology & Basic Medical Sciences, Soochow University, Suzhou 215101, China
2. Suzhou Chien-Shiung Institute of Technology, Suzhou 215101, China
3. Key Laboratory of Functional Genomic and Molecular Diagnosis of Gansu Province, Lanzhou 730030, China
* Correspondence: shensongdong@suda.edu.cn; Tel.: +86-0512-65880276
† These authors contributed equally to this work.

Abstract: *Ulva prolifera*, a type of green algae that can be consumed, was utilized in the production of an angiotensin-I converting enzyme (ACE) inhibitory peptide. The protein from the algae was isolated and subsequently hydrolyzed using a neutral protease. The resulting hydrolysate underwent several processes including Sephadex-G100 filtration chromatography, ultrafiltration, HPLC-Q-TOF-MS analysis, ADMET screening, UV spectrum detection test, molecular docking, and molecular dynamic simulation. Then, the ACE inhibitory peptide named KAF (IC$_{50}$, 0.63 ± 0.26 μM) was identified. The effectiveness of this peptide in inhibiting ACE can be primarily attributed to two conventional hydrogen bonds. Additionally, it could activate endothelial nitric oxide synthase (eNOS) activity to promote the generation of nitric oxide (NO). Additionally, KAF primarily increased the intracellular calcium (Ca^{2+}) level by acting on L-type Ca^{2+} channel (LTCC) and the ryanodine receptor (RyR) in the endoplasmic reticulum, and completed the activation of eNOS under the mediation of protein kinase B (Akt) signaling pathway. Our study has confirmed that KAF has the potential to be processed into pharmaceutical candidate functions on vasoconstriction.

Keywords: *Ulva prolifera* protein; ACE inhibitory peptide; Akt; vasodilation mechanism

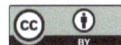

1. Introduction

Hypertension has emerged as a global health concern, affecting more than 1.13 billion people worldwide, according to a survey conducted by the World Health Organization [1]. The renin–angiotensin–aldosterone regulatory system (RAAS) plays a crucial role in the regulation of blood pressure [2]. Within this system, ACE is one of the key enzymes, catalyzes the conversion of inactive Angiotensin I (Ang I) into the potent vasoconstrictor Angiotensin II (Ang II), thereby deactivating the vasodilator bradykinin [3]; this highlights the effectiveness of ACE inhibitors as an important therapeutic approach for the treatment of hypertension. Small molecules can enter the active pocket and inhibit the activity of ACE [4]. Currently, bioactive peptides with ACE inhibitory activity and no side effects have garnered significant attention. Various animal and plant proteins, such as *Mytilus edulis* [5], sea cucumber (*Apostichopus japonicus*) gonads [6], skipjack tuna (*Katsuwonus pelamis*) muscle [7], and *Takifugu flavidus* [8] have been reported to contain ACE inhibitory peptides. These peptides hold promise as natural alternatives for managing hypertension.

Ulva prolifera, an edible green alga, thrives in the coastal areas of China. However, over the past decade, excessive nutrients in the water have caused recurring outbreaks of green tides dominated by *U. prolifera*. These tides lead to the accumulation of algae on the seabed, resulting in water hypoxia and the subsequent death of aquatic organisms [9]. Cleaning up excessive *U. prolifera* requires significant manpower and resources. Therefore, it is essential to explore ways to transform this alga into a valuable resource. A previous study indicated that *Enteromorpha spp.* (one of *U. prolifera*) boasts a substantial biomass and possesses an excellent nutritional composition, including proteins (9–14%), ether extract (2–3.6%), ash (32–36%), and a total fatty acid content of 10.9 g/100 g [10]. These characteristics make *U. prolifera* a promising candidate for various commercial applications. Previous studies have shown that the enzymatic hydrolysis of *U. prolifera* proteins can generate small-molecule peptides with ACE inhibitory activity [11]. However, the mechanism behind the vasodilation effects of *U. prolifera* peptides has not been reported before.

The endothelium, a cellular monolayer lining the blood vessel wall, plays a crucial role in maintaining overall health and homeostasis in multiple organs [12]. Endothelial cells are involved in regulating blood pressure through the secretion of various cytokines. However, metabolic disorders can lead to endothelial dysfunction and damage in the body. Therefore, in vitro cultivation of vascular endothelial cells is an important method of studying the mechanism of ACE inhibitory peptides [13,14]. Nitric oxide (NO), produced by various organs and tissues, has a blood-pressure-lowering effect and enhances male sexual function. Previous studies have reported that small molecules can activate the phosphorylation of eNOS in endothelial cells, thereby promoting NO synthesis [15]. Therefore, it is important to explore the function of eNOS activation and NO production by *U. prolifera* peptides.

The objective of this study was to develop a promising ACE inhibitory peptide from *U. prolifera*. Additionally, the inhibitory pattern and molecular interaction mechanism of the peptide were investigated. Furthermore, the cellular mechanism by which the purified peptide regulates blood pressure was explored using human umbilical vein endothelial cells (HUVECs).

2. Results and Discussion

2.1. Purification and Identification of ACE Inhibitory Peptides from U. prolifera Protein Hydrolysate

Some proteins can produce ACE inhibitory peptides in the digestion of neutral protease, such as Pacific saury [16], tuna processing by-products [17], and Bovine casein [18]. It has also been reported that *U. prolifera* protein contains peptides with ACE inhibitory activity [11]. Therefore, in this study, *U. prolifera* protein was hydrolyzed using neutral protease under optimal conditions.

Then, a hydrolysate with ACE inhibitory activity was obtained, with degrees of hydrolysisi (DH) and IC_{50} of 33.59% and 1471.92 μg/mL, respectively (Figure 1). DH is a parameter that describes the degree of *U. prolifera* protein hydrolysis, which is higher than in the previous report [11]. The result indicates that a large amounts of peptides and amino acids were released from *U. prolifera* protein.

To obtain a more efficient fraction, the hydrolysate was separated using the Sephadex-G100. The separation range of Sephadex-G100 is 4000–15,000 Da, and it can exclude undecomposed proteins. Additionally, peptides larger than the gel mesh of Sephadex-G100 flow out of the gap quickly. But, instead, peptides smaller than the gel mesh can be repeatedly shuttled through each gel particle before eventually exiting the column. Fraction 2 has a longer separation time and therefore contains more small peptides. Subsequently, Fraction 2 with the highest ACE inhibitory activity was further purified by an ultrafiltration membrane (Figure 1). Among the three fractions, the one with a molecular weight less than 3 kDa showed the highest ACE inhibitory activity, with an IC_{50} value of 26.36 μg/mL (Table 1). These findings support the notion that smaller peptides are more likely to enter the active center and possess stronger ACE inhibitory activity [11]. To determine the amino acid sequences of this fraction (<3 kDa), HPLC-MS/MS analysis was performed, resulting in the identification of 2257 peptides by comparing the data with those available in the NCBI database (Table S1).

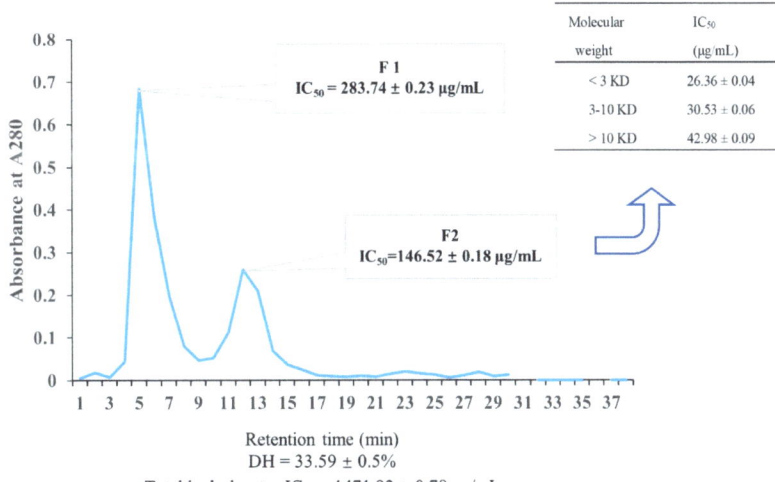

Figure 1. Purification of ACE inhibitory peptides. Sephadex G-100 gel chromatography of fractions from hydrolysates (neutral protease); the IC$_{50}$ value of different fractions from the ultrafiltration of Fraction 2 (F2) are exhibited in the inserted table. Data are presented as mean ± SD.

Table 1. Potential ACE inhibitory peptides form protease hydrolysis.

Peptide	Peptide Ranker	WS	Toxin	HIA	BBB	-C Dock Energy	IC$_{50}$ (µM)
DRW	0.88931	GOOD	NO	0.7047	−0.8101	fail	
GMR	0.884249	GOOD	NO	0.6327	−0.6948	fail	
MGR	0.860347	GOOD	NO	0.6327	−0.6948	fail	
RYFR	0.846704	GOOD	NO	0.4488	0.8791	fail	
KWY	0.794787	GOOD	NO	0.9434	−0.8790	fail	
RWK	0.774831	GOOD	NO	0.8444	−0.8040	fail	
LGSFR	0.737369	GOOD	NO	0.8291	−0.7994	fail	
EGRW	0.734044	GOOD	NO	0.8291	−0.7994	fail	
WRAA	0.702731	GOOD	NO	0.9124	−0.8063	fail	
KAF	0.682106	GOOD	NO	0.7042	−0.8181	88.967	0.63 ± 0.26
DFT	0.600067	GOOD	NO	0.4747	−0.8839	fail	
ERFY	0.464208	GOOD	NO	0.6018	−0.8872	fail	
PAMK	0.419096	GOOD	NO	0.774	−0.7314	fail	
Captopril						46.94	0.017 [19]

Note: Peptide ranker, >0.5 represents of high biological activity; WS, water solubility; Toxin, water-solubility HIA+, high human intestinal absorptivity (>30%); BBB+, high blood–brain barrier permeability (>0.1); -CE score, the score of -C Docker energy (kcal/moL). Fail represents of docking failure between candidates and ACE. Data are presented as mean ± SD.

2.2. Screening of the Potential ACE Inhibitory Peptides

ADMET has been widely used to screen the highest ACE inhibitory peptides [4]. As shown in Table 1, thirteen peptides exhibited desirable ADMET parameters, including non-toxicity, good water solubility, high biological activity, high human intestinal absorptivity, and high blood–brain barrier permeability. However, among these peptides, only KAF can dock with ACE according to molecular docking. The MS/MS spectra of this peptide is shown in Figure 2. In vitro ACE inhibitory assay revealed that KAF exhibited an IC$_{50}$ value of 0.63 ± 0.26 µM. Interestingly, KAF had a higher -C Dock Energy than captopril (0.025 µM) but less ACE inhibitory activity [19]. This discrepancy may be attributed to the fact that captopril, with its smaller molecular size, is more likely to interact with the ACE enzyme.

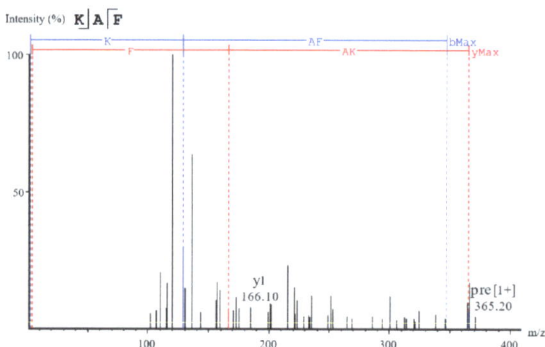

Figure 2. MS/MS spectra of the selected peptide.

2.3. Inhibition Pattern of Peptide against ACE

To investigate the inhibition mechanism of KAF, it was co-incubated with the substrate (HHL) and ACE under the optimum conditions. Lineweaver–Burk plots suggested KAF was a competitive inhibitor (Figure 3). Similarly, other peptides from natural product protein, such as EACF [4], QDVL [15], and AEYLCEAC [20], also exhibited competitive inhibition. These peptides interacted with the active site of ACE, preventing the generation of products.

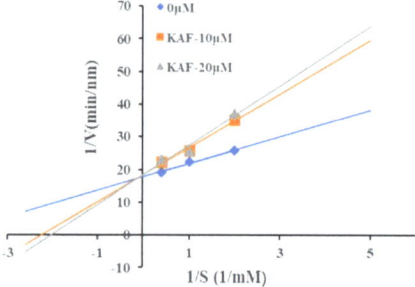

Figure 3. Lineweaver–Burk plots of ACE inhibition by KAF.

2.4. Molecular Docking and Dynamics Simulation

Molecular docking was performed to explore the interaction mechanism between candidates and ACE. As shown in Figure 4, the stabilized poses of KAF are attributable to five types of bonds: attractive charge, conventional hydrogen, carbon hydrogen, pi-alkyl, and metal-acceptor bonds. Among these, the three conditional hydrogen bonds and the key binding sites Ala354 and Asp415 played an important role in stabilizing KAF-ACE complex (Figure 4). Additionally, KAF was able to bind the active site Zn701 of ACE by attractive charge and metal-acceptor bonds, which aligns with the kinetics result indicating that KAF, as a competitive inhibitor, can enter the active pocket of ACE. In comparison, the control group Captopril formed one hydrogen bond with ACE and Captopril (Figure 4). However, Captopril (IC$_{50}$, 0.025 μM) has a smaller molecular weight (217.28 Da), and it exhibited higher ACE inhibitory activity than KAF [19]. This may be attributed to the fact that Captopril, with its smaller molecular size, is more likely to enter the active pocket and inhibit ACE activity. Similarly, Captopril can enter the S1 active pockets according to the bind site Ala 354 according to the result of docking result (Table 2). Additionally, both KAF and Captopril can bind with ACE at several sites as follows: Arg522, Ala354, and Zn701 (Figure 4).

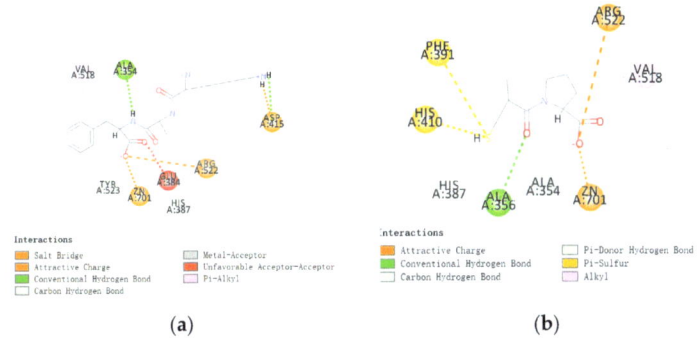

(a)   (b)

Figure 4. Docking simulation of candidates with ACE. Two-dimensional interaction of KAF–ACE (**a**) and Captopril–ACE (**b**).

Table 2. Interaction information.

Candidates	Bond Position	Distance(Å)	Type	Number
KAF	A: ASP415:OD2-KAF:H22 A: ARG522:NH1-KAF: O44 A: ZN701: ZN-KAF: O44	2.16146 4.49144 2.24177	Attractive Charge	3
	A: ASP415:OD1-KAF: H21 A: ALA354:O-KAF: H36	2.26404 2.3907	Conventional Hydrogen Bond	2
	A: HIS387:HD2-KAF: O44 A: TYR423: OH-KAF: H38	3.01083 2.3496	Carbon Hydrogen Bond	2
	A: VAL418-KAF	4.90944	Pi-Alkyl	1
	A: ZN701: ZN-KAF: O34	3.0144	Metal-Acceptor	1
Captopril (Cap)	A: ARG522:NH1-Cap: O11 A: ZN701: ZN-Cap: O11	4.49391 2.27274	Attractive Charge	2
	A: ALA356:HN-Cap: O1	2.89368	Conventional Hydrogen Bond	1
	A: ALA354:O-Cap: H22	2.91634	Carbon Hydrogen Bond	1
	A: HIS387-Cap:H18	2.76629	Pi-Donor Hydrogen Bond; Pi-Sulfur	1
	A: VAL518-Cap	4.64702	Alkyl	1
	A: PHE391-Cap: S4 A: HIS410-Cap: S4	4.77799 4.40347	Pi-Sulfur	2

In order to validate the docking results, an MD simulation was conducted to analyze the dynamic behavior of complexes where atoms and molecules interact as a function of time [21]. Structural parameters including the root mean square deviation (RMSD), the root mean square fluctuation (RMSF), radius of gyration (Rg) and accessible surface area (SASA) were important factors when analyzing the flexibility and conformations of peptide–ACE complex in solution [22]. As shown in Figure 5a, the lower RMSD value of KAF-ACE exhibited a higher stability than Captopril-ACE before 20 ns. Similarly, the lower SAS value indicated the better stability of KAF-ACE before 10 ns. However, Captopril-ACE exhibited better stability according to RMSD, Rg and SAS value in plateau phase. RMSF calculates the fluctuations of each atom relative to its average position and is an indicator of the degree of freedom of atomic motion. In this study, there were five similar flexible areas (motion amplitude) (100–108; 150–161; 286–319; 430–445 ns and 496–520) in both KAF–ACE and Captopril–ACE complex (Figure 5c). Interestingly, these flexible regions were located far from the hydrogen bond sites between KAF and ACE (Asp415 and Ala354), which explains the affinity between the peptides and ACE.

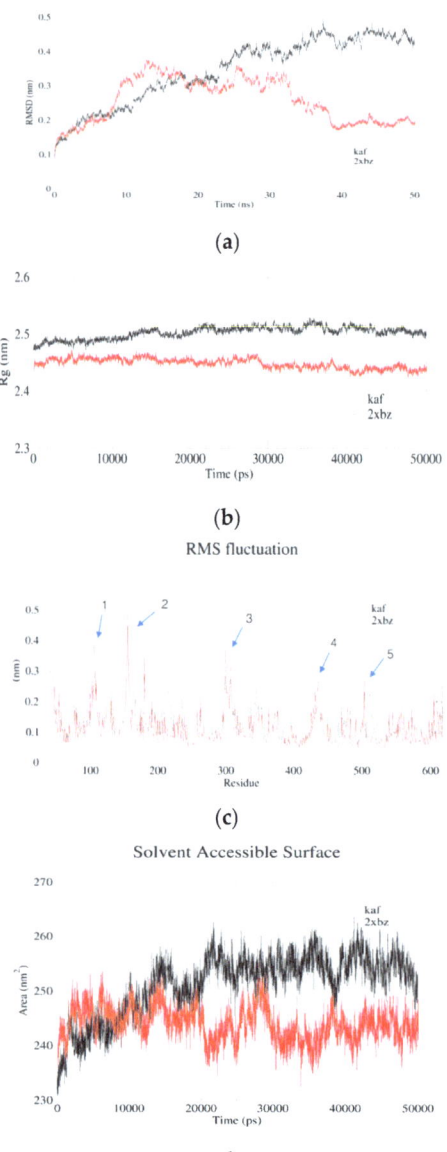

Figure 5. The result of molecular dynamics simulation (kaf: KAF; 2xbz: Captopril; (**a**) RMSD; (**b**) Rg; (**c**) RMSF (the number represents of flexible areas); (**d**) SASA.

2.5. Effect of Synthetic Peptides on NO Production, eNOS Activity in HUVECs

In vitro HUVEC incubation has been widely used to investigate the potential antihypertensive mechanism of drug-candidates [15]. In this study, KAF has no effect on HUVEC proliferation in the concentration of 0–100 μM (Figure 6a). NO, an endothelium-derived relaxing factor, is produced by eNOS in HUVECs. The phosphorylation of eNOS is known to enhance NO production, leading to vasodilation [23]. As shown in Figure 6b, KAF was found to enhance eNOS activity, resulting in increased NO production at a concentration of 100 μM. Previous studies have reported the involvement of several cytokines, such as Akt [24], AMP-activated protein kinase (AMPK) [25] and mitogen-activated protein kinase (P38, Jun) [26] in the phosphorylation of eNOS. In order to study explore the activation mechanism of peptides on eNOS. Some commercial protease inhibitors, such as Compound C (AMPK inhibitor), SB203580 (P38 inhibitor), LY294002 (Akt inhibitor), and SP600125 (Jun inhibitor), were used to interfere eNOS phosphorylation induced by peptide. Western blot shown that only LY294002 can prevent eNOS phosphorylation ($p < 0.05$) (Figure 7). This suggests that Akt may be involved in KAF-dependent eNOS phosphorylation. Furthermore, KAF treatment was found to significantly increase the intracellular Ca^{2+} content in HUVECs compared to the untreated peptide group (Figure 8). Ca^{2+} and calmodulin kinases were important in eNOS phosphorylation and NO production [27]. Previous studies have reported the existence of channels proteins and their function of increasing Ca^{2+} level in endothelial cells [28].

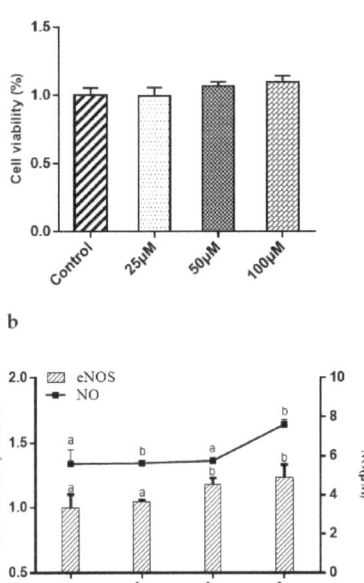

Figure 6. Effect of this *Ulva prolifera* peptide (KAF) on HUVECs. (**a**) Effect of peptide on HUVECs viability; (**b**) effect of peptide on eNOS activity and NO production in HUVECs. The cells were treated with peptides at 0, 25, 50, and 100 μM for 24 h; values that do not share a common superscript lowercase letter within a column differ significantly, $p < 0.05$.

Additionally, the involvement of Ca^{2+}/calmodulin kinases, such as CaMKII, in increasing intracellular Ca^{2+} levels and facilitating Ca^{2+}/calmodulin-mediated eNOS activation has been reported [29]. In this study, calcium chelators (EGTA), CaMK-II inhibitor (KN93), LTCC blockade (Tetracaine) and RyR inhibition (Nifedipine) attenuated the KAF-induced eNOS phosphorylation, which indicated that Ca^{2+} and Ca^{2+} channels were also involved in KAF-induced eNOS phosphorylation (Figure 9). A similar situation has been reported in Betulinic acid, which activates eNOS phosphorylation and NO synthesis via the Ca^{2+}/calmodulin-dependent protein kinase kinase/AMPK pathways [25]. Therefore, it can be concluded that KAF may activate LTCC and RyR, leading to an increase in intracellular Ca^{2+} levels. This rise in Ca^{2+} serves as a signaling molecule that promotes Akt-dependent eNOS phosphorylation and subsequent NO production. These results suggest that KAF has various beneficial effects on HUVECs.

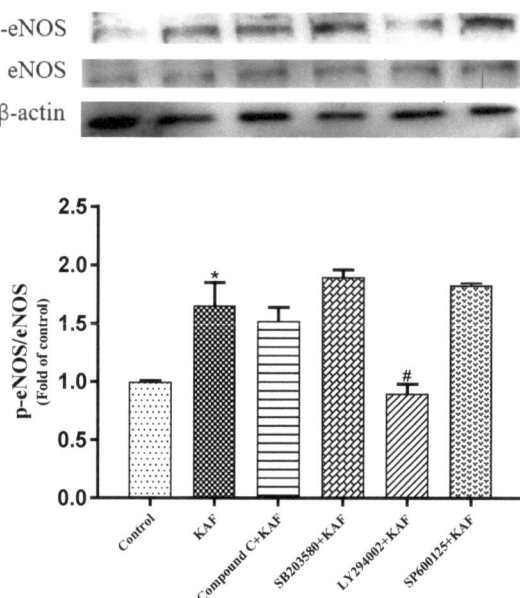

Figure 7. The effect of *U. prolifera* peptide (KAF) *on* eNOS phosphorylation. Control, Cells were cultured by medium for 24 h; KAF, cells were cultured by 100 μM KAF for 18 h; Compound C (AMPK inhibitor) + KAF, cells were cultured by 100 μM KAF for 12 h and then, adding 10 μM Compound C for another 6 h; SB203580 (P38 inhibitor) + KAF, cells were cultured by 100 μM KAF for 12 h and then, adding 10 μM SB203580 for another 6 h; LY294002 (Akt inhibitor) + KAF, cells were cultured by 100 μM KAF for 12 h and then, adding 10 μM LY294002 for another 6 h; SP600125 (Jun inhibitor) + KAF, cells were cultured by 100 μM KAF for 12 h and then, adding 10 μM SP600125 for another 6 h; * $p < 0.05$, compared with control; # $p < 0.05$, compared with KAF treatment.

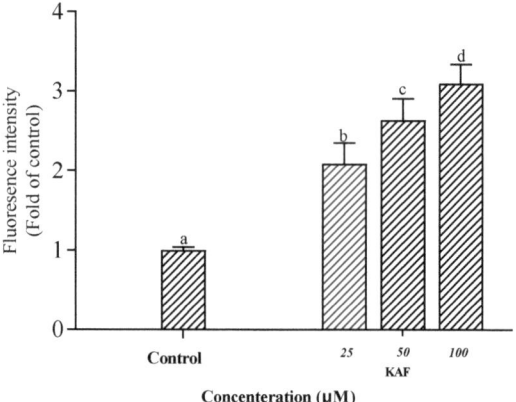

Figure 8. Effect of *U. prolifera* peptide (KAF) on Ca^{2+} content in HUVECs (values that do not share a common superscript lowercase letter within a column differ significantly, $p < 0.05$).

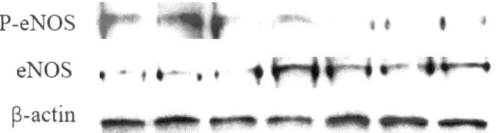

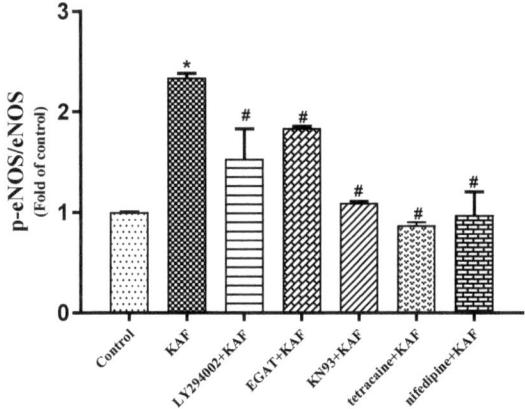

Figure 9. Role of Ca^{2+} channels on *Ulva prolifera* peptide (KAF)-induced eNOS phosphorylation. Control, Cells were cultured by medium for 24 h; KAF, cells were cultured by 100 μM KAF for 18 h; LY294002 (Akt inhibitor) + KAF, cells were cultured by 100 μM KAF for 12 h and then, adding 10 μM LY294002 for another 6 h; EGTA (calcium chelators) + KAF, cells were cultured by 100 μM KAF for 12 h and then, adding 500 nM EGTA for another 6 h; KN93 (CaMK-II inhibitor) + KAF, cells were cultured by 100 μM KAF for 12 h and then, adding 10 μM KN93 for another 6 h; Tetracaine (LTCC blockade) + KAF, cells were cultured by 100 μM KAF for 12 h and then, adding 60 μM Tetracaine for another 6 h; Nifedipine (RyR inhibition) + KAF, cells were cultured by 100 μM KAF for 12 h and then, adding 60 μM Nifedipine for another 6 h; * $p < 0.05$, compared with control; # $p < 0.05$, compared with KAF treatment.

3. Materials and Methods

3.1. Materials and Reagents

U. prolifera was obtained from the Institute of Oceanography, Chinese Academy of Sciences (Qingdao, China). Angiotensin I-converting enzyme (from rabbit lung), N-hippuril-L-histidy-L-leucine (HHL), Ang II, Neutral protease was purchased from Sangon Biotech (Shanghai, China). Sephadex G-100 were purchased from Auyoo Biotechnology Co. (Shanghai, China). Ultrafiltration membrane was purchased form Merck Millipore (Burlington, VT, USA). LY294002, SB203580, LY294002 SP600125, PD 98059, tetracaine, Compound C were purchased from Merck (Darmstadt, Germany). Nitric Oxide Assay Kit was purchased from Beyotime (Shanghai, China). MTT cell proliferation and cytotoxicity assay kits were purchased from Sigma-Aldrich (St. Louis, MO, USA). HUVEC cell line was purchased from Sangon Biotech (Shanghai, China). All other reagents were of analytical reagent grade.

3.2. Preparation of U. prolifera Protein Hydrolysate

The protein from *U. prolifera* was extracted, and the concentration of peptides was determined as described in our previous report [30]. The enzymatic hydrolysis condition accorded with the reported method with some modifications [11]. The protein was then dissolved in deionized water at a concentration of 10% (w/v). The pH and temperature of the solution were adjusted to the appropriate levels. Neutral proteases were added to the solution at a pH of 7.4, temperature of 47 °C, and an enzyme-to-substrate ratio of 3500 U/g (1% enzyme/substrate, w/w extracted protein powder). The hydrolysis reaction was carried out for 1 h and then terminated using a boiling water bath. The DH and ACE inhibitory activity of the *U. prolifera* protein hydrolysate was measured according to the previous report [11].

3.3. Determination of ACE Inhibitory Activity

The ACE inhibitory rate was explored according to a previous report [11]. Briefly, 80 μL of 5 mM HHL solution was mixed with 10 μL of peptide solution, followed by incubation for 5 min at 37 °C. Subsequently, 10 μL of ACE solution (0.1 U/mL) was added, followed by incubation at 37 °C for 60 min. The reaction was terminated by 200 μL HCl (1 M). In the blank group, peptide solution was replaced by 0.1 M sodium borate buffer. The reaction production was extracted with 1500 μL of ethyl acetate with slight oscillation for 1 min. Then, the mixture was centrifuged at 4000 rpm for 15 min, 1 mL of supernatant was transferred to another test tube, mixed with 1000 μL of acetic anhydride and 2000 μL of 0.5% (v/v) p-dimethyl amino benzaldehyde in pyridine, and then incubated at 40 °C for 30 min prior to spectrophotometric measurement at 459 nm. The degree of ACE inhibition (in percentage) was calculated according to Equation (1):

$$\text{The inhibition of ACE (\%)} = (Ab - Aa)/(Ab - Ac) \times 100\% \qquad (1)$$

where Aa represents the mixture of HHL, peptide and ACE; Ab represents the mixture of HHL and ACE; and Ac represents the mixture of HHL and inactive ACE. The IC50 value was defined as the inhibitor concentration inhibiting 50% activity of ACE.

3.4. Purification and Identification of ACE-Inhibitory Peptides from Hydrolysates

The hydrolysates were first purified by Sephadex-G100 column (2.5 cm × 70 cm) with deionized water as the elution at a flow rate of 1.0 mL/min. Fractions were collected at 2 min intervals, and each fraction was tested for ACE inhibitory activity. The fraction with the highest ACE inhibitory activity was further fractionated using an ultrafiltration membrane, resulting in three fractions: <3 kDa, 3–10 kDa, and >10 kDa. The purified fractions were then analyzed using online nano-flow liquid chromatography tandem mass spectrometry, following the methods described in our previous report [30].

3.5. Screening and Synthesis of the Potential ACE Inhibitory Peptides

The identified peptides were determined by BIOPEP (https://biochemia.uwm.edu.pl/biopep-uwm/, accessed on 15 July 2022) to remove the reported peptides [4]. The peptides were then evaluated for various biological parameters such as biological activity potential, solubility, toxicity, and human intestinal absorption (HIA) using Peptide Ranker, Innovagen, and admetSAR (ecust.edu.cn; accessed on 15 July 2022) tools, respectively. Additionally, the affinities between the selected peptides and ACE were assessed through molecular docking using Discovery Studio 2022 software with the ACE crystal structure (ID: 1O8A) chosen as the receptor. Finally, the selected peptide was synthetized by China peptides (Shanghai, China) (peptide purity 98%).

3.6. Inhibition Kinetics

The kinetics of the peptide on ACE was explored using the Lineweaver–Burke plot. The protocol was the same as in the ACE inhibition assay. The experimental procedure was similar to the ACE inhibition assay. ACE was preincubated with peptides of different concentrations ranging from 0 to 100 μM, and then reacted with hippuryl-L-histidyl-L-leucine (HHL) at various concentrations ranging from 1 to 5 mM. The Michaelis–Menten constant (Km) and maximum initial velocity (Vmax) were calculated based on the y- and x-axis intercepts of the primary plot, respectively.

3.7. Molecular Dynamics (MD) Simulation

To validate the docking results, a 50 ns MD simulation was conducted for ACE in complex with selected peptide and the control group (Captopril). The MD simulation was performed using the GROMACS program (version 2020) and the Amber ff12SB force field, following a previously reported protocol [31].

3.8. Cell Culture of HUVEC

The cytotoxicity assay of HUVECs was performed using the MTT Cell Proliferation and Cytotoxicity Assay Kit [32]. NO production and eNOS activity in HUVECs treated with peptides were measured by Total Nitric Oxide Assay Kit and Nitric Oxide Synthase Assay Kit. HUVECs with a content of 1×10^6 cells/bottle were seeded in T25 cell cultured bottle for 24 h. Subsequently, the cells were treated with peptides at 100 μM for 24 h. After that, the cell culture medium containing peptides and specific protease inhibitors at appropriate final concentrations (EGTA, 500 nM; KN93, 10 μM; Nifedipine, 60 μM; Tetracaine, 60 μM; Compound C, 10 μM; SB203580, 10 μM; LY294002, 10 μM; SP600125, 10 μM) were used to culture HUVECs for additional 6 h [25].

3.9. Statistical Analysis

All experiments were performed in triplicate and the results reported as the mean ± standard deviation (SD). Data were analyzed by one-way analysis of variance (ANOVA), and then Dunnett multiple tests were performed using GraphPad Prism Version 9 (San Diego, CA, USA). Significance level was set at p less than 0.05.

4. Conclusions

In the above-presented work, a novel anti-ACE peptide KAF (0.63 ± 0.26 μM) was separated and identified from *U. prolifera* protein. This peptide effectively inhibits ACE activity through competitive bind, primarily due to the formation of two conventional hydrogen bonds. In HUVECs, KAF can activate the eNOS activity in the generation of NO. KAF can increased the intracellular Ca^{2+} level through the LTCC and the RyR in endoplasmic reticulum, and completed the activation of eNOS under the mediation of Akt signaling pathway. These findings supported that KAF has the potential to be a safe candidate against ACE and relax blood vessel. Subsequently, the antihypertension activity of KAF on hypertension rat will be performed.

Supplementary Materials: The following supporting information can be downloaded at: https://www.mdpi.com/article/10.3390/md22090398/s1, Table S1: Peptides pool.

Author Contributions: Conceptualization, methodology, writing—original draft, Z.L.; writing—review and editing, H.H.; validation, J.L.; investigation, H.G.; formal analysis, C.F.; data curation, A.Z.; project administration, T.C.; funding acquisition, supervision, S.S. All authors have read and agreed to the published version of the manuscript.

Funding: This research was funded by National Natural Science Foundation of China, (grant number: 42276100) and Project Funded by the Priority Academic Program Development of Jiangsu Higher Education Institutions (PAPD).

Data Availability Statement: The data presented in this study are available on request from the corresponding author.

Conflicts of Interest: The authors declare no conflict of interest.

Abbreviations

ACE, angiotensin-I converting enzyme; HPLC-Q-TOF-MS, ultra high performance liquid chromatography quadrupole time-of-flight mass spectrometry; UV, ultraviolet and visible spectrum; KAF, Lys-Ala-Phe; IC_{50}, half maximal inhibitory concentration; eNOS, endothelial nitric oxide synthase; NO, nitric oxide; LTCC, L-type Ca^{2+} channel; RyR, ryanodine receptor; RAAS, renin-angiotensin-aldosterone regulatory system; Ang I, Angiotensin I; Ang II, Angiotensin II; Akt, protein kinase B; AMPK, AMP-activated protein kinase; P38, P38 mitogen-activated protein kinase; Jun, Jun proto-oncogene; HUVECS, human umbilical vein endothelial cells; CaMKII, Ca^{2+}/calmodulin-dependent kinase II. HHL, N-hippuril-L-histidy-L-leucine; Km, Michaelis–Menten constant; MTT, 3-(4,5-Dimethylthiazol-2yl)-2,5 dip-henyltetrazolium bromide; Cap, captopril.

References

1. Rapsomaniki, E.; Timmis, A.; George, J.; Pujades-Rodriguez, M.; Shah, A.D.; Denaxas, S.; White, I.R.; Caulfield, M.J.; Deanfield, J.E.; Smeeth, L.; et al. Blood pressure and incidence of twelve cardiovascular diseases: Lifetime risks, healthy life-years lost, and age-specific associations in 1.25 million people. *Lancet* **2014**, *383*, 1899–1911. [CrossRef] [PubMed]
2. Azushima, K.; Morisawa, N.; Tamura, K.; Nishiyama, A. Recent Research Advances in Renin-Angiotensin-Aldosterone System Receptors. *Curr. Hypertens. Rep.* **2020**, *22*, 22. [CrossRef] [PubMed]
3. Raghavan, S.; Kristinsson, H.G. ACE-inhibitory activity of tilapia protein hydrolysates. *Food Chem.* **2009**, *117*, 582–588. [CrossRef]
4. Chen, J.; Yu, X.; Chen, Q.; Wu, Q.; He, Q. Screening and mechanisms of novel angiotensin-I-converting enzyme inhibitory peptides from rabbit meat proteins: A combined in silico and in vitro study. *Food Chem.* **2022**, *370*, 131070. [CrossRef] [PubMed]
5. Suo, S.-K.; Zhao, Y.-Q.; Wang, Y.-M.; Pan, X.-Y.; Chi, C.-F.; Wang, B. Seventeen novel angiotensin converting enzyme (ACE) inhibitory peptides from the protein hydrolysate of Mytilus edulis: Isolation, identification, molecular docking study, and protective function on HUVECs. *Food Funct.* **2022**, *13*, 7831–7846. [CrossRef]
6. Wang, Y.; Chen, S.; Shi, W.; Liu, S.; Chen, X.; Pan, N.; Wang, X.; Su, Y.; Liu, Z. Targeted Affinity Purification and Mechanism of Action of Angiotensin-Converting Enzyme (ACE) Inhibitory Peptides from Sea Cucumber Gonads. *Mar. Drugs* **2024**, *22*, 90. [CrossRef]
7. Zheng, S.-L.; Luo, Q.-B.; Suo, S.-K.; Zhao, Y.-Q.; Chi, C.-F.; Wang, B. Preparation, Identification, Molecular Docking Study and Protective Function on HUVECs of Novel ACE Inhibitory Peptides from Protein Hydrolysate of Skipjack Tuna Muscle. *Mar. Drugs* **2022**, *20*, 176. [CrossRef]
8. Su, Y.; Chen, S.; Cai, S.; Liu, S.; Pan, N.; Su, J.; Qiao, K.; Xu, M.; Chen, B.; Yang, S.; et al. A Novel Angiotensin-I-Converting Enzyme (ACE) Inhibitory Peptide from Takifugu flavidus. *Mar. Drugs* **2021**, *19*, 651. [CrossRef]
9. Ye, N.-H.; Zhang, X.-W.; Mao, Y.-Z.; Liang, C.-W.; Xu, D.; Zou, J.; Zhuang, Z.-M.; Wang, Q.-Y. 'Green tides' are overwhelming the coastline of our blue planet: Taking the world's largest example. *Ecol. Res.* **2011**, *26*, 477–485. [CrossRef]
10. Aguilera-Morales, M.; Casas-Valdez, M.; Carrillo-Domínguez, S.; González-Acosta, B.; Pérez-Gil, F. Chemical composition and microbiological assays of marine algae Enteromorpha spp. as a potential food source. *J. Food Compos. Anal.* **2005**, *18*, 79–88. [CrossRef]
11. Pan, S.; Wang, S.; Jing, L.; Yao, D. Purification and characterisation of a novel angiotensin-I converting enzyme (ACE)-inhibitory peptide derived from the enzymatic hydrolysate of Enteromorpha clathrata protein. *Food Chem.* **2016**, *211*, 423–430. [CrossRef]
12. Xu, S.; Ilyas, I.; Little, P.J.; Li, H.; Kamato, D.; Zheng, X.; Luo, S.; Li, Z.; Liu, P.; Han, J.; et al. Endothelial Dysfunction in Atherosclerotic Cardiovascular Diseases and Beyond: From Mechanism to Pharmacotherapies. *Pharmacol. Rev.* **2021**, *73*, 924–967. [CrossRef] [PubMed]
13. Li, Q.; Liu, K.; Gao, Z.; Tayyab Rashid, M. An ACE-inhibitory peptide derived from maize germ antagonizes the Angiotensin II-induced dysfunction of HUVECs via the PI3K/Akt/eNOS signaling pathway. *J. Funct. Foods* **2024**, *112*, 105967. [CrossRef]
14. Cai, S.; Pan, N.; Xu, M.; Su, Y.; Qiao, K.; Chen, B.; Zheng, B.; Xiao, M.; Liu, Z. ACE Inhibitory Peptide from Skin Collagen Hydrolysate of Takifugu bimaculatus as Potential for Protecting HUVECs Injury. *Mar. Drugs* **2021**, *19*, 655. [CrossRef]
15. Wu, Q.; Li, Y.; Peng, K.; Wang, X.L.; Ding, Z.; Liu, L.; Xu, P.; Liu, G.Q. Isolation and Characterization of Three Antihypertension Peptides from the Mycelia of Ganoderma lucidum (Agaricycetes). *J. Agric. Food Chem.* **2019**, *67*, 8149–8159. [CrossRef]
16. Wang, S.; Zhang, L.; Wang, H.; Hu, Z.; Xie, X.; Chen, H.; Tu, Z. Identification of novel angiotensin converting enzyme (ACE) inhibitory peptides from Pacific saury: In vivo antihypertensive effect and transport route. *Int. J. Biol. Macromol.* **2024**, *254*, 127196. [CrossRef]
17. Qiao, Q.-Q.; Luo, Q.-B.; Suo, S.-K.; Zhao, Y.-Q.; Chi, C.-F.; Wang, B. Preparation, Characterization, and Cytoprotective Effects on HUVECs of Fourteen Novel Angiotensin-I-Converting Enzyme Inhibitory Peptides From Protein Hydrolysate of Tuna Processing By-Products. *Front. Nutr.* **2022**, *9*, 868681. [CrossRef]
18. Wu, Z.; Pan, D.; Zhen, X.; Cao, J. Angiotensin I-converting enzyme inhibitory peptides derived from bovine casein and identified by MALDI-TOF-MS/MS. *J. Sci. Food Agric.* **2012**, *93*, 1331–1337. [CrossRef] [PubMed]
19. Afrin, S.; Rakib, M.A.; Kim, B.H.; Kim, J.O.; Ha, Y.L. Eritadenine from Edible Mushrooms Inhibits Activity of Angiotensin Converting Enzyme in Vitro. *J. Agric. Food Chem.* **2016**, *64*, 2263–2268. [CrossRef]
20. Chen, H.; Chen, Y.; Zheng, H.; Xiang, X.; Xu, L. A novel angiotensin-I-converting enzyme inhibitory peptide from oyster: Simulated gastro-intestinal digestion, molecular docking, inhibition kinetics and antihypertensive effects in rats. *Front. Nutr.* **2022**, *9*, 981163. [CrossRef]
21. Esam, Z.; Akhavan, M.; Lotfi, M.; Bekhradnia, A. Molecular docking and dynamics studies of Nicotinamide Riboside as a potential multi-target nutraceutical against SARS-CoV-2 entry, replication, and transcription: A new insight. *J. Mol. Struct.* **2022**, *1247*, 131394. [CrossRef] [PubMed]

22. Qi, C.Y.; Zhang, R.; Huang, G.D.; Wu, W.J. Studies on the conformations and hydrogen bonding of ACE inhibitory tripeptide VEF by all-atom molecular dynamics simulations and molecular docking. *Chin. J. Struct. Chem.* **2017**, *36*, 189–196. [CrossRef]
23. Joy, S.; Siow, R.; Rowlands, D.; Becker, M.; Wyatt, A.; Aaronson, P.; Coen, C.; Kalló, I.; Jacob, R.; Mann, G. The isoflavone Equol mediates rapid vascular relaxation: Ca^{2+}-independent activation of endothelial nitric-oxide synthase/Hsp90 involving ERK1/2 and Akt phosphorylation in human endothelial cells. *J. Biol. Chem.* **2006**, *281*, 27335–27345. [CrossRef]
24. Wang, Y.; Cui, L.; Xu, H.; Liu, S.; Zhu, F.; Yan, F.; Shen, S.; Zhu, M. TRPV1 agonism inhibits endothelial cell inflammation via activation of eNOS/NO pathway. *Atherosclerosis* **2017**, *260*, 9–13. [CrossRef]
25. Jin, S.W.; Choi, C.Y.; Hwang, Y.P.; Kim, H.G.; Kim, S.J.; Chung, Y.C.; Lee, K.J.; Jeong, T.C.; Jeong, H.G. Betulinic Acid Increases eNOS Phosphorylation and NO Synthesis via the Calcium-Signaling. *J. Agric. Food Chem.* **2016**, *64*, 785–791. [CrossRef]
26. Jin, S.W.; Pham, H.T.; Choi, J.H.; Lee, G.H.; Han, E.H.; Cho, Y.H.; Chung, Y.C.; Kim, Y.H.; Jeong, H.G. Impressic Acid, a Lupane-Type Triterpenoid from Acanthopanax koreanum, Attenuates TNF-α-Induced Endothelial Dysfunction via Activation of eNOS/NO Pathway. *Int. J. Mol. Sci.* **2019**, *20*, 5772. [CrossRef]
27. Takata, T.; Kimura, J.; Tsuchiya, Y.; Naito, Y.; Watanabe, Y. Calcium/calmodulin-dependent protein kinases as potential targets of nitric oxide. *Nitric Oxide* **2011**, *25*, 145–152. [CrossRef] [PubMed]
28. Steinkamp-Fenske, K.; Bollinger, L.; Xu, H.; Yao, Y.; Horke, S.; Förstermann, U.; Li, H. Reciprocal regulation of endothelial nitric-oxide synthase and NADPH oxidase by betulinic acid in human endothelial cells. *J. Pharmacol. Exp. Ther.* **2007**, *322*, 836–842. [CrossRef]
29. Schneider, J.-C.; Kebir, D.E.; Chéreau, C.; Lanone, S.; Huang, X.-L.; Roessingh, A.S.D.B.; Mercier, J.-C.; Dall'Ava-Santucci, J.; Dinh-Xuan, A.T. Involvement of Ca^{2+}/calmodulin-dependent protein kinase II in endothelial NO production and endothelium-dependent relaxation. *Am. J. Physiol.-Heart Circ. Physiol.* **2003**, *284*, H2311–H2319. [CrossRef]
30. Li, Z.; He, Y.; He, H.; Zhou, W.; Li, M.; Lu, A.; Che, T.; Shen, S. Purification identification and function analysis of ACE inhibitory peptide from Ulva prolifera protein. *Food Chem.* **2023**, *401*, 134127. [CrossRef]
31. Mirza, S.B.; Ekhteiari Salmas, R.; Fatmi, M.Q.; Durdagi, S. Discovery of Klotho peptide antagonists against Wnt3 and Wnt3a target proteins using combination of protein engineering, protein–protein docking, peptide docking and molecular dynamics simulations. *J. Enzym. Inhib. Med. Chem.* **2016**, *32*, 84–98. [CrossRef] [PubMed]
32. Hu, Y.-D.; Xi, Q.-H.; Kong, J.; Zhao, Y.-Q.; Chi, C.-F.; Wang, B. Angiotensin-I-Converting Enzyme (ACE)-Inhibitory Peptides from the Collagens of Monkfish (*Lophius litulon*) Swim Bladders: Isolation, Characterization, Molecular Docking Analysis and Activity Evaluation. *Mar. Drugs* **2023**, *21*, 516. [CrossRef] [PubMed]

Disclaimer/Publisher's Note: The statements, opinions and data contained in all publications are solely those of the individual author(s) and contributor(s) and not of MDPI and/or the editor(s). MDPI and/or the editor(s) disclaim responsibility for any injury to people or property resulting from any ideas, methods, instructions or products referred to in the content.

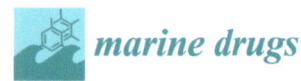

Article

Peptides from *Harpadon nehereus* Bone Ameliorate Sodium Palmitate-Induced HepG2 Lipotoxicity by Regulating Oxidative Stress and Lipid Metabolism

Siyi Song, Wei Zhao, Qianxia Lin, Jinfeng Pei * and Huoxi Jin *

School of Food and Pharmacy, Zhejiang Ocean University, Zhoushan 316022, China; song18234214689@163.com (S.S.); zhaoweiolivia@163.com (W.Z.); linqianxia_zjou@163.com (Q.L.)
* Correspondence: pffzjut@163.com (J.P.); jinhuoxi@163.com (H.J.)

Abstract: Antioxidant peptides are a well-known functional food exhibiting multiple biological activities in health and disease. This study investigated the effects of three peptides, LR-7 (LALFVPR), KA-8 (KLHDEEVA), and PG-7 (PSRILYG), from *Harpadon nehereus* bone on sodium palmitate (PANa)-induced HepG2. The findings indicated that all three peptides significantly reduced the oxidative damage and fat accumulation in the HepG2 cells while also normalizing the abnormal blood lipid levels caused by PANa. Furthermore, treatment with LR-7 resulted in a more than 100% increase in catalase (CAT), glutathione peroxidase (GSH-Px), and nuclear factor erythroid 2-related factor 2 (Nrf2) levels within the HepG2 cells ($p < 0.001$). Western blot analysis showed that LR-7 treatment significantly lowered the expression of fatty acid synthase (FASN) by 59.6% ($p < 0.001$) while enhancing carnitine palmitoyl transferase 1 (CPT1) by 134.7% ($p < 0.001$) and adipose triglyceride lipase (ATGL) by 148.1% ($p < 0.001$). Additionally, these peptides effectively inhibited the pancreatic lipase activity. Notably, LR-7 demonstrated superior effectiveness across all of the evaluated parameters, likely due to its greater hydrophobicity. In summary, LR-7, KA-8, and PG-7 are effective at mitigating oxidative stress as well as regulating lipid metabolism, thus protecting HepG2 cells from PANa-induced injury and lipid buildup. This research indicates that these collagen-derived peptides, especially LR-7, show promise as natural agents for managing hyperlipidemia.

Keywords: sodium palmitate; HepG2; hyperlipidemia; oxidative stress; lipid metabolism

1. Introduction

Lipotoxicity is a pathological feature of chronic liver disease. It is characterized by the accumulation of lipids, which in turn leads to cell dysfunction and injury [1]. Saturated fatty acids (SFAs), as essential dietary components, play a crucial role in maintaining human physiological structure and function. However, excessive circulating lipids and subsequent cellular uptake can induce lipotoxicity, which has been implicated in the pathogenesis of various metabolic disorders and contributes to the progression of non-alcoholic fatty liver disease (NAFLD) [2,3]. Distinct effects on cell survival and death are exerted by saturated versus unsaturated fatty acids; however, the mechanisms behind these differences remain poorly understood. Numerous studies have shown that free fatty acids can lead to liver cell damage and apoptosis [4]. High concentrations of free fatty acids result in fat accumulation within the liver, prompting inflammatory factor release and cellular dysfunction [5]. Palmitic acid (PA), a prevalent saturated fatty acid constituting about 20–30% of total body fats, can be ingested through diet or synthesized endogenously via de novo lipogenesis (DNL) [6]. PA ranks among the most abundant saturated fatty acids found in plasma and has been implicated in toxicity affecting pancreatic beta cells as well as hepatocytes, among other cell types [7]. HepG2 cells are frequently utilized in vitro to study hyperlipidemia due to their capacity to accumulate intracellular lipids when exposed to free fatty acids like oleic acid and palmitic acid [8].

Numerous studies have shown that oxidative stress is a primary mechanism responsible for inducing abnormal lipid metabolism [9]. Oxidative stress causes lipid peroxidation and the formation of oxidized low-density lipoprotein (ox-LDL), which exacerbates hyperlipidemia [10]. Elevated blood lipid levels, combined with the buildup of lipid metabolism by-products, contribute to the onset of oxidative stress [11]. A promising approach to managing hyperlipidemia involves reducing the blood lipid and oxidative stress levels. Recent studies have highlighted the potential role of food protein peptides in treating hyperlipidemia [12]. Evidence suggests that peptides derived from animal proteins exert anti-lipidemic and antioxidant activity [13]. These beneficial effects are partly attributed to the specific amino acid compositions of the peptides [14]. For instance, peptides rich in hydrophobic amino acids, such as leucine, isoleucine, and proline, have shown efficacy in combating oxidative stress and hyperlipidemia [15]. Due to its high proline content, collagen is likely to exhibit significant antioxidant and anti-hyperlipidemic activity. Marine collagen peptides have gained significant attention as a research focus because of their diverse bioactive functions, safety, and lack of toxicity [13,16]. Collagen peptides derived from the skin of the great hammerhead shark (*Sphyrna mokarran*) have been found to mitigate hyperlipidemia by enhancing antioxidant enzyme activities and downregulating the expression of fatty acid synthase and 3-hydroxy-3-methylglutaryl-CoA reductase [17]. However, there is still limited research on the hypolipidemic activities of peptides derived from marine bone collagen and their underlying mechanisms.

Harpadon nehereus, a nutrient-rich marine species indigenous to the Indo-Pacific region, remains underexploited despite its significant collagen content (18–22% wet weight) [18]. *Harpadon nehereus* serves as an economical source that is rich in protein and trace elements. Its proteins and derived peptides offer numerous health benefits including immune enhancement, blood pressure reduction, cardiovascular protection, and inflammation mitigation [19]. In prior research, we successfully isolated three novel peptides LALFVPR (LR-7), KLHDEEVA (KA-8), and PSRILYG (PG-7) from the enzymatic hydrolysates of *Harpadon nehereus* bone collagen [20]. Notably, PG-7 was observed to improve angiotensin II-induced dysfunctions within HUVECs [21], while LR-7 exhibited protective qualities against cardiovascular injuries in hypertensive mice [22]. However, the anti-hyperlipidemic activity of these three peptides remain unreported. This study aimed to investigate the antioxidant and lipid metabolism regulatory effects of these peptides on HepG2 cells induced by sodium palmitate (PANa) to assess their potential utility in combating hyperlipidemia.

2. Results

2.1. Cytoprotective Effects of LR-7, KA-8, and PG-7 on HepG2 Cells

The impact of peptides LR-7, KA-8, and PG-7 on the viability of HepG2 cells stimulated by PANa was examined. To investigate whether peptides KA-8, LR-7, and PG-7 affected cell apoptosis, HepG2 cells were treated with different concentrations of each peptide (50, 100, 200 μM) for 24 h. As shown in Figure 1a, compared with those of the untreated cells with peptides, the cell proliferation rates were not significantly reduced with the three peptide treatments at concentrations up to 200 μM for 24 h. These results indicated that peptides KA-8, LR-7, and PG-7 had no effect on the apoptosis of HepG2 cells at concentrations below 200 μM. Based on systematic evaluation, a concentration of 100 μM was selected for all three oligopeptides (KA-8, LR-7, and PG-7) in subsequent experimental procedures. As illustrated in Figure 1b, the cell viability decreased from 100% at 0 μM PANa to 33.3% ($p < 0.0001$) at 1000 μM. Based on a comprehensive evaluation, a concentration of 350 μM, an intermediate between 250 and 500 μM, was selected as the optimal concentration for model establishment. Figure 1c demonstrates that treatment with LR-7, KA-8, and PG-7 notably enhanced the cell viability in HepG2 cells exposed to 350 μM PANa. To directly evaluate the protective effects of these peptides on the PANa-treated HepG2 cells, their morphology was observed under a microscope. In Figure 1d, it can be seen that the normal cells (Con) adhered well to the surface and displayed a polygonal shape. Conversely, those in the PANa group appeared loose, with a marked decrease in cell count and showed signs of apoptosis. However, following treatment with all three peptides, clusters formed among the cells along with a considerable increase in their numbers.

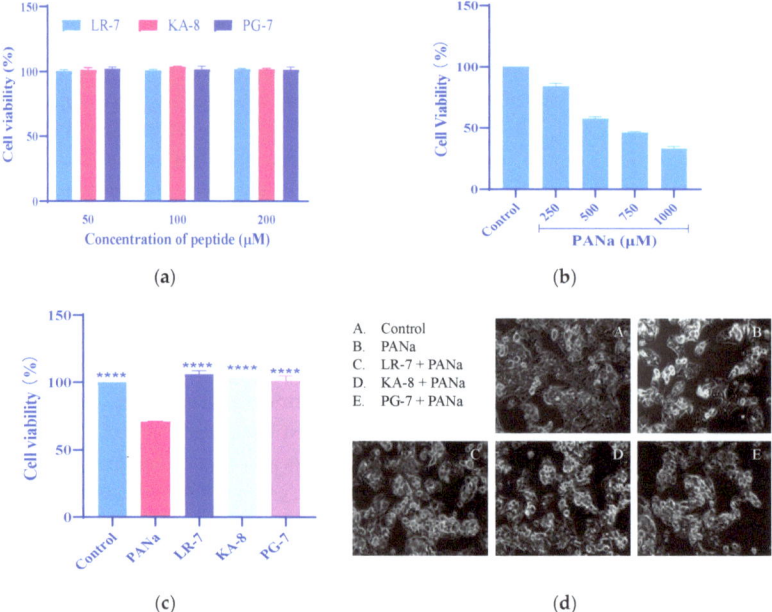

Figure 1. Protective effects of LR-7, KA-8, and PG-7 on HepG2 cells. (**a**) HepG2 cell proliferation after three oligopeptide (50, 100, 200 μM) treatments. (**b**) Effects of PANa on HepG2 cell viability. (**c**) Effects of three peptides (100 μM) on the cell viability of HepG2 induced by 350 μM PANa. (**d**) Morphology of HepG2 (200×). Con: normal control; PANa: HepG2 was treated with 350 μM PANa for 24 h. HepG2 was incubated with 100 μM KA-8 (KA-8 group), LR-7 (LR-7 group), and PG-7 (PG-7 group) for 4 h, followed by 350 μM PANa treatment for 24 h. **** represents $p < 0.0001$ compared with the PANa group.

2.2. Effects of LR-7, KA-8, and PG-7 on Antioxidant Capacity of HepG2 Cells

The mitigation of PANa-induced HepG2 damage by the three peptides in Figure 1 may be related to their reduction of oxidative stress. Research indicates that intracellular antioxidant enzymes play vital roles protecting against oxidative stress damage [23]. To evaluate the antioxidant potential of LR-7, KA-8, and PG-7, we examined their impact on the levels of catalase (CAT), glutathione peroxidase (GSH-Px), superoxide dismutase (SOD), and malondialdehyde (MDA) in the HepG2 cells. Figure 2 illustrates that the activities of CAT and GSH-Px were significantly diminished by more than 20% ($p < 0.001$) in the PANa group when compared with the Con group, while the MDA levels showed a notable increase by 105% ($p < 0.0001$). Treatment with LR-7, KA-8, and PG-7 effectively reversed the reduction in CAT, SOD, and GSH-Px activities induced by PANa. Remarkably, in the LR-7

(100 μM) treatment group, the CAT and GSH-Px activities increased by over 100% than those in the PANa group ($p < 0.0001$). Furthermore, the MDA concentrations within this same group decreased to values similar to those observed in the Con group. These findings indicate that all three peptides, especially LR-7, substantially improved the antioxidant enzyme activity in the HepG2 cells affected by PANa exposure.

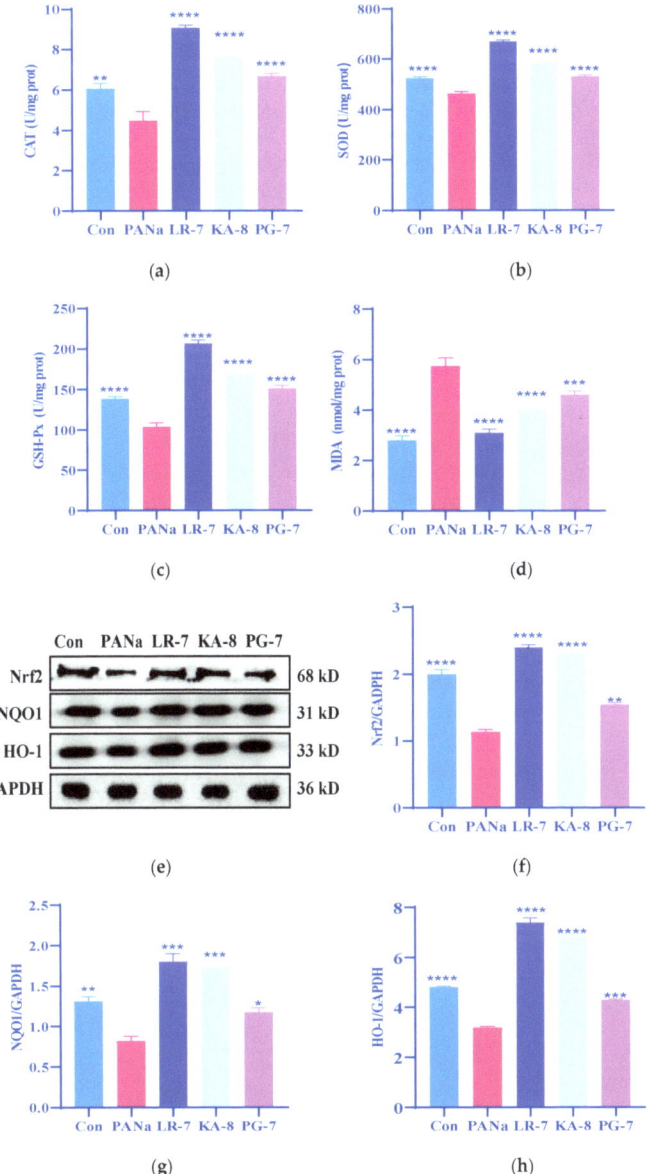

Figure 2. Effects of LR-7, KA-8, and PG-7 on the antioxidant capacity of HepG2 cells. The levels of CAT (**a**), SOD (**b**), GSH-Px (**c**), MDA (**d**), Nrf2 (**e**,**f**), NQO1 (**e**,**g**), and HO-1 (**e**,**h**) in HepG2 cells were measured. Con: normal control; PANa: HepG2 was treated with 350 μM PANa for 24 h. HepG2 was incubated with 100 μM KA-8 (KA-8 group), LR-7 (LR-7 group), and PG-7 (PG-7 group) for 4 h, followed by 350 μM PANa treatment for 24 h. *, **, ***, and **** represent $p < 0.05$, <0.01, <0.001, and <0.0001 compared with the PANa group, respectively.

Nuclear factor erythroid 2-related factor 2 (Nrf2) is a critical transcription factor that regulates the expression of antioxidant enzymes and plays an essential role in disease prevention. To assess whether LR-7, KA-8, and PG-7 could activate the Nrf2 signaling pathways within the HepG2 cells, we analyzed the protein expressions related specifically to Nrf-2, HO-1, and NQO-1. Figure 2e–h revealed a significant reduction regarding the expression levels of these proteins in the PANa group compared with the Con group. In contrast, following treatment with LR-7, the levels of Nrf2, HO-1, and NQO1 were significantly elevated by 111.5%, 131.7%, and 120% ($p < 0.0001$), respectively. These findings suggest that LR-7, KA-8, and PG-7 enhanced the antioxidant activity of PANa-induced HepG2 by activating the Nrf2 signaling pathway.

2.3. Effects of LR-7, KA-8, and PG-7 on Levels of Lipid in HepG2

In addition to reducing oxidative stress, lowering blood lipids is at the core of treating hyperlipidemia. Therefore, we investigated the effects of the three peptides on the fat accumulation and lipid levels in PANa-treated HepG2. Oil Red O (ORO) is a fat-soluble dye specifically used for staining neutral fats like triglycerides, resulting in red-stained lipid droplets within the stained cells [24]. As shown in Figure 3a, compared with the Con group, there was an evident rise in fat droplet formation and accumulation within the PANa group. Among the treatments with these three peptides, LR-7 exhibited the most significant reduction in fat accumulation relative to the PANa group. These findings suggest that all three peptides, especially LR-7, effectively diminished the intracellular fat droplet buildup within the HepG2 cells induced by PANa.

Triacylglycerol (TG), total cholesterol (TCHO), low-density lipoprotein cholesterol (LDL-C), and high-density lipoprotein cholesterol (HDL-C) are standard indicators for lipids. To analyze the negative effects of LR-7, KA-8, and PG-7 on the lipid levels in the PANA-induced HepG2, the TG, TCHO, LDL-C, and HDL-C levels were measured, respectively. Figure 3b–e revealed that the TG, TCHO, and LDL-C levels in the PANa group were significantly increased by 124.1%, 48.4%, and 58.3% ($p < 0.0001$), respectively, while HDL-C decreased markedly by 51.7% ($p < 0.001$) when compared with the Con group. Treatment with LR-7, KA-8, and PG-7 notably reversed the PANa-induced increases in TG, TCHO, and LDL-C, and the decrease in HDL-C. Among the three peptides, LR-7 demonstrated the most effective lipid-lowering impact.

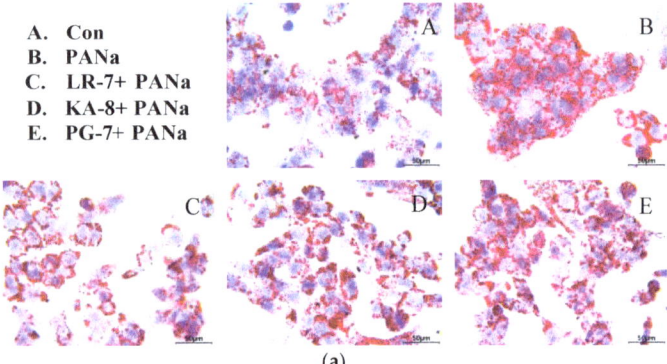

A. Con
B. PANa
C. LR-7+ PANa
D. KA-8+ PANa
E. PG-7+ PANa

(a)

Figure 3. *Cont.*

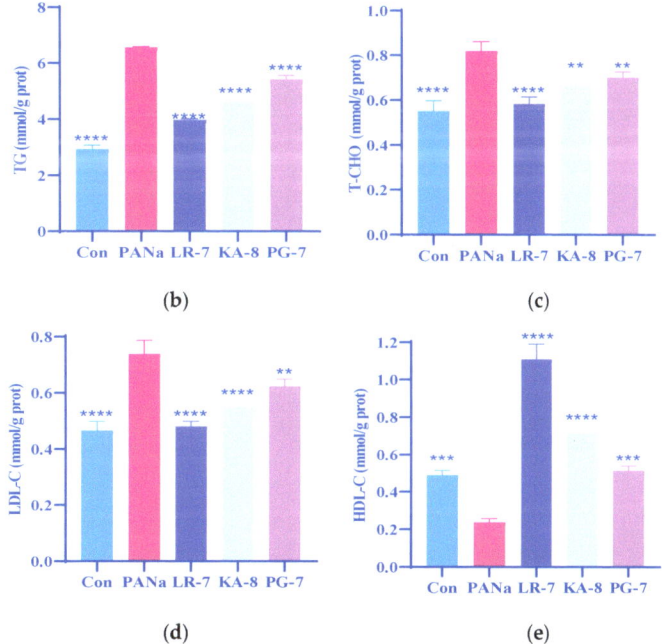

Figure 3. Effects of LR-7, KA-8, and PG-7 on the fat accumulation ((**a**), 200×) and levels of TG (**b**), TCHO (**c**), LDL-C (**d**), and HDL-C (**e**) in the HepG2 cells. Con: normal control; PANa: HepG2 was treated with 350 µM PANa for 24 h. HepG2 was incubated with 100 µM KA-8 (KA-8 group), LR-7 (LR-7 group), and PG-7 (PG-7 group) for 4 h, followed by 350 µM PANa treatment for 24 h. **, ***, and **** represent $p < 0.01$, <0.001, and <0.0001 compared with the PANa group, respectively.

2.4. Effects of LR-7, KA-8, and PG-7 on the Lipid Metabolism in PANa-Induced HepG2 Cells

The results presented in Figure 3 demonstrated that the three peptides inhibited fat accumulation and alleviated dyslipidemia induced by PANa treatment, suggesting that their mechanism of action may involve the regulation of lipid metabolism. Fatty acid synthase (FASN), a crucial enzyme involved in fatty acid synthesis, is vital for lipid metabolism [25]. Acetyl-CoA carboxylase (ACC), as one of the primary lipogenic enzymes, plays a significant role in lipid accumulation [26]. To investigate how LR-7, KA-8, and PG-7 influence lipogenesis in HepG2 cells induced by PANa, we measured the levels of FASN and phosphorylated ACC1 (p-ACC1). As depicted in Figure 4, there was a notable increase in FASN expression within the PANa group compared with the Con group while the p-ACC1 levels were significantly reduced ($p < 0.01$). After treatment with LR-7, KA-8, and PG-7, the p-ACC1 levels increased significantly while FASN expression decreased when compared with the PANa group. Among these peptides, LR-7 demonstrated superior efficacy in reducing the FASN levels (59.6%) while enhancing the p-ACC1 concentrations (293.7%).

Carnitine palmitoyl transferase 1 (CPT1) serves as a pivotal enzyme in the process of fatty acid oxidation, whereas adipose triglyceride lipase (ATGL) plays a crucial role in the hydrolysis of triglycerides into fatty acids. Consequently, both CPT1 and ATGL are vital enzymes in lipolysis and are indispensable for the reduction in blood lipids. The findings presented in Figure 4b indicate that the expression levels of ATGL and CPT1 were markedly diminished in the PANa group relative to the Con group ($p < 0.05$). Conversely, these protein levels exhibited a substantial elevation across all three peptide intervention groups when compared with the PANa group. Notably, among these peptides, LR-7 demonstrated the most significant enhancement in ATGL (148.1%) and CPT1 (134.7%) levels ($p < 0.0001$).

AMP-activated protein kinase (AMPK) exerts an inhibitory effect on acetyl-CoA carboxylase (ACC), thereby suppressing the synthesis of fatty acids and triglycerides. Moreover, AMPK mitigates the inhibition of CPT1 activity by decreasing the concentration of malonyl-CoA, thus facilitating fatty acid oxidation. AMPK is recognized as a critical upstream regulator of lipid metabolism [27].

In the present study, PANa was found to attenuate the phosphorylation of AMPKα (p-AMPKα) in HepG2; however, the administration of the three peptides notably ameliorated the reduced levels of p-AMPKα induced by PANa.

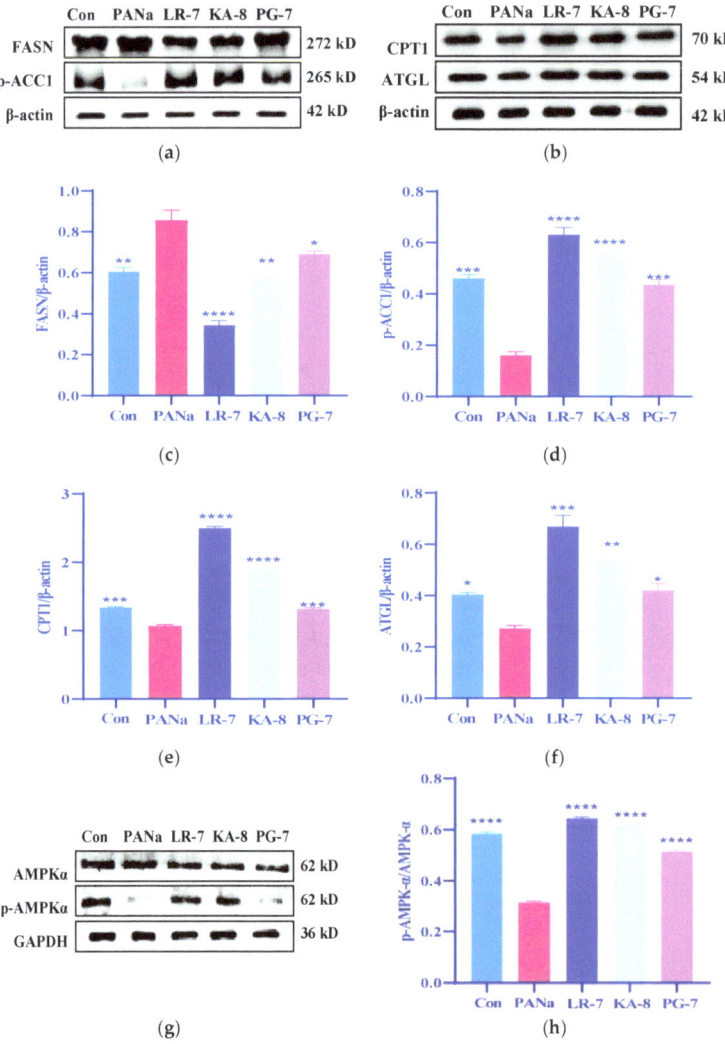

Figure 4. Effects of LR-7, KA-8, and PG-7 on the lipid metabolism in PANa-induced HepG2 cells. The expression of FANS, p-ACC1, CPT1, ATGL, and AMPKα were evaluated (a,b,g). The levels of FASN (c), p-ACC1 (d), CPT1 (e), ATGL (f), and p-AMPKα (h) were analyzed in PANa-stimulated HepG2. Con: normal control; PANa: HepG2 was treated with 350 μM PANa for 24 h. HepG2 was incubated with 100 μM KA-8 (KA-8 group), LR-7 (LR-7 group), and PG-7 (PG-7 group) for 4 h, followed by 350 μM PANa treatment for 24 h. *, **, ***, and **** represent $p < 0.05$, <0.01, <0.001, and <0.0001 compared with the PANa group, respectively.

2.5. Effects of LR-7, KA-8, and PG-7 on Pancreatic Lipase Activity

Pancreatic lipase is an enzyme produced by the pancreas, and plays a crucial role in fat digestion. By inhibiting pancreatic lipase activity, it is possible to decrease dietary triglyceride digestion and absorption, thereby promoting lipid reduction [28]. This study assessed the pancreatic lipase activity inhibition rates to confirm the lipid-lowering effects of the three peptides. As illustrated in Figure 5, LR-7 exhibited superior inhibitory effects compared with orlistat (the positive control), while KA-8 showed comparable results to orlistat; however, PG-7 was less effective than orlistat. These three peptides showed an inhibition in pancreatic lipase activity, which effectively reduced the digestion and absorption of dietary fat, thereby reducing the level of blood lipids.

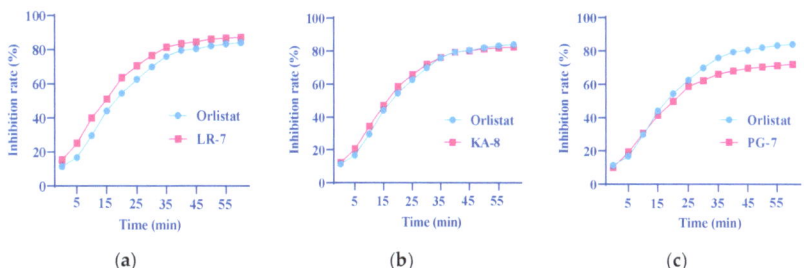

Figure 5. Inhibition of LR-7 (**a**), KA-8 (**b**), and PG-7 (**c**) on pancreatic lipase activity.

3. Discussion

Studies have confirmed that oxidative stress and lipid metabolism disorders are significant factors in the occurrence and development of hyperlipidemia Dietary intervention is a crucial auxiliary strategy for the management of hyperlipidemia. Collagen peptides have been extensively used as a nutritional intervention in the treatment of various diseases due to their notable antioxidant, anti-inflammatory, and hypolipidemic activities [17,29]. Our previous study showed that HNCP, an oligopeptide derived from *Harpadon nehereus* bone, attenuated oxidative stress and lowered blood glucose. Another oligopeptide (HNBC), also isolated from *Harpadon nehereus*, was protective against Ang II-stimulated HUVEC injury. Notably, the activation of Nrf2 and AMPK was consistent across all models, suggesting a unified antioxidant pathway, while newly identified lipid-specific targets (e.g., FASN, pancreatic lipase) emphasized the multifunctionality of the peptide. These findings collectively position *Harpadon nehereus* peptides as versatile candidates for managing metabolic syndromes. Therefore, this study aimed to investigate whether three collagen peptides (LR-7, KA-8, and PG-7) extracted from *Harpadon nehereus* bone could ameliorate oxidative stress and lipid metabolism disorders in HepG2 cells, thereby assessing their potential for hyperlipidemia intervention.

Exposure to PANa resulted in a notable decrease in cell viability and increased apoptosis rates; however, treatment with these three peptides led to a substantial recovery in cell numbers. These results indicate that LR-7, KA-8, and PG-7 provide protective benefits against HepG2 cell injury caused by PANa. PANa triggers the buildup of reactive oxygen species (ROS) within cells, resulting in oxidative stress and subsequent cellular injury. Antioxidant enzymes are essential for alleviating oxidative stress [30]. The findings revealed that LR-7, KA-8, and PG-7 significantly decreased the MDA levels while enhancing the activities of SOD, CAT, and GSH-Px. These results suggest that these peptides effectively mitigate oxidative stress in PANa-treated HepG2 cells. Numerous studies have indicated that various peptides can lower oxidative stress by boosting antioxidant enzyme activity in HepG2 cells; those with a higher proportion of hydrophobic amino acids were particularly successful at enhancing this activity [31,32]. Therefore, the higher antioxidant enzyme activities observed in the LR-7 group may be related to the presence of hydrophobic amino acids such as proline (Pro), leucine (Leu), and phenylalanine (Phe). The transcription factor Nrf2 serves as a vital regulator for genes involved in antioxidant responses and electrophilic reactions [33]. Research has shown that hesperetin can reduce hepatic steatosis, alleviate oxidative stress, decrease inflammatory cell infiltration, and mitigate fibrosis through activation of the Nrf2 pathway [34]. In our investigation, we observed a decline in the expression levels of Nrf2, HO-1, and NQO1 following PANa treatment; however, the administration of LR-7, KA-8, and PG-7 led to significant increases in the levels of these proteins. Our findings indicate that LR-7, KA-8, and PG-7 enhance antioxidative capabilities by activating the Nrf2 signaling pathway.

Hyperlipidemia is defined as a metabolic disorder marked by excessive fat accumulation along with elevated levels of TC, TG, and LDL-C [35]. Treatment with PANa significantly enhanced lipid droplet formation alongside a rise in the TG, TCHO, and LDL-C levels. Among the tested peptides, LR-7 notably decreased lipid accumulation while lowering the TG, TCHO, and LDL-C levels in HepG2 cells treated with PANa. These findings validated the lipid-lowering potential of all three peptides but highlighted LR-7 as having the most significant impact. Previous studies have indicated that higher proportions of hydrophobic amino acids within peptides are positively associated with their lipid-lowering capabilities [36]. Therefore, the observed reductions in TG, TCHO, and LDL-C levels within the LR-7 group may also be linked to the presence of Pro, Leu, and Phe.

Lipid metabolism, including lipolysis, lipogenesis, and lipid transport, determines the lipid levels in the body [37]. FASN and ACC are two significant lipid synthetases that play a key role in lipid accumulation. PANa primarily influences hepatic lipogenesis through the modulation of FASN and ACC1 expression [38]. Research has indicated that sesamol (SEM), a kind of natural lignan extracted from sesame oil, can influence lipid accumulation by decreasing the expression levels of FASN and ACC1 [39]. CPT1 and ATGL are closely linked to lipolysis and are crucial for regulating lipid levels. Iso-alpha acids, which are derived from *Humulus lupulus*, a plant cultivated on a large scale across the globe for its use as a raw material in the brewing industry, have been shown to reduce lipid levels by enhancing CPT1 expression in mice with non-alcoholic fatty liver disease (NAFLD) [40]. Recent studies have shown that AMPK regulates both lipolysis and lipogenesis via phosphorylation processes in healthy hepatocytes [41]. In the present study, PANa treatment led to an increase in FASN while simultaneously reducing the ATGL, CPT1, and p-AMPKα levels. Notably, the abnormal expression of proteins associated with lipid metabolism by PANa treatment was significantly reversed by LR-7, KA-8, or PG-7 treatment. Our findings indicate that LR-7, KA-8, and PG-7 modulate lipid metabolism effectively through promoting lipolysis and inhibiting lipogenesis associated with the AMPK pathway, thereby diminishing fat accumulation in HepG2 cells induced by PANa.

Pancreatic lipase, a major enzyme in the breakdown of lipids, is essential for the digestion and absorption of dietary fats [42]. This enzyme gradually converts triglycerides into 2-monoacylglycerol and free fatty acids, which aids in the thorough digestion and absorption of dietary fats [43]. Therefore, the inhibition of pancreatic lipase can reduce the intestinal absorption of triglycerides, thereby preventing hyperlipidemia and obesity [44]. It has been proposed that blocking pancreatic lipase would hinder triglyceride degradation and slow down the entry of fatty acids into systemic circulation and adipose tissue [43]. In this study, we compared the pancreatic lipase inhibitory effects of three peptides with those of orlistat. The results indicated that LR-7 exhibited a stronger inhibitory effect on pancreatic lipase than orlistat, while PG-7 showed less effectiveness compared with orlistat. In summary, these three peptides, particularly LR-7, may lower lipid levels by inhibiting pancreatic lipase activity as well as modulating protein expression related to lipid metabolism. In conclusion, LR-7 exhibits significant antioxidant, lipid metabolism regulation, and lipase activity inhibition, and could be used as a nutritional intervention in the management of hyperlipidemia.

4. Materials and Methods

4.1. Materials

(PSRILYG, PG-7), (KLHDEEVA, KA-8), and (LALFVPR, LR-7) were isolated and identified in our previous research [20]. HepG2 cells were obtained from the Chinese Academy of Sciences (Shanghai, China). Sodium palmitate (PANa) was sourced from Kunchuang Technology Development Co., Ltd. (Xi'an, China). DMEM was acquired from Gibco Co., Ltd. (Carlsbad, CA, USA). The Oil Red O staining solution along with assay kits for the antioxidant enzymes were purchased from Beyotime Biotechnology (Shanghai, China). Assay kits for blood lipid levels as well as all antibodies used in this study were procured from Nanjing JianCheng Bioengineering Institute (Nanjing, China). All other reagents utilized were of analytical grade.

4.2. Cell Cultures

HepG2 cells were cultured in DMEM supplemented with penicillin at a concentration of 100 U/mL, streptomycin at 100 µg/mL, and fetal bovine serum at a volume ratio of 10% under conditions of 37 °C and 5% CO_2. A total of 2×10^4 cells per well were seeded into a 96-well plate for overnight culture. The upper layer of medium was carefully aspirated, and 200 µL of different concentrations of oligopeptide solution (50 µM, 100 µM, 200 µM) prepared with cell complete medium was added to each well. Twenty-four hours later, the proliferation rate of the cells was measured according to the instructions of the CCK-8 kit, and the appropriate concentration of oligopeptide was screened out.

After incubation, different concentrations (250, 500, 750, 1000 µmol/L) of PANa were added and treated for 24 h. The cell proliferation rates were measured according to the CCK-8 assay instructions.

4.3. Cell Viability Assay

A total of 2×10^4 cells/well were inoculated in 96-well plates for culture at 37 °C and 5% CO_2. Following this period, the cells received treatment with 200 µL medium containing 100 µM LR-7, KA-8, or PG-7 for 4 h before adding 350 µM PANa to each well. After incubation for an additional 24 h, the cell proliferation rates were assessed using the CCK-8 assay protocols.

4.4. Observation of Cell Morphology

Cells grown in culture flasks underwent digestion to create a single-cell suspension that was then diluted with fresh medium before being transferred into six-well plates at a final concentration of 4×10^5/well (2 mL/well). Peptides at concentrations of 100 µM were introduced prior to adding PANa for a 4 h incubation. Following another 24 h culture period, cells were examined and photographed using an inverted microscope.

4.5. Oil Red O Staining

After incubation, the supernatants were discarded, and 2 mL of Oil Red O stationary solution was added to each well for 20–30 min. The stationary solution was subsequently washed away with 60% isopropyl alcohol. A freshly prepared Oil Red O staining solution was then applied for immersion dyeing lasting 10–20 min. After removing the staining solution with water, a Mayer hematoxylin staining solution was added for counterstaining the nucleus for 1–2 min before being discarded. An Oil Red O buffer solution was applied for 1 min and then discarded. Stained cells were photographed using an Olympus BX41 microscope (Tokyo, Japan) at 100× magnification. The emission wavelength of fluorescence detection was 600 nm.

4.6. Determination of Antioxidant Enzymes and Lipid-Related Indexes

After incubation, cells were treated with 100 μM of peptides for 4 h. After removing the media, PANa was added for 24 h of incubation. The levels of catalase (CAT), superoxide dismutase (SOD), glutathione peroxidase (GSH-Px), malondialdehyde (MDA), triacylglycerol (TG), total cholesterol (TCHO), low-density lipoprotein cholesterol (LDL-C), and high-density lipoprotein cholesterol (HDL-C) in the supernatant were determined according to the kit instructions [45].

4.7. Western Blot Assay

After treatment, cells were washed with pre-chilled PBS and lysed with ice-cold lysis buffer for 30 min. The supernatant was collected after centrifugation at 12,000× g for 10 min and stored at −80 °C. Protein concentration was determined using a BCA protein assay kit. Equal amounts of protein (20–40 μg) were subjected to 10% sodium dodecyl sulfate-polyacrylamide gel electrophoresis (SDS-PAGE) and transferred to PVDF membranes (Polyvinylidene Fluoride, Merck, Darmstadt, Germany). Non-specific binding sites were blocked with 5% bovine serum albumin (BSA) solution at room temperature for 1 h, followed by incubation with the primary antibody at 4 °C overnight. After washing with TBST (3 times, 10 min/time), the membrane was incubated with the secondary antibody at room temperature for 1 h. Following further washing with TBST (3 times, 10 min/time), antibody signals were detected using a Western blot development system. The dilution ratios for the internal reference protein, vascular endothelial injury-related proteins, and oxidative stress-related pathway proteins were prepared according to the manufacturer's instructions.

4.8. Determination of Pancreatic Lipase Activity

A working substrate solution consisting of 4-nitrophenyl palmitate dissolved in sodium acetate solution (containing 1% Triton-X 100, 100 mL, 5 mM, pH 5.0) was prepared. Enzyme powder was dissolved in Tris-HCl buffer (pH 8.0, 37 °C). This mixture was incubated at 4 °C for 2 h before centrifugation at 5000 r/min for 5 min, yielding the supernatant used to prepare a pancreatic lipase solution of 1.2 mg/mL. Orlistat at a concentration of 1 mg/mL in Tris-HCl buffer (pH 8.0; 37 °C) was prepared alongside DMSO to reach a concentration of 350 μg/mL peptide solution. The peptide solution of 100 μM was prepared with Tris-HCl buffer (pH = 8.0, 37 °C). The absorbance was measured at 405 nm, and the inhibition rate was measured in parallel with three holes due to the methodology of Franco et al. [46].

4.9. Data Analysis

All experiments were performed three times, and the results were expressed as the mean ± SD. GraphPad Prism 8.0 software was used for one-way ANOVA and comparison between groups.

5. Conclusions

This research investigated the effects of three peptides (LR-7, KA-8, and PG-7) derived from bone collagen on PANa-induced hyperlipidemia in HepG2 cells. Our study indicated that all three peptides, particularly LR-7, mitigated the cell damage caused by PANa by enhancing the antioxidant enzyme levels through Nrf2 upregulation. LR-7 demonstrated superior effectiveness in reducing oxidative stress and lipid accumulation compared with

KA-8 and PG-7 by modulating the expression of proteins associated with lipid metabolism (FASN, ACC1, ATGL, and CPT1). LR-7 exhibited a stronger inhibitory effect on pancreatic lipase activity than orlistat. Collectively, these results may offer new insights into the potential use of marine peptides from bone collagen as functional foods or therapeutic agents for managing hyperlipidemia. Future studies will aim to further investigate the effects and mechanisms of these three peptides in mice with hyperlipidemia.

Author Contributions: Conceptualization, S.S., W.Z., H.J., and J.P.; Methodology, W.Z. and Q.L.; Validation, S.S., W.Z., and Q.L.; Investigation, S.S. and W.Z.; Writing—original draft preparation, Q.L.; Writing—review and editing, J.P. and H.J.; Supervision, H.J. All authors have read and agreed to the published version of the manuscript.

Funding: This research was supported by the Zhejiang Provincial Natural Science Foundation of China under grant no. LTGY24D060001.

Institutional Review Board Statement: Not applicable.

Informed Consent Statement: Not applicable.

Data Availability Statement: Data are contained within the article.

Conflicts of Interest: The authors declare no conflicts of interest.

References

1. Hsu, J.-Y.; Lin, H.-H.; Chyau, C.-C.; Wang, Z.-H.; Chen, J.-H. Aqueous Extract of Pepino Leaves Ameliorates Palmitic Acid-Induced Hepatocellular Lipotoxicity via Inhibition of Endoplasmic Reticulum Stress and Apoptosis. *Antioxidants* **2021**, *10*, 903. [CrossRef]
2. Piccolis, M.; Bond, L.M.; Kampmann, M.; Pulimeno, P.; Chitraju, C.; Jayson, C.B.K.; Vaites, L.P.; Boland, S.; Lai, Z.W.; Gabriel, K.R.; et al. Probing the Global Cellular Responses to Lipotoxicity Caused by Saturated Fatty Acids. *Mol. Cell* **2019**, *74*, 32–44.e8. [CrossRef]
3. Terry, A.R.; Nogueira, V.; Rho, H.; Ramakrishnan, G.; Li, J.; Kang, S.; Pathmasiri, K.C.; Bhat, S.A.; Jiang, L.; Kuchay, S.; et al. CD36 maintains lipid homeostasis via selective uptake of monounsaturated fatty acids during matrix detachment and tumor progression. *Cell Metab.* **2023**, *35*, 2060–2076.e9. [CrossRef] [PubMed]
4. Zheng, X.; Zhang, X.; Liu, Y.; Zhu, L.; Liang, X.; Jiang, H.; Shi, G.; Zhao, Y.; Zhao, Z.; Teng, Y.; et al. Arjunolic acid from Cyclocarya paliurus ameliorates nonalcoholic fatty liver disease in mice via activating Sirt1/AMPK, triggering autophagy and improving gut barrier function. *J. Funct. Foods* **2021**, *86*, 104686. [CrossRef]
5. Cazanave, S.C.; Wang, X.; Zhou, H.; Rahmani, M.; Grant, S.; Durrant, D.E.; Klaassen, C.D.; Yamamoto, M.; Sanyal, A.J. Degradation of Keap1 activates BH3-only proteins Bim and PUMA during hepatocyte lipoapoptosis. *Cell Death Differ.* **2014**, *21*, 1303–1312. [CrossRef] [PubMed]
6. Murru, E.; Manca, C.; Carta, G.; Banni, S. Impact of Dietary Palmitic Acid on Lipid Metabolism. *Front. Nutr.* **2022**, *9*, 861664. [CrossRef]
7. Plötz, T.; Krümmel, B.; Laporte, A.; Pingitore, A.; Persaud, S.J.; Jörns, A.; Elsner, M.; Mehmeti, I.; Lenzen, S. The monounsaturated fatty acid oleate is the major physiological toxic free fatty acid for human beta cells. *Nutr. Diabetes* **2017**, *7*, 305. [CrossRef]
8. Guo, X.; Yin, X.; Liu, Z.; Wang, J. Non-Alcoholic Fatty Liver Disease (NAFLD) Pathogenesis and Natural Products for Prevention and Treatment. *Int. J. Mol. Sci.* **2022**, *23*, 15489. [CrossRef]
9. Liu, L.N.; Chen, Y.H.; Chen, B.; Xu, M.; Liu, S.J.; Su, Y.C.; Qiao, K.; Liu, Z.Y. Advances in Research on Marine-Derived Lipid-Lowering Active Substances and Their Molecular Mechanisms. *Nutrients* **2023**, *15*, 5118. [CrossRef]
10. Manso, M.A.; Miguel, M.; Even, J.; Hernández, R.; Aleixandre, A.; López-Fandiño, R. Effect of the long-term intake of an egg white hydrolysate on the oxidative status and blood lipid profile of spontaneously hypertensive rats. *Food Chem.* **2008**, *109*, 361–367. [CrossRef]
11. Firdous, S.M.; Hazra, S.; Gopinath, S.C.B.; El-Desouky, G.E.; Aboul-Soud, M.A.M. Antihyperlipidemic potential of diosmin in Swiss Albino mice with high-fat diet induced hyperlipidemia. *Saudi J. Biol. Sci.* **2021**, *28*, 109–115. [CrossRef] [PubMed]
12. Tacherfiout, M.; Petrov, P.D.; Mattonai, M.; Ribechini, E.; Ribot, J.; Bonet, M.L.; Khettal, B. Antihyperlipidemic effect of a Rhamnus alaternus leaf extract in Triton-induced hyperlipidemic rats and human HepG2 cells. *Biomed. Pharmacother.* **2018**, *101*, 501–509. [CrossRef] [PubMed]
13. Fernando, I.P.; Jayawardena, T.U.; Wu, J. Marine proteins and peptides: Production, biological activities, and potential applications. *Food Innov. Adv.* **2023**, *2*, 69–84. [CrossRef]

14. Lee, H.; Shin, E.; Kang, H.; Youn, H.; Youn, B. Soybean-Derived Peptides Attenuate Hyperlipidemia by Regulating Trans-Intestinal Cholesterol Excretion and Bile Acid Synthesis. *Nutrients* **2022**, *14*, 95. [CrossRef]
15. Takeshita, T.; Okochi, M.; Kato, R.; Kaga, C.; Tomita, Y.; Nagaoka, S.; Honda, H. Screening of peptides with a high affinity to bile acids using peptide arrays and a computational analysis. *J. Biosci. Bioeng.* **2011**, *112*, 92–97. [CrossRef]
16. Lin, Q.; Song, S.; Pei, J.; Zhang, L.; Chen, X.; Jin, H. Preparation and characterization of cysteine-rich collagen peptide and its antagonistic effect on microplastic induced damage to HK-2 cells. *Food Biosci.* **2024**, *61*, 104647. [CrossRef]
17. Vijayan, D.K.; Raman, S.P.; Dara, P.K.; Jacob, R.M.; Mathew, S.; Rangasamy, A.; Nagarajarao, R.C. In vivo anti-lipidemic and antioxidant potential of collagen peptides obtained from great hammerhead shark skin waste. *J. Food Sci. Tech. Mys* **2022**, *59*, 1140–1151. [CrossRef]
18. Féral, J.-P. How useful are the genetic markers in attempts to understand and manage marine biodiversity? *J. Exp. Mar. Biol. Ecol.* **2002**, *268*, 121–145. [CrossRef]
19. Yang, T.; Huang, X.; Ning, Z.; Gao, T. Genome-Wide Survey Reveals the Microsatellite Characteristics and Phylogenetic Relationships of Harpadon nehereus. *Curr. Issues Mol. Biol.* **2021**, *43*, 1282–1292. [CrossRef]
20. He, S.; Xu, Z.; Li, J.; Guo, Y.; Lin, Q.; Jin, H. Peptides from *Harpadon nehereus* protect against hyperglycemia-induced HepG2 via oxidative stress and glycolipid metabolism regulation. *J. Funct. Foods* **2023**, *108*, 105723. [CrossRef]
21. Shao, M.; Zhao, W.; Shen, K.; Jin, H. Peptides from Harpadon nehereus Bone Ameliorate Angiotensin II-Induced HUVEC Injury and Dysfunction through Activation of the AKT/eNOS and Nrf2 Pathway. *ACS Omega* **2023**, *8*, 41655–41663. [CrossRef] [PubMed]
22. Song, S.; He, S.; Lin, Q.; Jin, H. Synergistic effect of collagen peptide LR-7 and taurine on the prevention of cardiovascular injury in high salt-induced hypertensive mice. *Food Biosci.* **2024**, *61*, 104907. [CrossRef]
23. Tao, L.; Gu, F.; Liu, Y.; Yang, M.; Wu, X.Z.; Sheng, J.; Tian, Y. Preparation of antioxidant peptides from Moringa oleifera leaves and their protection against oxidative damage in HepG2 cells. *Front. Nutr.* **2022**, *9*, 1062671. [CrossRef]
24. Liu, Y.; Chen, Z. New role of oil red O in detection of double stranded DNA. *Talanta* **2019**, *204*, 337–343. [CrossRef]
25. Zhang, J.; Song, Y.; Shi, Q.; Fu, L. Research progress on FASN and MGLL in the regulation of abnormal lipid metabolism and the relationship between tumor invasion and metastasis. *Front. Med.* **2021**, *15*, 649–656. [CrossRef]
26. Liu, D.; Pang, Q.; Han, Q.; Shi, Q.; Zhang, Q.; Yu, H. Wnt10b Participates in Regulating Fatty Acid Synthesis in the Muscle of Zebrafish. *Cells* **2019**, *8*, 1011. [CrossRef]
27. Liu, Y.-C.; Wei, G.; Liao, Z.; Wang, F.; Zong, C.; Qiu, J.; Le, Y.; Yu, Z.; Yang, S.Y.; Wang, H.; et al. Design and Synthesis of Novel Indole Ethylamine Derivatives as a Lipid Metabolism Regulator Targeting PPARα/CPT1 in AML12 Cells. *Molecules* **2024**, *29*, 12. [CrossRef] [PubMed]
28. Rocha, S.; Rufino, A.T.; Freitas, M.; Silva, A.M.S.; Carvalho, F.; Fernandes, E. Methodologies for Assessing Pancreatic Lipase Catalytic Activity: A Review. *Crit. Rev. Anal. Chem.* **2023**, *54*, 3038–3065. [CrossRef]
29. Jiang, N.; Zhang, S.; Zhu, J.; Shang, J.; Gao, X. Hypoglycemic, Hypolipidemic and Antioxidant Effects of Peptides from Red Deer Antlers in Streptozotocin-Induced Diabetic Mice. *Tohoku J. Exp. Med.* **2015**, *236*, 71–79. [CrossRef]
30. Engin, A. Non-Alcoholic Fatty Liver Disease. *Adv. Exp. Med. Biol.* **2017**, *960*, 443–467.
31. Hu, Y.M.; Lu, S.Z.; Li, Y.S.; Wang, H.; Shi, Y.; Zhang, L.; Tu, Z.C. Protective effect of antioxidant peptides from grass carp scale gelatin on the H2O2-mediated oxidative injured HepG2 cells. *Food Chem.* **2022**, *373*, 131539. [CrossRef] [PubMed]
32. Wang, J.; Wu, T.; Fang, L.; Liu, C.L.; Liu, X.T.; Li, H.M.; Shi, J.H.; Li, M.H.; Min, W.H. Peptides from walnut (*Juglans mandshurica* Maxim.) protect hepatic HepG2 cells from high glucose-induced insulin resistance and oxidative stress. *Food Funct.* **2020**, *11*, 8112–8121. [CrossRef]
33. Wang, C.; Li, X.; Xue, B.; Yu, C.; Wang, L.; Deng, R.; Liu, H.; Chen, Z.; Zhang, Y.; Fan, S.; et al. RasGRP1 promotes the acute inflammatory response and restricts inflammation-associated cancer cell growth. *Nat. Commun.* **2022**, *13*, 7001. [CrossRef] [PubMed]
34. Li, J.; Wang, T.; Liu, P.; Yang, F.; Wang, X.; Zheng, W.; Sun, W. Hesperetin ameliorates hepatic oxidative stress and inflammation via the PI3K/AKT-Nrf2-ARE pathway in oleic acid-induced HepG2 cells and a rat model of high-fat diet-induced NAFLD. *Food Funct.* **2021**, *12*, 3898–3918. [CrossRef] [PubMed]
35. Birger, M.; Kaldjian, A.S.; Roth, G.A.; Moran, A.E.; Bellows, B.K. Spending on Cardiovascular Disease and Cardiovascular Risk Factors in the United States: 1996–2016. *Circulation* **2021**, *144*, 271–282. [CrossRef]
36. Saito, M.; Kiyose, C.; Higuchi, T.; Uchida, N.; Suzuki, H. Effect of Collagen Hydrolysates from Salmon and Trout Skins on the Lipid Profile in Rats. *J. Agric. Food Chem.* **2009**, *57*, 10477–10482. [CrossRef]
37. Zeng, S.; Chen, Y.; Wei, C.; Tan, L.; Li, C.; Zhang, Y.; Xu, F.; Zhu, K.; Wu, G.; Cao, J. Protective effects of polysaccharide from *Artocarpus heterophyllus* Lam. (jackfruit) pulp on non-alcoholic fatty liver disease in high-fat diet rats via PPAR and AMPK signaling pathways. *J. Funct. Foods* **2022**, *95*, 105195. [CrossRef]
38. Qiu, L.; Cai, C.; Zhao, X.; Fang, Y.; Tang, W.; Guo, C. Inhibition of aldose reductase ameliorates ethanol-induced steatosis in HepG2 cells. *Mol. Med. Rep.* **2017**, *15*, 2732–2736. [CrossRef]

39. Xu, H.; Yu, L.; Chen, J.; Yang, L.; Lin, C.; Shi, X.; Qin, H. Sesamol Alleviates Obesity-Related Hepatic Steatosis via Activating Hepatic PKA Pathway. *Nutrients* **2020**, *12*, 329. [CrossRef]
40. Mahli, A.; Koch, A.; Fresse, K.; Schiergens, T.; Thasler, W.E.; Schönberger, C.; Bergheim, I.; Bosserhoff, A.; Hellerbrand, C. Iso-alpha acids from hops (*Humulus lupulus*) inhibit hepatic steatosis, inflammation, and fibrosis. *Lab. Investig.* **2018**, *98*, 1614–1626. [CrossRef]
41. Kim, M.; Seong, J.; Huh, J.; Bae, Y.; Lee, H.; Lee, D. Peroxiredoxin 5 ameliorates obesity-induced non-alcoholic fatty liver disease through the regulation of oxidative stress and AMP-activated protein kinase signaling. *Redox Biol.* **2020**, *28*, 101315. [CrossRef] [PubMed]
42. de Camargo, A.C.; de Souza Silva, A.P.; Soares, J.C.; de Alencar, S.M.; Handa, C.L.; Cordeiro, K.S.; Figueira, M.S.; Sampaio, G.R.; Torres, E.A.F.S.; Shahidi, F.; et al. Do Flavonoids from Durum Wheat Contribute to Its Bioactive Properties? A Prospective Study. *Molecules* **2021**, *26*, 463. [CrossRef] [PubMed]
43. Rajan, L.; Palaniswamy, D.; Mohankumar, S.K. Targeting obesity with plant-derived pancreatic lipase inhibitors: A comprehensive review. *Pharmacol. Res.* **2020**, *155*, 104681. [CrossRef] [PubMed]
44. Pu, Y.; Chen, L.; He, X.; Cao, J.; Jiang, W. Soluble polysaccharides decrease inhibitory activity of banana condensed tannins against porcine pancreatic lipase. *Food Chem.* **2023**, *418*, 136013. [CrossRef]
45. Liu, W.; Ren, J.; Wu, H.; Zhang, X.; Han, L.; Gu, R. Inhibitory effects and action mechanism of five antioxidant peptides derived from wheat gluten on cells oxidative stress injury. *Food Biosci.* **2023**, *56*, 103236. [CrossRef]
46. Franco, R.R.; Mota Alves, V.H.; Ribeiro Zabisky, L.F.; Justino, A.B.; Martins, M.M.; Saraiva, A.L.; Goulart, L.R.; Espindola, F.S. Antidiabetic potential of Bauhinia forficata Link leaves: A non-cytotoxic source of lipase and glycoside hydrolases inhibitors and molecules with antioxidant and antiglycation properties. *Biomed. Pharmacother.* **2020**, *123*, 109798. [CrossRef]

Disclaimer/Publisher's Note: The statements, opinions and data contained in all publications are solely those of the individual author(s) and contributor(s) and not of MDPI and/or the editor(s). MDPI and/or the editor(s) disclaim responsibility for any injury to people or property resulting from any ideas, methods, instructions or products referred to in the content.

MDPI AG
Grosspeteranlage 5
4052 Basel
Switzerland
Tel.: +41 61 683 77 34

Marine Drugs Editorial Office
E-mail: marinedrugs@mdpi.com
www.mdpi.com/journal/marinedrugs

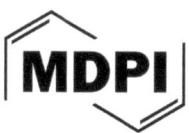

Disclaimer/Publisher's Note: The title and front matter of this reprint are at the discretion of the Guest Editors. The publisher is not responsible for their content or any associated concerns. The statements, opinions and data contained in all individual articles are solely those of the individual Editors and contributors and not of MDPI. MDPI disclaims responsibility for any injury to people or property resulting from any ideas, methods, instructions or products referred to in the content.

www.ingramcontent.com/pod-product-compliance
Lightning Source LLC
LaVergne TN
LVHW072349090526
838202LV00019B/2507